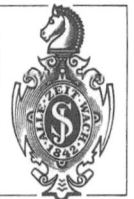

Archives of Toxicology, Supplement 11

Mechanisms and Models in Toxicology

Proceedings of the
European Society of Toxicology
Meeting Held in Harrogate, May 27–29, 1986

Edited by
Philip L. Chambers, Claire M. Chambers and Donald S. Davies

With 99 Figures

Springer-Verlag Berlin Heidelberg New York
London Paris Tokyo

CLAIRE M. CHAMBERS and PHILIP L. CHAMBERS
University of Dublin, Department of Pharmacology and Therapeutics,
Trinity College, Dublin 2, Ireland

D. S. Davies
Royal Postgraduate Medical School, Du Cane Road, London W12 OHS,
United Kingdom

ISBN-13: 978-3-540-17614-5   e-ISBN-13: 978-3-642-72558-6
DOI: 10.1007/978-3-642-72558-6

Library of Congress Cataloging in Publication Data. European Society of Toxicology. Meeting (1986 May 27–29: Harrogate, North Yorkshire) Mechanisms and models in toxicology. (Archives of toxicology. Supplement; 11) Includes index. 1. Toxicology, Experimental – Congresses. 2. Toxicology – Animal models – Congresses. I. Chambers, P. L. (Philip L.), 1931– . II. Chambers, C. M. (Claire M.) III. Davies, Donald S. IV. Title. V. Series. [DNLM: 1. Models, Biological – congresses. 2. Toxicology – methods – congresses. W1 AR49GA v.11/ QV 600 E897m 1986]
RA1190.E8 Suppl., vol. 11   615.9 s   87-12695   [RA1199]   [615.9]
ISBN 0-387-17614.4 (U.S.)

Typesetting, printing and bookbinding: Brühlsche Universitätsdruckerei, Giessen
2127/3020-543210

Contents

Contents VII

Mechanisms of Cell Injury

Mechanisms and Models in Toxicology
Arch. Toxicol., Suppl. 11, 3–10 (1987)

Apoptosis: Cell Death Under Homeostatic Control

A. H. Wyllie

Department of Pathology, University of Edinburgh Medical School,
Teviot Place, Edinburgh, EH8 9AG, Scotland, UK

Introduction

The purpose of this paper is to present a concept of cell death which differs from, but complements, the classical toxicological view. Evidence will be reviewed which shows that cells can (and in most cases eventually do) die in response to physiological stimuli. Physiological cell death will be seen to be mediated by certain intracellular events, which can be defined in molecular terms, and which are themselves internally regulated.

Cell Death is a Physiological Event

Physiological cell death is a phylogenetically ancient process. In planaria, periods of starvation are accompanied by loss of cells (Bowen and Ryder 1974; Bowen et al. 1976). In the developing nervous system of the nematode *Caenorhabditis elegans*, certain cells are deleted while others differentiate or proliferate, according to a well-defined genetically determined programme (Hedgecock 1985). Physiological cell death is essential for the swift removal of cells in the metamorphosis of insects and amphibia. Normal development in all vertebrates is as dependent upon programmed cell death as it is upon cell differentiation and proliferation. In later postnatal life also, cell death occurs in the physiological turnover of cells in tissues. Particularly well-documented examples exist in endocrine-dependent tissues, in which cell loss swiftly follows changes in trophic hormone drive (Kerr and Searle 1973; Wyllie et al. 1973; Hopwood and Levison 1974; Sandow et al. 1979; O'Shea et al. 1978; Ferguson and Anderson 1981). It appears that at all stages in the life of multicellular organisms, cell number homeostasis is maintained not only by regulation of cell birth rate, but also by control of cell death rate.

The fact that physiological cell death exists does not necessarily mean that it is always achieved by identical cellular processes. Indeed, the morphology of cell death in planaria differs from that in nematodes (Robertson and Thomson 1982),

Presented at the Joint Symposium of the European Society of Toxicology and the Society of Toxicology.

and neither is identical to that observed in the other circumstances cited above (Wyllie 1981). Remarkably, however, there is very close similarity in the morphology of physiological cell death, induced by a wide variety of stimuli, in insects and vertebrates (Wyllie et al. 1980; Wyllie 1981). Some, but not all of the characteristic features are present also in the programmed death of neurones in the developing nematode. This similarity of morphology led to the belief that a common mechanism might be involved. It was therefore of interest to attempt to define the structural changes in such dying cells more precisely.

The Morphology of Physiological Cell Death

The central features of physiological cell death in insects and vertebrates include contraction of cell volume, nuclear chromatin condensation, cellular fragmentation, and swift recognition and phagocytosis by adjacent cells (Wyllie et al. 1980; Wyllie 1981). Cytoplasmic organelles are well preserved and the dying cell or cell fragments retain intact membranes. Functionally, these membranes exclude trypan blue, nigrosine and ethidium bromide.

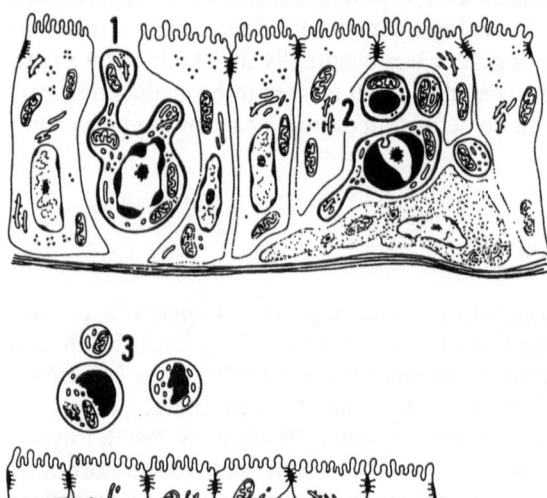

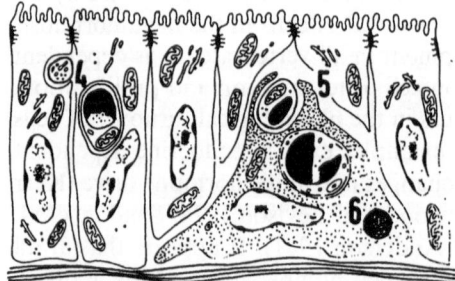

Fig. 1. Scheme of events in apoptosis. The dying cell loses contact with its neighbours (*1*), rounding up and undergoing chromatin condensation. It may separate into a cluster of membrane-bounded bodies (*2*). These are sometimes voided from the tissue, for example, into a lumen (*3*) where they undergo secondary degenerative changes. More usually they are phagocytosed either by adjacent parenchymal cells (*4*) or specialised mononuclear phagocytes (*5*), to undergo digestion and degradation to lysosomal residual bodies (*6*). (Reprinted with permission from Wyllie et al. 1980)

This series of changes is characteristic of physiological cell death in vertebrates, but differs in many respects from the cell death induced by high concentrations of toxins. In order to distinguish it from other forms of death and draw attention to its role complementary to mitosis in tissue homeostasis, it is designated *apoptosis* (Kerr et al. 1972; Wyllie et al. 1980; Wyllie 1981), a term derived from the Greek for the falling off of leaves from trees in autumn (Fig. 1).

Cells undergoing apoptosis within tissues do not elicit an inflammatory reaction. Phagocytosis by their viable neighbours ensures that the cells are deleted with minimum disturbance to tissue structure. Apoptotic cells can be identified in the light microscope by their condensed, fragmented chromatin, and sometimes by their sharply defined rounded cell contours, but they quickly vanish as a result of digestion within the phagosomes of the ingesting cell. Estimates of the half-time for which apoptotic cells remain visible in the light microscope are under 9 h (Wyllie et al. 1980; Ijiri and Potten 1983). These features fit the process well for playing a role in physiological involution and atrophy, and make study of the biochemical basis of apoptosis difficult, since the dying cells are greatly outnumbered by their surrounding, viable neighbours. It proved possible, however, to purify thymocytes, rendered apoptotic by exposure to glucocorticoid hormones in culture, using density gradient centrifugation (Wyllie and Morris 1982). Unlike cells dying as a result of membrane damage, apoptotic thymocytes have higher than normal density. Using cells purified in this way, molecular events were identified underlying the recognition of apoptotic cells by their neighbours, and responsible for the characteristic chromatin changes.

Recognition of Apoptotic Cells by Their Neighbours

Although the recognition and phagocytosis of apoptotic cells is not in itself part of the lethal process, it plays a significant role in the efficient removal of dying cells from involuting tissues. The existing literature on recognition of dying "self" cells is meagre, although endogenous lectins with specificities for desialylated glycoproteins have been implicated in the removal of damaged proteins from the circulation by cells of the reticulo-endothelial system (Hudgin et al. 1974; Stockert et al. 1976; Priels et al. 1978). In vitro, monolayers of murine peritoneal macrophages were found to bind apoptotic isogeneic thymocytes in preference to non-apoptotic cells. The binding took place at 4 °C in the absence of serum factors, and was inhibited by monosaccharides in a selective way (Morris et al. 1984; Duvall et al. 1985). Thus mannose, fucose and N-acetyl neuraminic acid had little effect on binding, whereas N-acetyl glucosamine reduced the binding of apoptotic cells to the background observed with normal cells, Galactose and N-acetyl galactosamine had a lesser inhibitory effect, whereas inhibition was strongest with the dimer of N-acetyl glucosamine, N,N'-diacetyl chitobiose. The inhibition was established as dependent upon a lectin-like molecule on the monocyte and not on the thymocyte, as preincubation of monocytes with diacetyl chitobiose, with washing before exposure to thymocytes, still inhibited binding.

These experiments suggested that monocytes posses an endogenous lectin-like molecule capable of binding to sugar residues exposed preferentially on the surface of apoptotic cells. Interestingly, the sugar specificity of this presumed lectin differs from that of previously described mammalian endogenous lectins (Duvall et al. 1985).

The question arises as to how novel sugar residues might become exposed on the surface of apoptotic cells. Exposure of N-acetyl glucosamine would require selective loss of the terminal sialyl groups, and there is some evidence for this from cell electrophoretic data (Morris et al. 1984). These show that the migration rate of apoptotic cells is less than that of their normal neighbours, a result most easily interpreted to mean that the surface density of charged N-acetyl neuraminic acid groups is reduced in apoptosis. The reduction in mobility is small, however, relative to that achieved by exhaustive digestion of normal cells by neuraminidase. A selective loss of exposed acid groups could be achieved by several mechanisms which have been discussed elsewhere (Wyllie et al. 1984; Duvall and Wyllie 1986), but one of them includes the premature fusion of endoplasmic reticulum membranes with the cell surface, a phenomenon well-documented in apoptotic cells (Yamada and Ohyama 1980; Galili et al. 1982; Morris et al. 1984).

Chromatin Changes in Apoptosis

The morphological changes in the nucleus of apoptotic cells are consistently associated with evidence of cleavage of chromatin at internucleosomal sites, apparently by an endogenous endonuclease (Skalka et al. 1976; Wyllie 1980; Suciu and Bojan 1981; Umansky et al. 1981; Yamada et al. 1981; Zvonareva et al. 1983; Wyllie et al. 1984). The nature of the products of the cleavage reaction suggests that they result from endonuclease activation in the absence of concurrent protease activity. Thus, the fragments show all the features of well-organized chromatin: in terms of buoyant density, sedimentation velocity and digestion kinetics when exposed to exogenous nucleases in vitro, the fragments of chromatin from apoptotic cells behaved in an exactly similar manner to chromatin extracted from normal cells (Wyllie, Morris, and Arends, unpublished work). Moreover, morphological changes closely similar to those observed in apoptosis can be induced in isolated nuclei by exposing them to purified nucleases, such as micrococcal nuclease, in the presence of high concentrations of protease inhibitors.

Recently, there have been attempts in this laboratory and elsewhere to extract the nuclease responsible for these changes from the nuclei of thymocytes and lymphoma cells. Thymocyte nuclei contain an endonuclease which requires the coincident presence of calcium and magnesium for activity, is active at neutral pH, and cleaves chromatin at internucleosomal sites in the same manner as that observed in apoptosis (Duke et al. 1983; Cohen and Duke 1984; Wyllie et al. 1986). The enzyme does not appear to have the ability to digest purified DNA to completion, although there is no evidence of restriction of the cleavage sites to particular base sequences. This activity is present in normal thymocytes, but it is absent from many cultured cell lines, including lymphoma cells remotely derived from murine thymus and human leukaemia. In some of these cell lines, however, treatment with glucocorticoid in vitro results in apoptosis, together with the characteristic chromatin cleavage, and appearance of the calcium plus magnesium endonuclease. The time-course of the induction of the enzyme is entirely compatible with the view that it is responsible for the cleavage observed.

The data thus support the hypothesis that synthesis of the endonuclease, under glucocorticoid induction, is a prerequisite for apoptosis in these proliferating lymphoma cells. In the terminally differentiated, nondividing thymocytes, by contrast, the enzyme is present, but presumably requires activation by glucocorticoid-dependent or other mechanisms. Such mechanisms might include relatively nonspecific injury stimuli, capable of increasing calcium concentration in the nucleus. The ionophore A23 187, for example, activates the endonuclease (in the absence of steroid) although the density shift described above does not occur (Wyllie et al. 1984). Even in thymocytes, however, the endonucleases may undergo constant replenishment, as inhibitors of protein synthesis abrogate apoptosis caused by both glucocorticoid and ionophore, and reduce the quantity of endogenous nuclease recovered from treated cells.

Apoptosis and Toxicology

Although this account has concentrated on the role of apoptosis in the mediation of physiological cell death, there is good evidence that apoptosis may also occur in tissues subjected to injury by a variety of nonphysiological stimuli, including viruses, ionizing radiation, and many toxic substances (Table 1). Although the data are incomplete, two general points appear to be valid. First, apoptosis is in-

Table 1. Topography of apoptosis after cell injury

Tissue	Injury	Location of apoptosis	Reference
Adrenal cortex	DMBA	Z fascic and z retic	Currie et al. (1962)
	ACTH deficiency	Z retic	Wyllie et al. (1973)
	None	Z retic	Wyllie et al. (1973)
Thymus	Glucocorticoid	Cortex	Van Haelst (1967)
	Irradiation	Cortex	Umansky et al. (1981)
	Polyoma virus	Cortex	Inamura et al. (1971)
	Thioacetamide	Cortex	Barker and Smuckler (1973)
	Zinc deficiency	Cortex	Fraker et al. (1977)
	None	Cortex	Van Haelst (1967)
Lymph node	AD, MC, ara C	Reactive centre	Searle et al. (1975)
	None	Reactive centre	Kerr et al. (1972)
GI epithelium	Irradiation	Crypt posn 4–5	Ijiri and Potten (1983)
	NM	Crypt posn 6–7	Ijiri and Potten (1983)
	5FU	Crypt posn 7–9	Ijiri and Potten (1983)
	VCR HU	Crypt posn 10–11	Ijiri and Potten (1983)
	Zinc deficiency	Mid crypt	Elmes (1977)
	None	Crypt	Searle et al. (1975)
Liver	Hypoxia	Centrilobular	Kerr (1971)
	None	? Centrilobular	Zajicek et al. (1985)

AD, actinomycin D; ara C, cytosine arabinoside; DMBA, dimethylbenzanthracine; 5FU, 5 fluorouracil; HU, hydroxyurea; MC, mitomycin C; NM, nitrogen mustard; VCR, vincristine.

duced in susceptible tissues by injurious stimuli of smaller amplitude than those which cause necrosis in the same tissues. Secondly, the cells undergoing toxin-induced apoptosis appear to be within the same tissue subpopulation that is susceptible to apoptosis under physiological circumstances. The last point suggests that, at relatively low concentrations, toxic stimuli may trigger endogenous lethal mechanisms in certain tissue cells which are already primed to undergo apoptosis. Other cells, not so primed, presumably die by different mechanisms, requiring higher toxin concentrations. There is some direct evidence in support of this from work on cells damaged by ionizing radiation (Umansky et al. 1981; Afanas'ev et al. 1986). The endonuclease described in the preceding section may be one of the endogenous lethal mechanisms, triggered by specific regulatory stimuli such as glucocorticoids, and also by other, less specific injury stimuli.

Acknowledgement. This work is supported by the Cancer Research Campaign and the Wellcome Trust.

References

Afanas'ev VN, Korol' BA, Mantsygin YA, Nelipovich PA, Pechatnikov VA, Umansky SR (1986) Flow cytometry and biochemical analysis of DNA degradation characteristic of two types of cell death. FEBS Letters 194:347–350

Barker EA, Smuckler EA (1973) Nonhepatic thioacetamide injury. I.Thymic cortical necrosis. Am J Pathol 71:409–418

Bowen ID, Ryder TA (1974) Cell autolysis and deletion in the planarian *Polycelis tenuis* Iijima. Cell Tiss Res 154:265–274

Bowen ID, Ryder TA, Dark C (1986) The effects of starvation on the planarian worm *Polycelis tenuis* Iijima. Cell Tiss Res 169:193–209

Cohen JJ, Duke RC (1984) Glucocorticoid activation of a calcium-dependent endonuclease in thymic nuclei leads to cell death. J Immunol 132:38–42

Currie AR, Helfenstein JE, Young S (1962) Massive adrenal necrosis in rats caused by 9,10-dimethyl-1,2-benzanthrene and its inhibition by methyrapone. Lancet 2:1199–1200

Duke RC, Cherniak R, Cohen JJ (1983) Endogenous endonuclease-induced DNA fragmentation: an early event in cell-mediated cytolysis. Proc Natl Acad Sci USA 80:6361–6365

Duvall E, Wyllie AH (1986) Death and the cell. Immunology Today 7:115–119

Duvall E, Wyllie AH, Morris RG (1985) Macrophage recognition of cells undergoing programmed cell death (apoptosis). Immunology 56:351–358

Elmes ME (1977) Apoptosis in the small intestine of zinc-deficient and fasted rats. J Pathol 123:219–223

Ferguson DJP, Anderson TJ (1981) Ultrastructural observations on cell death by apoptosis in the "resting" human breast. Virchows Arch [A] 393:193–203

Fraker PJ, Haas SM, Luecke RW (1977) Effect of zinc deficiency on the immune response of the young adult A/J mouse. J Nutr 107:1889–1895

Galili U, Leizerowitz R, Moreb J, Gamliel H, Gurfel D, Polliack A (1982) Metabolic and ultrastructural aspects of the in vitro lysis of chronic lymphocytic leukaemia cells by glucocorticoids. Cancer Res 42:1433–1440

Hedgecock EM (1985) Cell lineage mutants in the nematode *Caenorhabditis elegans*. Trends in Neurosciences 8:288–293

Hopwood D, Levison DA (1974) Atrophy and apoptosis in the cyclical human endometrium. J Pathol 119:159–166

Hudgin RL, Pricer WE, Ashwell G, Stockert RJ, Morell AG (1974) The isolation and properties of a rat liver binding protein specific for asialoglycoproteins. J Biol Chem 249:5536–5543

Ijiri K, Potten CS (1983) Response of intestinal cells of differing topographical and hierarchical status to ten cytotoxic drugs and five sources of radiation. Br J Cancer 47:175–185

Imamura M, Matsuyama T, Toh K, Okuyama T (1971) Electron microscopic study on acute thymic involution induced by polyoma virus infection. J Natl Canc Inst 47:289–299

Kerr JFR (1971) Shrinkage necrosis: a definite mode of cellular death. J Pathol 105:13–20

Kerr JFR, Searle J (1973) Deletion of cells by apoptosis during castration-induced involution of the rat prostate. Virchows Arch [B] 13:87–102

Kerr JFR, Wyllie AH, Currie AR (1972) Apoptosis: a basic biological phenomenon with wide-ranging implications in tissue kinetics. Br J Cancer 26:239–257

Morris RG, Hargreaves AD, Duvall E, Wyllie AH (1984) Hormone-induced cell death: II. Surface changes in thymocytes undergoing apoptosis. Am J Pathol 115:426–436

O'Shea JD, Hay MF, Cran DG (1978) Ultrastructural changes in the theca interna during follicular atresia in sheep. J Reprod Fertil 54:183–187

Priels JP, Pizzo S, Glasgow LR, Paulson JC, Hill RL (1978) Hepatic receptor that specifically binds oligosaccharides containing fucosyl 1-3 N-acetylglucosamine linkages. Proc Natl Acad Sci USA 75:2215–2219

Robertson AMG, Thomson JN (1982) Morphology of programmed cell death in the ventral nerve cord of Caenorhabditis elegans larvae. J Embryol Exp Morph 67:89–100

Sandow BA, West NB, Norman RJ, Brenner RM (1979) Hormonal control of apoptosis in hamster uterine luminal epithelium. Am J Anat 156:15–35

Searle J, Lawson TA, Abbott PJ, Harmon B, Kerr JFR (1975) An electron microscope study of the mode of cell death induced by cancer chemotherapeutic agents in populations of proliferating normal and neoplastic cells. J Pathol 116:129–138

Skalka M, Matyasova J, Cejkova M (1981) DNA in chromatin of irradiated lymphoid tissues degrades in vivo into regular fragments. FEBS Letters 72:271–274

Stockert RH, Morell AB, Scheinberg IH (1976) The existence of a second route for the transfer of certain glycoproteins from the circulation into the liver. Biochem Biophys Res Commun 68:988–993

Suciu D, Bojan O (1981) Autodigestion of chromatin in some radiosensitive and radioresistant mouse cells. Role of proteolysis and endonucleolysis. Int J Radiat Biol 39:273–279

Umansky SR, Korol BA, Nelipovich PA (1981) In vivo DNA degradation in thymocytes of γ-irradiated or hydrocortisone-treated rats. Biochim Biophys Acta 655:9–17

van Haelst U (1967) Light and electron microscopic study of the normal and pathological thymus of the rat. I. The normal thymus. Z Zellforsch 77:534–553

van Haelst U (1967) Light and electron microscopic study of the normal and pathological thymus of the rat. II. The acute thymic involution. Z Zellforsch Mikrosk Anat 80:153–182

Wyllie AH (1980) Glucocorticoid-induced thymocyte apoptosis is associated with endogenous endonuclease activation. Nature 284:555–556

Wyllie AH (1981) Cell death: a new classification separating apoptosis from necrosis. In: Bowen ID, Lockshin RA (eds) Cell death in biology and pathology. Chapman and Hall, London, pp 9–34

Wyllie AH, Morris RG (1982) Hormone-induced cell death. Purification and properties of thymocytes undergoing apoptosis after glucocorticoid treatment. Am J Pathol 109:78–87

Wyllie AH, Kerr JFR, Currie AR (1973 a) Cell death in the normal neonatal rat adrenal cortex. J Pathol 111:255–261

Wyllie AH, Kerr JFR, Macaskill IAM, Currie AR (1973 b) Adrenocortical cell deletion: the role of ACTH. J Pathol 111:85–94

Wyllie AH, Kerr JFR, Currie AR (1980) Cell death: the significance of apoptosis. Int Rev Cytol 68:251–306

Wyllie AH, Duvall E, Blow JJ (1984 a) Intracellular mechanisms in cell death in normal and pathological tissues. In: Davies I, Sigee DC (eds) Cell ageing and cell death. Cambridge University Press, Cambridge, pp 269–294

Wyllie AH, Morris RG, Smith AL, Dunlop D (1984 b) Chromatin cleavage in apoptosis: association with condensed chromatin morphology and dependence on macromolecular synthesis. J Pathol 142:67–77

Wyllie AH, Morris RG, Watt AE (1986) Terminally differentiated and dying cells contain nuclear endonuclease potentially responsible for chromatin changes of apoptosis. J Pathol 148:94A

Yamada T, Ohyama H (1980) Changes in surface morphology of rat thymocytes accompanying inter-
phase death. J Radiat Res 21:190–196
Yamada T, Ohyama H, Kinjo Y, Watanabe M (1981) Evidence for the internucleosomal breakage of
chromatin in rat thymocytes irradiated in vitro. Radiat Res 85:544–553
Zajicek G, Oren R, Weinreb M (1985) The streaming liver. Liver 5:293–300
Zvonareva NB, Zhivotovsky BD, Hanson KP (1983) Distribution of nuclease attack sites and complex-
ity of DNA in the products of post-irradiation degradation of rat thymus chromatin. Int J Radiat
Biol 44:261–266

Mechanisms and Models in Toxicology
Arch. Toxicol., Suppl. 11, 11–19 (1987)

On the Role of Calcium in Chemical Toxicity

S. Orrenius and P. Nicotera

Department of Toxicology, Karolinska Institutet, PO Box 60400, S-104 01 Stockholm, Sweden

Introduction

It is now well established that the toxic effects of a variety of chemicals are mediated by reactive products formed during their biotransformation in the organism. It is equally clear that there exist protective systems which can trap or inactivate toxic metabolites and thereby prevent their accumulation within the tissues and subsequent toxicity. Although phase I reactions, in particular those mediated by the cytochrome P_{450}-linked monooxygenase system, are most often responsible for the production of toxic metabolites, there are now many examples of metabolic activation via phase II reactions, despite the fact that the latter normally serve a protective function (Jakoby 1980). It therefore follows that the formation of toxic metabolites cannot be attributed to any single enzyme or enzyme system, and that the balance between metabolic activation and inactivation is critical in deciding whether exposure to a potentially toxic compound will result in toxicity or not.

Glutathione plays a unique role in the cellular defense against toxic chemicals. It is present at high concentrations in most mammalian cells and almost entirely in its reduced form (GSH), with glutathione disulfide (GSSG), mixed disulfides, and thioethers constituting minor fractions of the total glutathione pool (Larsson et al. 1983). Depletion of intracellular GSH is known to be one of the most detrimental effects of toxic injury, since loss of glutathione protection against reactive intermediates rapidly leads to the failure of vital cell functions and cell death.

During the past several years this laboratory has been actively engaged in studies of the role of thiol depletion in toxic cell injury. Using freshly isolated hepatocytes and subcellular fractions, it has been shown that GSH depletion and modification of protein thiols can result in a perturbation of intracellular Ca^{2+} homeostasis, alteration of hepatocyte morphology and cell death. The following is a brief discussion of the mechanisms responsible for the perturbation of thiol and Ca^{2+} homeostasis following the metabolism of toxic agents by isolated hepatocytes.

Presented at the Joint Symposium of the European Society of Toxicology and the Society of Toxicology.

Mechanisms of Glutathione Depletion

Conjugation with GSH represents the most important protective mechanism against the toxicity of a wide variety of reactive electrophiles. Although GSH can react nonenzymatically with many electrophilic compounds, this process is normally catalyzed by the glutathione transferases (Jakoby 1980; Larsson et al. 1983). Under extreme conditions, the formation of glutathione conjugates can result in GSH depletion and tissue toxicity.

The selenoprotein glutathione peroxidase provides protection against hydrogen peroxide and a variety of organic hydroperoxides (Jakoby 1980). GSH serves as the electron donor, and the GSSG formed in the reaction is subsequently reduced back to GSH by glutathione reductase at the expense of NADPH. Under conditions of oxidative stress, when the cell must cope with large amounts of hydroperoxides, the glutathione reductase is unable to keep up with the rate of glutathione oxidation, and GSSG accumulates. In an apparent effort to avoid the detrimental effects of increased intracellular levels of GSSG, the cell actively excretes the disulfide which can lead to a depletion of the intracellular glutathione pool.

As mentioned above, the toxicity of many xenobiotics is preceded by depletion of intracellular GSH. Any process resulting in GSH consumption at a rate which exceeds the capacity of the cell to replenish its thiol pool will lead to GSH depletion. Although depletion of GSH as a result of oxidation would appear to be a reversible process due to the presence of glutathione reductase, it is clear from the discussion above that this is not always the case. Therefore, both conjugate formation and oxidation may result in the depletion of intracellular GSH and subsequent toxicity.

Role of Protein Thiol Modification

Although the presence of free sulfhydryl groups in proteins has been recognized since the beginning of this century, interest in the role they may play as highly reactive functional groups in biological systems arose only after the discovery of glutathione. A large number of enzymes, catalyzing a wide variety of reactions, are now known to depend on free sulfhydryl groups for their activity, and it is therefore not surprising that modification of protein thiols can result in severe functional damage in biological systems.

Thiol groups are highly reactive and participate in several different reactions, such as alkylation, arylation, oxidation, thiol-disulfide exchange, etc. All of these reactions may be involved in the modification of protein thiols resulting from the interaction with reactive intermediates formed during the metabolism of toxic chemicals. Thus, although the toxicological implications of 'covalent binding' (i.e., alkylation, arylation) of reactive intermediates to various proteins have often been emphasized, it is clear that thiol oxidation and mixed disulfide formation may also interfere with normal protein function. Such modifications of protein thiols may be particularly important during oxidative stress (Di Monte et al. 1984).

Appearance of Surface Blebs in Hepatocytes Exposed to Toxic Agents

Incubation of hepatocytes with a variety of toxic agents results in alterations in surface morphology characterized by a loss of microvilli and appearance of multiple blebs on the surface of the hepatocytes (Jewell et al. 1982). These changes usually appear before any signs of increased plasma membrane permeability are observed and seem to be reversible initially, i.e., they disappear when the toxic agent is removed from the incubation. The formation of surface blebs does not seem to be related to cell swelling caused by increased plasma membrane permeability, since it is not affected by changes in the osmolarity of the incubation medium.

Cell surface morphology is thought to be determined by organization of cortical microfilaments associated with the plasma membrane (Cheung 1980, and references therein). This assumption is supported by the finding that two classes of compounds, the cytochalasins and phalloidins, which disrupt cortical microfilament structure, cause bleb formation on the surface of hepatocytes similar to that observed with other toxic agents. However, with most toxic agents there is no evidence for a direct interaction of the reactive metabolites with cytoskeletal components, and it therefore appears more likely that the observed abnormalities are produced indirectly by alterations in levels of regulatory cofactors or ions.

The polymerization of monomeric to filamentous-form actin is dependent upon ATP; one mole of bound ATP is converted to ADP for every monomeric actin subunit polymerized. Thus, one would expect that, in the hepatocyte, ATP depletion would result in actin depolymerization, breakdown of the actomyosin network and plasma membrane blebbing. Indeed, inhibition of ATP synthesis by treatment of isolated hepatocytes with antimycin A is associated with extensive plasma membrane blebbing which precedes loss of cell viability. However, these alterations in surface morphology occur before ATP depletion does and are better correlated with alterations in intracellular Ca^{2+} distribution following antimycin A-induced release of mitochondrial Ca^{2+} (Smith et al. 1984). A change in intracellular Ca^{2+} distribution can alter hepatocyte cytoskeletal structure because Ca^{2+} and its associated binding proteins play a pivotal role in regulating cytoskeletal structure (Cheung 1980). Furthermore, the observation that the calcium ionophore A23187 produces plasma membrane blebbing in isolated hepatocytes supports the assumption that alterations in surface morphology observed during oxidative stress are related to perturbation of intracellular Ca^{2+} homeostasis (Jewell et al. 1982).

Disruption of Intracellular Ca^{2+} Homeostasis by Toxic Agents

The low resting concentration of Ca^{2+} in the cytosol of hepatocytes is maintained by active compartmentation processes and by calcium binding to specific proteins, including calmodulin. Mitochondrial Ca^{2+} homeostasis is regulated by a cyclic mechanism, involving Ca^{2+} uptake by an energy-dependent pathway and Ca^{2+} release which is probably mediated by a Ca^{2+}/H^+ antiporter. The latter appears to be regulated by the redox level of intramitochondrial pyridine nucleo-

Table 1. Effects of toxic agents on Ca^{2+} homeostasis in hepatocytes

Agent	Mitochondrial pool	Endoplasmic reticular pool	Cytosolic Ca^{2+}
Menadione	Decrease	Decrease	Increase
t-Butyl hydroperoxide	Decrease	Decrease	Increase
N-Acetyl-p-benzoquinone imine	Decrease	Decrease	Increase
Carbon tetrachloride	–	Decrease	Increase
Bromobenzene	–	Decrease	Increase
Extracellular ATP	Increase	Increase	Increase
Cystamine	Increase	Increase	Increase

tides (Lehninger et al. 1978), although membrane-bound protein thiols may also be important in modulating mitochondrial Ca^{2+} fluxes. The active transport of calcium ions through the endoplasmic reticular and plasma membrane is mediated by Ca^{2+}-stimulated, Mg^{2+}-dependent ATPases which appear to depend on free sulfhydryl groups for activity (Moore et al. 1975; Bellomo et al. 1983).

The availability of noninvasive techniques to measure Ca^{2+} content in intracellular compartments has made it possible to monitor alterations in Ca^{2+} compartmentation during the development of toxicity in hepatocytes (Bellomo et al. 1982). Under normal conditions freshly isolated rat hepatocytes contain approximately 3 nmol/10^6 cells of exchangeable Ca^{2+}; approximately 60% of this Ca^{2+} is sequestered in the mitochondria and approximately 40% in the endoplasmic reticulum. The concentration of cytosolic free Ca^{2+} is normally very low (~ 150 nM).

As shown in Table 1, incubation of hepatocytes with various toxic agents is associated with alterations in the intracellular Ca^{2+} pools. Common to all agents listed in the table is their ability to produce a sustained increase in cytosolic free Ca^{2+} concentration. This effect precedes the appearance of surface blebs and the loss of cell viability and seems to be a critical event in the development of toxicity.

As briefly mentioned above, the hepatic plasma membrane Ca^{2+}-ATPase contains functional sulfhydryl group(s), the modification of which is associated with inhibition of both Ca^{2+}-ATPase activity and Ca^{2+} extrusion from hepatocytes (Nicotera et al. 1985). In fact, it has been speculated that the impairment of Ca^{2+} efflux resulting from the interaction between electrophilic intermediates and a critical pool of plasma membrane protein thiols may represent a critical biochemical lesion in the development of hepatotoxicity (Nicotera et al. 1986a).

Mechanisms of Ca^{2+}-Mediated Toxicity

To further investigate the relationship between perturbation of intracellular Ca^{2+} homeostasis and cytotoxicity, isolated hepatocytes were exposed to agents that selectively interfere with the normal Ca^{2+} influx-efflux balance, thereby causing a sustained increase in cytosolic Ca^{2+} level (Nicotera et al. 1986a, b). As illustrated schematically in Fig. 1, incubation of hepatocytes with either extracellular

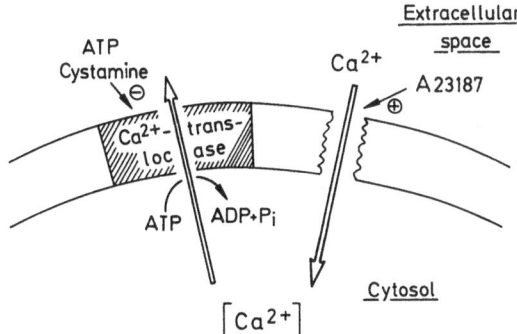

Fig. 1. Schematic illustration of the modulation of cytosolic Ca^{2+} concentration in hepatocytes by various agents, showing the inhibitory effects of extracellular ATP and cystamine on active Ca^{2+} extrusion and the extracellular Ca^{2+} permeation of the plasma membrane, facilitated by ionophore A23187

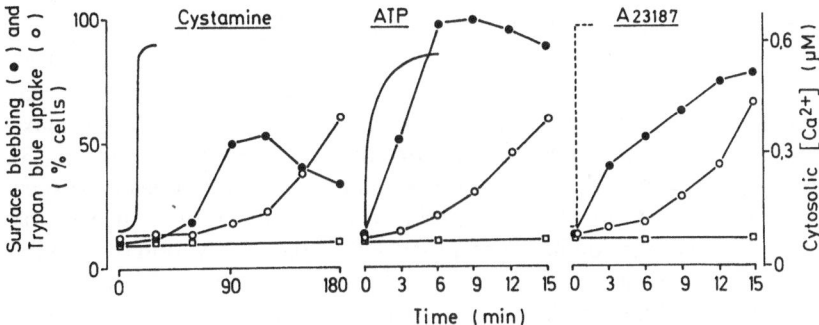

Fig. 2. Relationship between increase in cytosolic Ca^{2+} (*continuous line*), surface blebbing (●), and cell death (○) in hepatocytes untreated (■), or exposed to cystamine (1 mM), ATP (1 mM) and ionophore A 23187 (15 µM). Cytosolic Ca^{2+} was measured according to Cooper et al. (1985), while surface blebbing and cell death were determined as reported in Jewell et al. (1982)

ATP or cystamine is associated with an inhibition of Ca^{2+} efflux, whereas treatment of the cells with the cation ionophore A23187 results in enhanced influx of extracellular Ca^{2+}. All treatments resulted in a sustained increase in cytosolic Ca^{2+} concentration which was followed by the appearance of surface blebs and, subsequently, the loss of cell viability (Fig. 2). A previous study has shown that the effects of cystamine are caused by the selective inhibition of Ca^{2+} efflux associated with the formation of mixed disulfides between cystamine and a small pool of superficially located plasma membrane protein thiols (Nicotera et al. 1986 a). The mechanism by which extracellular ATP inhibits Ca^{2+} extrusion from hepatocytes is not yet well characterized (Bellomo et al. 1984).

The finding of a relationship between a sustained increase in cytosolic Ca^{2+} concentration and toxicity of several agents in hepatocytes has led to a search for mechanisms by which the increased cytosolic Ca^{2+} could trigger cytotoxicity. The formation of surface blebs is one of the earliest events associated with the increase in cytosolic Ca^{2+}, however, during the early phase blebbing is reversible, and it is difficult to assess whether the progression to irreversible damage may involve the same pathway as that responsible for bleb formation. It has been proposed

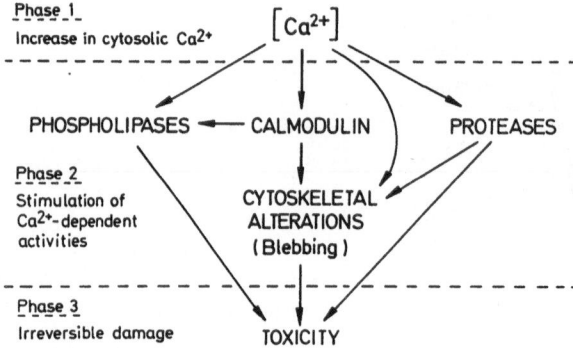

Fig. 3. Proposed pathways for Ca^{2+}-mediated cytotoxicity

that the sustained increase in Ca^{2+} concentration may cause abnormal stimulation of normal "physiological" processes, such as those dependent on calmodulin,
and it is conceivable that calmodulin may mediate some of the cytotoxic effects
of Ca^{2+}, although direct evidence is still lacking. On the other hand, Ca^{2+} may
activate catabolic enzymes, such as proteases and lipases, whose activity is maximally stimulated in the presence of high cytosolic Ca^{2+} concentrations (Fig. 3).
Phospholipases are widely distributed in mammalian cells, and it has been speculated that an enhanced rate of phospholipid hydrolysis may result in irreversible
cell damage. This assumption has been supported by the observation that inhibitors of phospholipases prevent ischemic cell death in liver and heart and by the
finding that phospholipid breakdown is enhanced during tissue injury (Chien et
al. 1977, 1979).

Recently it has been investigated whether phospholipase activation may contribute to cystamine toxicity in hepatocytes (Nicotera et al. 1986a). Indeed, cystamine exposure did enhance the rate of phospholipid hydrolysis, and this stimulation of phospholipid breakdown was apparent before any loss of cell viability
had occurred and was abolished by phospholipase inhibitors, including the calmodulin antagonist calmidazolium. However, neither phospholipase inhibitors
nor calmidazolium was able to prevent the cytotoxicity induced by cystamine in
isolated hepatocytes, suggesting that phospholipase activation and calmodulin-
dependent processes were not involved in cell killing.

It is now widely recognized that Ca^{2+} plays an important role in the control
of intracellular proteolysis in a number of tissues, and it has been speculated that
a rise in intracellular Ca^{2+} may lead to an enhanced rate of protein breakdown
which could result in lysis of cell structures and irreversible cell damage. Increases
in cytosolic Ca^{2+} induced by cystamine, ATP and ionophore A23187 did, in fact,
result in a stimulation of intracellular proteolysis in hepatocytes (Table 2). Further, it appears that a stimulation of cytosolic Ca^{2+}-dependent proteases was responsible for the enhanced rate of protein degradation. Several lines of evidence
support this conclusion:

1. Lysosomotropic agents, such as methylamine and chloroquine, did not prevent the Ca^{2+}-stimulated proteolysis.

Table 2. Relationship between stimulation of proteolysis and cytotoxic effects of agents which cause intracellular Ca^{2+} accumulation in hepatocytes[a]

Agent	Proteolysis (% change)	Surface blebbing (% cells)	Trypan blue uptake (% cells)
Control		6	9
ATP (1 mM)	+45	90	55
ATP plus leupeptin (100 µg/ml)	− 1	10	12
A23187 (15 µM)	+56	80	50
A23187 plus leupeptin (100 µg/ml)	+12	20	25
Cystamine (1 mM)	+59	60	58
Cystamine plus leupeptin (100 µg/ml)	− 2	15	12

[a] Incubation with ATP and ionophore A23187 was for 15 min and with cystamine for 120 min. Proteolysis was assayed according to Seglen et al. (1979). The labeling of proteins in vivo was achieved by intraperitoneal injection of 0.5 ml [^{14}C]-valine (50 µCi), 16 h prior to hepatocyte isolation. Blebbing and trypan blue uptake were monitored as previously described (Jewell et al. 1982).

2. 3-Methyladenine and a calmodulin inhibitor, calmidazolium, which, inhibit autophagic vacuole formation by different mechanisms, did not prevent the Ca^{2+}-activated proteolysis.
3. The inhibitors of Ca^{2+}-activated proteases, leupeptin and antipain, prevented the stimulation of proteolysis as well as the onset of toxicity in hepatocytes (Table 2).

The target proteins for cytosolic Ca^{2+}-activated proteases remain to be identified. However, the observation that the Ca^{2+}-induced formation of surface blebs was also prevented by antipain and leupeptin suggests that among the substrates for cytosolic Ca^{2+}-activated proteases are cytoskeletal proteins, as has been found previously in other systems (Collier and Wang 1982).

Thus, it appears that both plasma membrane blebbing and cytotoxicity induced by ATP, cystamine, and ionophore A23187 in hepatocytes are associated with the activation of intracellular proteolysis and prevented by antipain and leupeptin (Table 2). Other inhibitors of lysosomal proteases and a specific inhibitor of autophagy, 3-methyladenine, did not prevent either blebbing or toxicity, nor did they abolish the stimulation of proteolysis, indicating that a nonlysosomal system was responsible for the stimulation of proteolysis associated with toxicity.

Concluding Remarks

Thus, it is concluded that a sustained elevation of cytosolic Ca^{2+} may lead to cell death through the activation of a distinct catabolic process, i.e., intracellular proteolysis. Studies in our and other laboratories indicate that in some experimental systems cytotoxicity can be prevented by Ca^{2+} antagonists, including verapamil and nifedipine, further suggesting that elevation of cytosolic Ca^{2+} can be critical for the development of lethal cell injury. A sequence of events involved in Ca^{2+}-mediated cytotoxicity is proposed in Fig. 4.

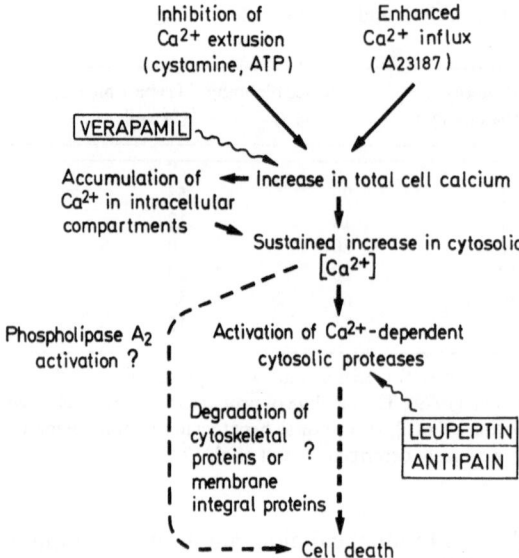

Fig. 4. Schematic illustration of proposed mechanisms of Ca^{2+} mediated cytotoxicity in isolated hepatocytes. Probable sites of action of protective agents are also shown

It remains to be established, however, whether this mechanism may apply to other toxic compounds and to different cell systems. Interestingly, it has been suggested that oxidative or covalent modification of proteins may render them more susceptible to enzymatic hydrolysis, and it has recently been shown that the proteolytic system responsible for the cleavage of oxidized proteins in neutrophils is dependent on Ca^{2+} for its activity (Rivett 1985). It is therefore likely that oxidative damage and/or changes in cytosolic Ca^{2+} may lead to enhanced proteolysis in tissues. However, since oxidation may also inactivate proteases and their inhibitors in the cell, it is at present difficult to draw any firm conclusions about the general toxicological importance of these processes.

References

Bellomo G, Jewell SA, Thor H., Orrenius S (1982) Regulation of intracellular calcium compartmentation; studies with isolated hepatocytes and *t*-butyl hydroperoxide. Proc Natl Acad Sci USA 79:6842–6846

Bellomo G, Mirabelli F. Richelmi P, Orrenius S (1983) Critical role of sulfhydryl group(s) in ATP-dependent Ca^{2+} sequestration by the plasma membrane fraction from rat liver. FEBS Letters 163:136–139

Bellomo G, Nicotera P, Orrenius S (1984) Alterations in intracellular Ca^{2+} compartmentation following inhibition of Ca^{2+} efflux from isolated hepatocytes. Eur J Biochem 144:19–23

Cheung WY (1980) Calmodulin plays a pivotal role in cellular regulation. Science 207:19–27

Chien KR, Abrams J, Pfau RG, Farber JL (1977) Prevention by chlorpromazine of ischemic liver cell death. Am J Pathol 88:539–558

Chien KR, Pfau RG, Farber JL (1979) Ischemic myocardial cell injury. Prevention by chlorpromazine of an accelerated phospholipid degradation and associated membrane dysfunction. Am J Pathol 97:505–530

Collier NC, Wang K (1982) Purification and properties of human platelet P235. J Biol Chem 257:6937–6943

Cooper RH, Coll KE, Williamson JR (1985) Differential effects of phorbol ester on phenylephrine and vasopressin-induced Ca^{2+} mobilization in isolated hepatocytes. J Biol Chem 260:3281–3288

Di Monte D, Bellomo G, Thor H, Nicotera P, Orrenius S (1984) Menadione-induced cytotoxicity is associated with protein thiol oxidation and alteration in intracellular Ca^{2+} homeostasis. Arch Biochem Biophys 235:343–350

Jakoby WB (1980) Enzymatic basis of detoxication, vols 1, 2. Academic, New York

Jewell SA, Bellomo G, Thor H, Orrenius S, Smith MT (1982) Bleb formation in hepatocytes during drug metabolism is caused by disturbances in thiol and calcium ion homeostasis. Science 217:1257–1259

Larsson A, Orrenius S, Holmgren A, Mannervik B (1983) Functions of glutathione: biochemical, physiological, toxicological and clinical aspects. Raven, New York

Lehninger AL, Vercesi A, Bababunmi E (1978) Regulation of Ca^{2+} release from mitochondria by the oxidation-reduction state of pyridine nucleotides. Proc Natl Acad Sci USA 75:1690–1694

Moore L, Chen T, Knapp HR, Landon E (1975) Energy-dependent calcium sequestration activity in rat liver microsomes. J Biol Chem 250:4562–4568

Nicotera P, Moore M, Mirabelli F, Bellomo G, Orrenius S (1985) Inhibition of hepatocyte plasma membrane Ca^{2+}-ATPase activity by menadione metabolism and its restoration by thiols. FEBS Letters 181:149–153

Nicotera P, Hartzell P, Baldi C, Svensson S-Å, Bellomo G, Orrenius S (1986a) Cystamine induces toxicity in hepatocytes through the elevation of cytosolic Ca^{2+} and the stimulation of a non-lysosomal proteolytic system. J Biol Chem 261:14628–14635

Nicotera P, Hartzell P, Davies G, Orrenius S (1986b) The formation of plasma membrane blebs in hepatocytes exposed to agents that increase cytosolic Ca^{2+} is mediated by the activation of a non-lysosomal proteolytic system. FEBS Letters 209:139–144

Rivett JA (1985) Preferential degradation of oxidatively modified form of glutamine synthetase by intracellular mammalian proteases. J Biol Chem 260:300–305

Seglen PO, Grinde B, Solheim AE (1979) Inhibition of the lysosomal pathway of protein degradation in isolated rat hepatocytes by ammonia, methylamine, chloroquine and leupeptin. Eur J Biochem 95:215–225

Smith MT, Thor H, Jewell SA, Bellomo G, Sandy MS, Orrenius S (1984) Free radical-induced changes in the surface morphology of isolated hepatocytes. In: Armstrong D, Sohal RS, Cutler RG, Slater TF (eds) Free radicals in molecular biology, aging and disease. Raven, New York, vol 27, pp 103–118

Mechanisms and Models in Toxicology
Arch. Toxicol., Suppl. 11, 20–33 (1987)

A Dynamic Liver Culture System:
A Tool for Studying Chemical Biotransformation and Toxicity

I. G. Sipes, R. L. Fisher, P. F. Smith, E. R. Stine, A. J. Gandolfi, and K. Brendel

Departments of Pharmacology and Toxicology, Pharmacology, and Anesthesiology,
University of Arizona Health Sciences Center, Tucson, Arizona 85721, USA

Introduction

The use of whole animal systems for toxicity testing has been extensively supplemented during the past several years with in vitro test systems. Such systems, through continued improvement and expanded versatility as research tools, hold great promise for the more rapid and less expensive evaluation of the potential toxicity of new and existing chemicals and pharmaceuticals. In addition, in vitro systems are useful in the elucidation of the mechanisms by which chemicals induce tissue damage. In in vitro systems the experimental system can be rigidly controlled. In vitro systems also provide opportunities to explore routes and rates of xenobiotic biotransformation, a factor which often determines the nature and degree of the observed toxicity.

There are a variety of in vitro test systems currently utilized for toxicity studies, each having a relatively specific set of applications. The major categories include systems that use microorganisms, cell/tissue culture, and organ culture. The use of mammalian cell/tissue culture systems for in vitro toxicology studies is seen as a valuable adjunct to whole animal studies. The most popular methods for in vitro hepatotoxicity evaluation employ suspensions of freshly isolated hepatocytes or cultures of hepatocytes. Hepatocytes are easily isolated and rapidly prepared. One liver can provide sufficient cells to permit carefully controlled experiments. Interindividual variation is greatly decreased because the cells are derived from a single tissue.

However, the cells are generally isolated by collagenase digestion, which may produce structural alterations and predispose the cells to toxicants. Also, with isolated hepatocytes (suspension or culture), the anatomical basis for the functional heterogeneity of the liver is destroyed. Therefore, a method for culturing liver tissue, under conditions where the architecture of the tissue and intercellular communication between the various cell types are maintained, while collagenase digestion is avoided, should provide significant additional information regarding the mechanism(s) of toxicity of xenobiotics. Cultured liver slices could theoreti-

---

Presented at the Joint Symposium of the European Society of Toxicology and the Society of Toxicology.

cally provide these advantages. However, the lack of a highly reproducible method for rapid production of precision-cut thin slices under minimally traumatic conditions has hindered their use for in vitro cytotoxicity studies (Smith et al. 1985). Furthermore, slices of adult mammalian liver have been difficult to maintain in culture because of apparent limitations in oxygen and nutrient diffusion (Campbell and Hales 1971). The problems result in the spontaneous and early occurrence of cellular degeneration (Grisham et al. 1978). Recently, a method was described for the rapid preparation of adult rat liver slices in large quantities under conditions which result in minimal tissue trauma (Krumdieck et al. 1983). To compliment this method, a dynamic tissue culture system was developed which allows for the biochemical maintenance of these slices for many hours (Smith et al. 1985, 1986 b).

In order for an in vitro liver slice system to be useful, it must provide the following: rapid production of precision-cut slices of consistent dimension under minimally traumatic conditions; viability and stability over time of incubation; integrated biotransformation capability; sequential progression of injury; morphological changes that correspond to in vivo effects; capacity to adapt to human tissue; and opportunities for the elucidation of the mechanisms by which chemicals produce hepatic injury. In what follows, some of the initial studies are described that demonstrate how the dynamic liver culture system meets many of these criteria.

Methods

Materials

Waymouth's MB752/1 powdered medium (without phenol red), L-glutamine and fetal calf serum were purchased from Gibco Laboratories (Grand Island, NY). Gentamycin sulfate, bovine serum albumin (fraction V), and the lactate dehydrogenase kit were obtained from Sigma Chemical (St. Louis, Mo). 1,2-Dichlorobenzene (1,2-DCB), 1,3-dichlorobenzene (1,3-DCB), 1,4-dichlorobenzene (1,4-DCB), and pyrazole were purchased from Aldrich Chemical (Milwaukee, Wis). Allyl alcohol and sodium phenobarbital were obtained from Mallinckrodt (St. Louis, Mo). [^{3}H]leucine (specific activity 5.0 Ci/mmol) was obtained from New England Nuclear (Boston, Mass). Betaphase liquid scintillation cocktail was from West Chem Products (San Diego, Calif). Dimethyl sulfoxide was purchased from Eastman Kodak (Rochester, NY). Bromobenzene was purchased from American Drug and Chemical (Culver City, Calif). All other chemicals used were of the purest analytical grade commercially available.

General

In the past, attempts to maintain rat liver explants in culture have proven extremely difficult. The high metabolic requirements of this tissue, coupled with limited oxygen and nutrient diffusion, often result in excessive degeneration of the cells except for a 200 µm band of cells at the gas-tissue interface (Hart et al. 1983). Therefore, a method developed by Smith et al. (1985) was used for preparation and culture of precision-cut liver slices. This system prepares slices from cores of liver by use of a mechanical slicer (Krumdieck et al. 1983). The slices are supported on a screen and placed in a rotating vial containing the appropriate culture medium. This system allows for the exposure of both sides of the slice to the gas phase.

The thinness of the sections (approximately 250 µm) allows for adequate diffusion of gas and nutrients. This results in a short-term (20 h) viable tissue culture that is uncompromised by cellular degeneration associated with limited oxygen or nutrient diffusion. The time of culture is long enough to demonstrate acute liver injury. The reader is referred to the following references which describe in greater detail this dynamic liver culture system (Smith et al. 1985, 1986a, b).

Preparation of the Slices

Male Fischer rats (250–350 g, Harlan Sprague-Dawley, Madison, Wis) were fed Wayne Lab Chow and water ad libitum and kept on wood shavings in 12-h light/ dark cycles. Animals were killed by cervical dislocation. Livers were excised through a midventral incision and immediately placed in cold Krebs-Henseleit buffer (4 °C, pH 7.4). Tissue cylinders were prepared with a sharpened metal tube of 1 cm outer diameter by slowly turning and advancing the metal tube into the liver lobes which were spread out on a wax support. Following the preparation of 8–10 cylinders, tissue slices (250 ± 25 µm) were prepared from the individual cylinders, using a modified version of a mechanical tissue slicer (Krumdieck et al. 1983), under ice-cold oxygenated (95% : 5% $O_2 : CO_2$) Krebs-Henseleit buffer (pH 7.4). The first and last slices, which contained the liver capsule, were discarded. Up to 100 slices were prepared within 15 min of liver isolation. The slices were placed in cold, oxygenated buffer until their incubation.

Slice Incubation

Rat liver slices were incubated according to the method of Smith et al. (1986b). Briefly, the liver slices in the Krebs-Henseleit buffer were floated on stainless steel mesh (260 µm pore size) cylinders (1.2 cm I.D.) equipped with two stainless steel wheels (1.6 cm O.D.). These inserts were then carefully blotted with tissue paper to remove any adhering buffer and loaded horizontally into glass scintillation vials containing 1.7 ml Waymouth's culture medium which had been gassed with $O_2 : CO_2$ (95% : 5%). The culture medium was supplemented with 10% fetal calf serum, 84 µg/ml gentamycin, and an additional 25 mM glucose. Vials were capped and placed on a heated (37 °C) vial rotator which was set so that the slice rotated through the medium at 3.5 rev/min. The vial rotator was housed in a black acrylic plastic box so that fluctuations in ambient temperature would not affect the temperature of incubation.

Treatment with Hepatotoxicants and Inhibitors

The toxicants (or vehicles) were added directly to the culture medium to achieve the final concentrations listed in the various tables and figures. In the studies with bromobenzene and the dichlorobenzenes, dimethylsulfoxide was used as the vehicle control and was present in the incubation media at 1% (v/v). Water was the vehicle for allyl alcohol.

Lactate Dehydrogenase Leakage

Aliquots of the culture medium were sampled for LDH activity using the method of Wroblewski and LaDue (1955). Results are expressed as units of LDH released per g of slice wet weight.

Intracellular Slice K^+ Content

Slices were removed from the incubation system, blotted, weighed and placed into 1.0 ml distilled water. Slices were then homogenized by sonication with a cell disrupter (10 pulses; Model 350, Branson Sonic Power, Danbury, Conn) and 20 µl perchloric acid (70%) was added to precipitate proteins. The homogenate was then centrifuged (5 min, 12000 × g) on a Beckman Microfuge B (Palo Alto, Calif) to pellet precipitable materials and the supernatant fraction was assayed for K^+ on a Perkin Elmer flame photometer (Model CA-51, Danbury, Conn). Results are expressed as µmol K^+ per g of slice wet weight.

Protein Synthesis/Secretion

The slices were incubated in the presence of 0.3 µCi [^{3}H]leucine/ml medium, for various lengths of time. They were then removed from the roller vials, immediately washed twice in buffer, and homogenized in 1.0 ml 1 N KOH. Aliquots (20 µl) of the homogenates were taken for protein determination (Lowry et al. 1951). Following the addition of an equal volume of 1.5 N acetic acid, the samples were centrifuged (3000 × g, 20 min). The pellets were washed by recentrifugation in 2 N acetic acid and dissolved by sonication in 0.5 ml 0.5 N NaOH. The incorporation of [^{3}H]leucine into acid-precipitable protein was determined by counting a 0.4-ml aliquot of the dissolved pellet after neutralization with 125 µl 2 N HCl. Results are expressed as dpm of [^{3}H]leucine incorporated per mg slice protein. Protein secretion was monitored by the appearance of [^{3}H]leucine in acid precipitable proteins that were secreted into the culture media.

Cytochrome P-450 Content

Following incubation slices were weighed, placed in microfuge tubes containing 1.0 ml cold buffer (0.05 mM Tris-KCl, 20% glycerol, pH 7.4) and sonicated to homogenize the tissue. The samples were diluted 1:1 with cold buffer. The carbon monoxide difference spectra was then determined following reduction of the heme with sodium dithionite (Omura and Sato 1964).

Statistical Analysis

The data are presented as the mean ± SEM for values compiled from three or more animals in which duplicate slices were used in each experiment. The dose-response curve for allyl alcohol was evaluated by a two-way ANOVA program and differences between control means and specific treatment means were determined using Dunnett's test for multiple comparisons (Dunnett 1964). The data from the enzyme inhibitor experiments involving bromobenzene or allyl alcohol toxicity were analyzed using a one-way ANOVA program and differences between specific means were compared using the Newman-Keul's post hoc test (Steel and Torrie 1960). All other comparisons were made using Student's two-tailed t-test for independent samples. Differences with $P < 0.05$ were considered significant.

In Vivo Hepatotoxicity Studies

Male Fischer rats (200–250 gm) were treated with various doses (0.9–4.5 mmol/kg, i.p.) of 1,2-DCB, 1,3-DCB, or 1,4-DCB to determine the hepatotoxic potential of these three isomers. At 24 h after dosing, the animals were killed and serum was obtained to determine the activity of glutamic-pyruvate transaminase as an indicator of liver injury.

In preliminary experiments male Sprague-Dawley rats (250–325 g), obtained from Harlan Sprague-Dawley) were administered the various DCBs (1.8 or 5.4 mmol/kg i.p.) to determine whether strain differences observed in vitro could be verified in vivo.

Results

K^+ and ATP Content

Following initial recovery periods, slice K^+ and ATP content of cultured liver slices rose to maximal levels, which were maintained for 16–20 h (Fig. 1). K^+ levels were maximal by 2 h, whereas the recovery of ATP to maximal levels took between 4 and 6 h. Between 16 and 20 h in culture, the slice ATP and K^+ content declined to approximately 80% of maximal. K^+ and ATP levels were normalized for slice DNA content (Kissane et al. 1958) and expressed as a percentage of the maximal values observed in the experiment.

Protein Synthesis and Secretion

Protein synthesis was evaluated by the incorporation of [^{3}H]leucine into slice protein. This incorporation into cultured liver slices was linear over 20 h in culture (Fig. 2). After a 2-h lag period, secretion of ^{3}H-labeled proteins from the liver slices increased at a linear rate for 16 h (Fig. 2).

Cytochrome P-450 Content

The cytochrome P_{450} content of cultured rat liver slices from either phenobarbital-induced or control animals was measured over a period of 8 h. In the slices obtained from phenobarbital-induced rats, the P_{450} content declined during the

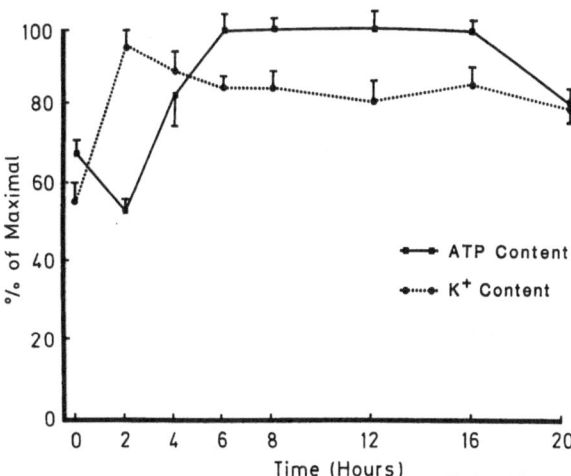

Fig. 1. Maintenance of slice K^+ and ATP content over 20 h of incubation in the dynamic liver culture system. Values given are the mean ± SEM from three or more animals. Maximal slice K^+ content corresponds to 100 µmol/g wet weight and maximal slice ATP content corresponds to 2.3 µmol/g wet weight. The zero time value was determined on slices directly after isolation at 4 °C

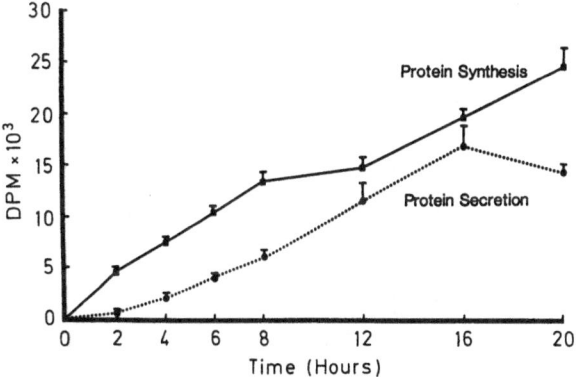

Fig. 2. Protein synthesis and secretion in rat liver slices cultured for 20 h in the dynamic liver culture system. Protein synthesis was determined by the incorporation of [³H]leucine into slice protein and protein secretion by incorporation of [³H]leucine into medium protein. The values for protein synthesis are expressed as DPM × 10³/mg protein and the values for protein secretion as DPM × 10³/total media (1.7 ml). Each point is the mean ± SEM from at least three animals

incubation period. Between 2 and 4 h, the P_{450} concentration decreased to 80% of the initial time point. This decrease continued to the end of the culture period and was 70% of the initial concentration at 8 h (Fig. 3). The P_{450} content of cultured slices obtained from control animals was two to three times lower than that in slices obtained from phenobarbital-induced animals. However, in the control slices, the P_{450} content was maintained for a longer period of time. After 8 h of culture, P_{450} content in the control slices was approximately 90% of the zero time point (Fig. 3). Data are expressed as nmol of cytochrome P_{450} per g of liver.

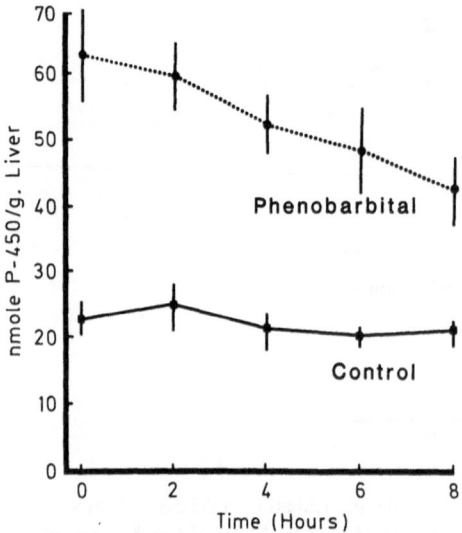

Fig. 3. Cytochrome P_{450} content of cultured rat liver slices. Liver slices from either phenobarbital-induced or control animals were incubated for up to 8 h and P_{450} content was determined in slice homogenates. Values given are the mean $\pm$ SEM from three or more animals

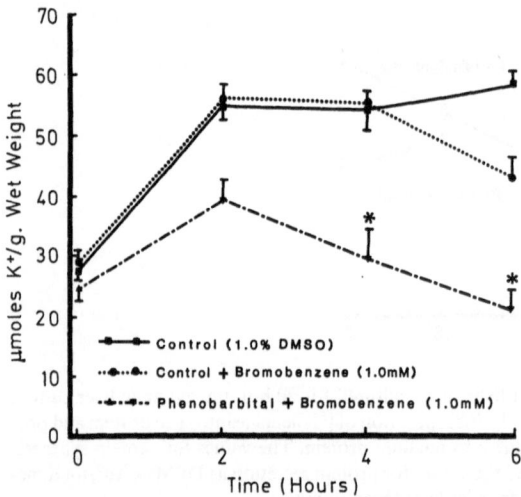

Fig. 4. Slice K^+ content of cultured rat liver slices from noninduced (control) animals and from phenobarbital-induced animals. Slices were incubated in the presence or absence of bromobenzene (1.0 mM). Values given are the mean $\pm$ SEM from three animals and differences between treated and control slices are indicated; $*p < 0.005$

Bromobenzene Toxicity and Inhibition

When rat liver slices from noninduced animals were exposed to 1.0 mM bromobenzene, slice K^+ content did not significantly differ from that of control slices. However, when slices from phenobarbital-induced animals were incubated with 1.0 mM bromobenzene, a significant drop in K^+ content was observed at 4 and

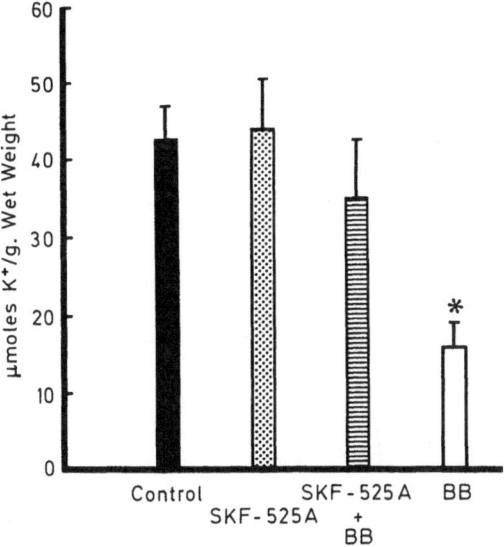

Fig. 5. SKF-525A (100 μM) was added to the incubation medium containing slices obtained from phenobarbital pretreated rats 0.5 h prior to the addition of 1.0 mM bromobenzene (BB). After 4 h the incubations were terminated and slice K^+ content was measured. Values are the mean $\pm$ SEM from three or more animals. Differences from control are indicated; $*p < 0.05$

6 h of incubation (Fig. 4). Preincubation (30 min) of the slices obtained from phenobarbital-treated rats with proadifen (SKF-525A; 100 μM) inhibited loss of K^+ from the slices (Fig. 5) as well as bromobenzene-induced changes in protein synthesis and LDH release (data not presented).

Allyl Alcohol Toxicity and Inhibition

Incubation of allyl alcohol with rat liver slices prepared from noninduced animals resulted in toxicity that was time- and dose-related. For example, dose-related decreases in intracellular K^+ were noted when slices were incubated with 0.5 and 1.0 mM allyl alcohol. The decreases were significantly different from control at 4 and 6 h of incubation with concentrations of 0.5 and 1.0 mM (Fig. 6). Significant allyl alcohol-induced inhibition of protein synthesis was evident after 2 h incubation of slices with 0.5 mM and at 4 h after incubation with 0.25 mM allyl alcohol. A 30-min preincubation of slices with pyrazole, an inhibitor of alcohol dehydrogenase, blocked the loss of K^+ produced by 1.0 mM allyl alcohol (Fig. 7). Pyrazole also inhibited allyl alcohol-induced decreases in protein synthesis and release of LDH into the media (data not presented).

Dichlorobenzene Toxicity

In vivo studies using Fischer rats indicate that the hepatotoxicity of the dichlorobenzenes (DCBs) can be ranked as follows: 1,2-DCB > 1,3-DCB > 1,4-DCB. These data are presented in Table 1. In order to determine whether the hepato-

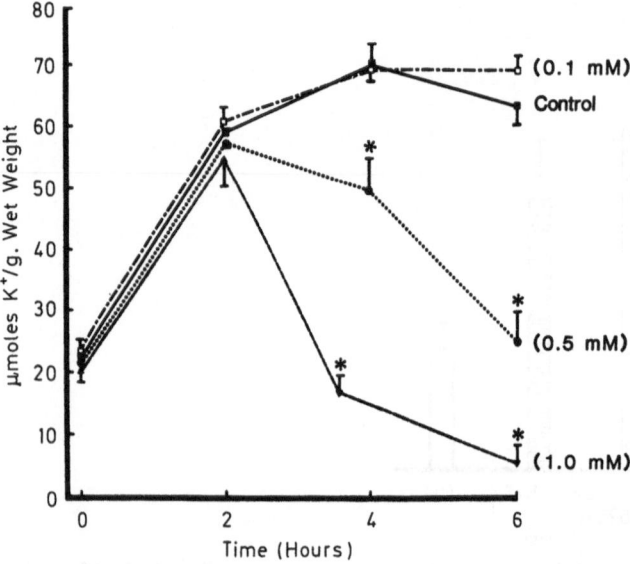

Fig. 6. Dose- and time-dependent loss of intracellular K$^+$ from cultured liver slices exposed to allyl alcohol. Values given are the mean $\pm$ SEM from three animals. Differences between control and allyl alcohol treated slices are indicated; *$p < 0.05$

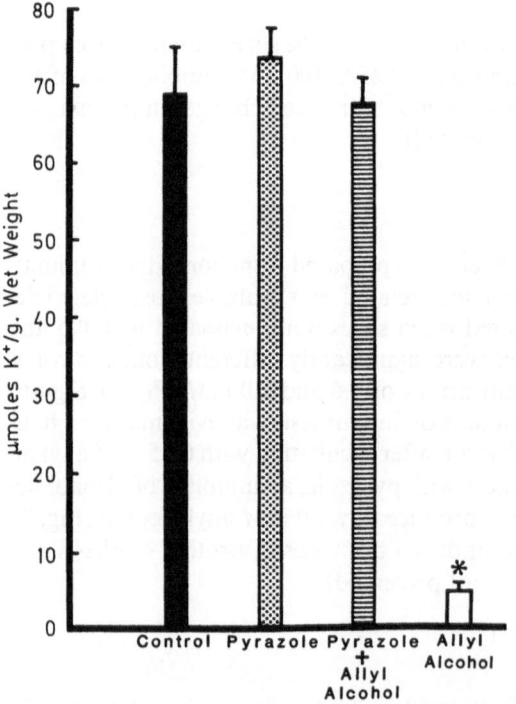

Fig. 7. Pyrazole (1.0 mM) was added to the incubation medium 0.5 h prior to the addition of 1.0 mM allyl alcohol. After 4 h, the incubation was terminated and intracellular K$^+$ measured. Values are the mean $\pm$ SEM from three or more animals. Differences from control are indicated; *$p < 0.05$

Table 1. Elevation of plasma GPT activity produced by various doses of each of the isomers of dichlorobenzene given to male Fischer 344 rats

	Dose (mmol/kg)				
	0.9	1.8	2.7	3.6	4.5
1,2-DCB	112±66	4083±961	7449±1224	5131±824	8525±1268
1,3-DCB	27± 1	43± 5	65± 8	255±101	306± 105
1,4-DCB	26± 2	29± 5	27± 3	23± 1	24± 2

Animals were killed 24 h after i.p. administration with the indicated dose of the isomer of DCB. Plasma was prepared and evaluated for GPT activity (expressed in Wroblewski-La Due units/ml). Dosing solutions were prepared by dissolving the indicated isomer of DCB in corn oil such that each animal received an injection volume of 2 ml/kg. Data are expressed as the mean±SEM ($n=4$–11).

toxic potential of these three DCBs would be expressed in this same rank order in the dynamic liver culture system, the DCBs were incubated with rat liver slices obtained from noninduced Fischer 344 rats for various times and at different concentrations. The indices for toxic injury were changes in intracellular K^+ content, protein synthesis, and LDH release. The data in Figs. 8 and 9 demonstrate that at 1.0 and 2.0 mM, 1,2-DCB results in an inhibition of protein synthesis and a more extensive loss of K^+ than does 1,3-DCB or 1,4-DCB. At 3.0 mM, 1,3-DCB inhibited protein synthesis and resulted in substantial K^+ loss, but to a lesser degree than 1,2-DCB (except at 6 h). Clearly, 1,4-DCB was less hepatotoxic than

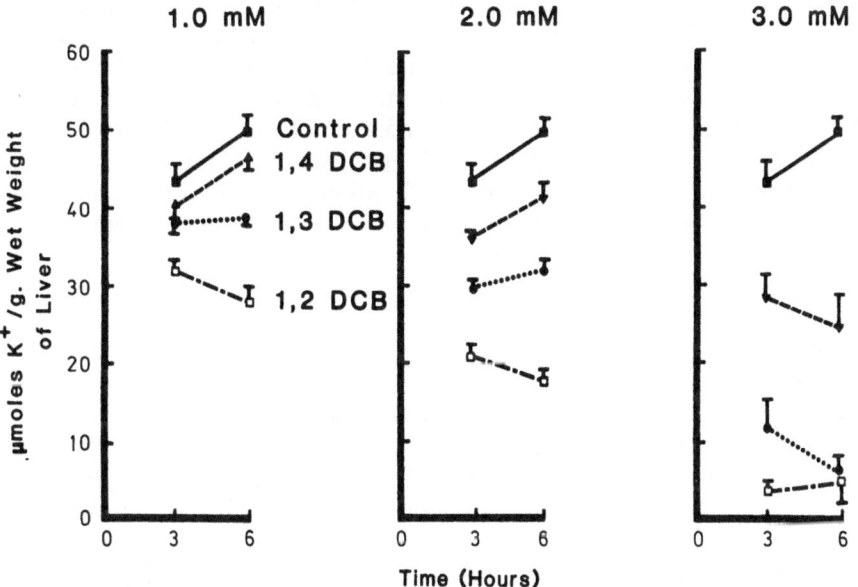

Fig. 8. Dose- and time-dependent loss of intracellular K^+ from cultured rat liver slices exposed to 1,2- 1,3-, or 1,4-dichlorobenzene (DCB). Values given are the mean±SEM for slices obtained from three different animals

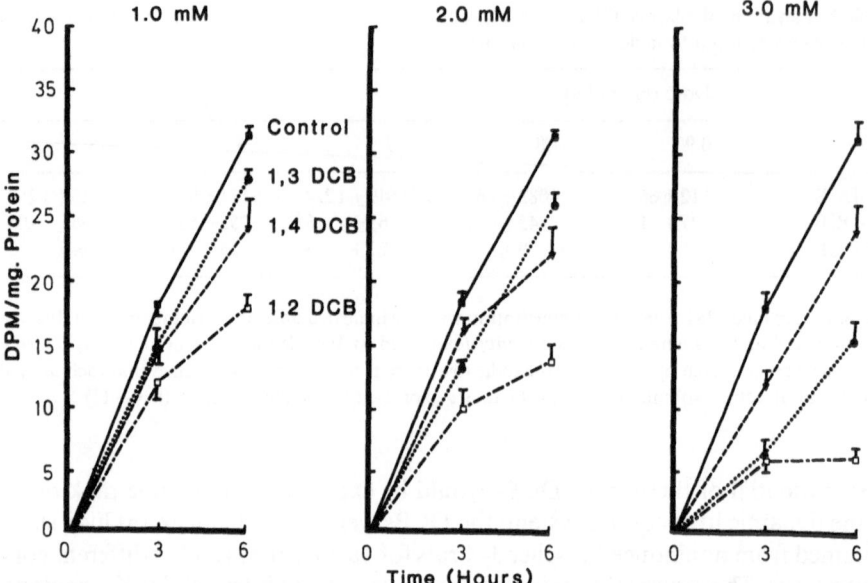

Fig. 9. Dose- and time-dependent inhibition of protein synthesis in cultured rat liver slices by 1,2-, 1,3-, or 1,4-dichlorobenzene. Protein synthesis was determined by the incorporation of [³H]leucine into slice protein. Values given are the mean ± SEM for slices obtained from three animals

1,2-DCB or 1,3-DCB. When release of LDH was used as a marker of hepatocellular injury, the rank order of hepatotoxicity of the DCBs was the same.

Preliminary studies using slices obtained from control Sprague-Dawley male rats indicate that the DCBs are less toxic in this strain than in the slices obtained from Fischer rats (data not presented). Similar findings were observed in vivo in that Sprague-Dawley rats are more resistant to the hepatotoxicity of the DCBs. At 24 h the respective SGPT values for 1.8 or 5.4 mmol/kg of the DCBs were: 1,2-DCB (260 ± 47, 90 ± 38); 1,3-DCB (48 ± 8, 71 ± 13); and 1,4-DCB (34 ± 3, 36 ± 2). These values are markedly lower than the elevations for 1,2-DCB seen in F-344 rats and the high doses of 1,3-DCB (Table 1). No evidence of hepatotoxicity is seen for 1,4-DCB in either strain of rat.

Discussion

In the Introduction several criteria were listed as necessary for establishment of an in vitro system to study the biotransformation and/or hepatotoxicity of chemicals. The data presented here indicate that the dynamic tissue culture system has the potential to meet these requirements, although further refinements and testing are necessary.

Use of the Krumdieck slicer provided a means of rapidly producing thin, uniform slices under conditions which result in minimal tissue injury. The slicer operates submerged in an appropriate medium. This allows for temperature control, adequate oxygenation, and prevention of osmotic changes and dehydration. The uniformity of the slices in thickness and weight is probably the major advantage offered by this mechanical slicer. Artifactual changes as a result of varying slice thickness are minimized.

The dynamic culture system also minimized culture-induced changes that are observed with static culture systems. In such systems, the cells that are immersed in the culture medium display pyknotic nuclei, cytoplasmic vacuolation, and abnormal staining, while the cells in the gas phase maintain normal morphological characteristics. Such changes may result from inadequate oxygen diffusion into those cells that are immersed (Campbell and Hales 1971). However, the design of the roller culture system allowed the slices to rotate out of the medium. This procedure provided sufficient oxygen to all cells and eliminated culture-induced change in the integrity of the slice. Elimination of these changes increases the sensitivity of biochemical markers to assess toxicant-induced injury. Potassium and LDH are not being lost from selected cells as a result of inadequate culture conditions. Clearly, the morphological changes observed by Smith et al. (1985), when they incubated slices in static culture, were prevented by the dynamic roller system.

Several parameters were assessed to determine the viability and stability of the dynamic liver slice system. These included loss of intracellular K^+, LDH and ATP; glycogen and protein synthesis; and responsiveness to hormones. After some initial loss of intracellular K^+ and ATP, the slices recovered and, at least according to these indicators, were stable and viable for 16–20 h of incubation. The liver slices prepared as described lost less ATP than those prepared by others (Krebs et al. 1974) and recovered the ATP levels more rapidly than hepatocytes maintained under monolayer conditions (Bissel et al. 1973). Therefore, it appears that the dynamic culture system described here offers numerous advantages over other in vitro "liver" systems. The fact that both protein synthesis and secretion are linear over time and that the tissues synthesize glycogen and respond to glucagon with glucose production are further evidence of the continued viability of the tissues maintained in culture (Smith et al. 1986b).

The parameters used to assess viability and stability over time of incubation also proved useful to assess toxicant-induced changes in the liver slices. Known hepatotoxicants produced changes in these parameters that were concentration dependent. Importantly, factors that are known to modify the toxicity of these chemicals in vivo, produced similar changes in the in vitro system. Phenobarbital pretreatment is known to enhance markedly the hepatotoxicity of bromobenzene (Brodie et al. 1971). Liver slices obtained from phenobarbital-pretreated rats lost K^+ earlier and at concentrations lower than those that produced changes in slices obtained from control rats. Prior exposure of the slices to SKF-525A inhibited bromobenzene-induced K^+ release from the slices, indicating that this agent effectively inhibited the biotransformation of bromobenzene to a reactive intermediate. Although the data are not presented here, phenobarbital and SKF-525A also enhanced or inhibited, respectively, bromobenzene-induced decreases in protein synthesis and increases in LDH release (Smith et al. 1986a). The allyl alcohol induced-decrease in protein synthesis and increases in K^+ and LDH leakage from the slices were dramatically reduced in the presence of pyrazole, an inhibitor on the enzyme which bioactivates allyl alcohol. Pyrazole also inhibits the hepatotoxicity of allyl alcohol in vivo (Reid 1972). Thus, it is concluded that the toxicity produced in these slices by allyl alcohol and bromobenzene results from a mechanism similar to that in vivo and does not merely reflect concentration-related solvent effects.

The findings with the DCBs provide further evidence that data derived in this in vitro culture system correlate well with the in vivo hepatotoxic potential of these three isomers. From these data it can be concluded that in Fischer male rats, 1,2-DCB is the most hepatotoxic of the three isomers and that 1,4-DCB is essentially nonhepatotoxic.1,3-DCB is intermediate in its ability to induce hepatotoxic injury. The interesting strain differences that were observed between the degree of liver injury produced by the DCBs in the Fischer and Sprague-Dawley rats were uncovered using the dynamic liver slice system. When slices from Sprague-Dawley rats were incubated with 1 or 2 mM of the DCBs, toxicity could not be demonstrated. Follow-up studies in vivo confirmed the relative lack of DCB-induced hepatotoxicity in this strain of rats. A future goal is to determine which of these two strains of rats best reflects the hepatotoxic potential of the DCBs in humans. Clearly, this is an important question. These two strains are widely used in toxicity studies, the results of which are often extrapolated to humans. Human data will be needed to address this question and can be obtained with parallel incubations of human and rat liver slices in the dynamic culture system.

Other criteria to help validate this system, that are under study but not reported here, include: integrated biotransformation of toxicants, sequential progression of injury, and morphological characterization of the toxicant-induced lesions. It is clear that the cultured liver slices can biotransform chemicals from the results of the toxicity studies with bromobenzene and allyl alcohol. Preliminary studies have demonstrated that the rat and human liver slices deethylate ethoxycoumarin to 7-hydroxycoumarin. The slices then convert this metabolite to the sulfate and glucuronic acid conjugate. This metabolic activity is maintained for at least 6 h of incubation. Chlorobenzene, p-nitroanisole, and halothane have also been shown to be metabolized in the liver culture system. There is concern that the activity of cytochrome P_{450} and other biotransformation enzymes will decrease over time incubation. This concern is underscored by the observed decrease in the content of cytochrome P_{450} in the slices obtained from phenobarbital pretreated rats. However, the activity of P_{450} and other enzymes may be sufficient at earlier times to permit comparison in the rates and routes of xenobiotic metabolism and to initiate the events that may ultimately be expressed as liver injury.

Of the toxicants reported here, the sequence of events that progress to liver injury would include: bioactivation, alterations in molecular and biochemical events, functional alterations, and, finally, morphological alterations. Although this sequence has not been studied in detail in the dynamic liver culture system, the results obtained do follow this general progression. Bioactivation was required to demonstrate toxicity at the lower concentrations of the toxicants. Following bioactivation of allyl alcohol, changes in protein synthesis were observed before the slices lost potassium or LDH. Studies are underway to better define the progression of toxicant-induced changes in the liver culture system as well as to describe the morphological changes that are produced. Description of chemically induced morphological changes has proved difficult because culture-induced changes are superimposed on chemically-induced changes. Also artifactual changes due to the processing of such thin slices have been observed. Modification in the fixation, embedding, and orientation of the slices during cutting may eliminate these artifactual changes.

In summary, a dynamic liver culture system has been described. This system is under development to help resolve the problems related to understanding mechanisms of liver injury and to aid in the extrapolation of in vitro data to the in vivo situation and animal data to humans. The systems has considerable potential, provided it is properly developed and provided its limitations are understood.

Acknowledgment. This work was supported in part by funds from NIEHS N01-ES-55112. The assistance of Leslie Auerbach and Lana Koepke in the preparation of the manuscript is gratefully appreciated.

References

Bissel DM, Hammaker LE, Meyer US (1973) Parenchymal cells from adult rat liver in nonproliferating monolayer culture. J Cell Biol 59:722–734

Brodie BB, Reid WD, Cho AK, Sipes IG, Krishna G, Gillette JR (1971) Possible mechanism of liver necrosis caused by aromatic organic compounds. Proc Natl Acad Sci USA 68:160–164

Campbell AK, Hales CN (1971) Maintenance of viable cells in an organ culture of mature rat liver. Exp Cell Res 68:33–42

Dunnett CW (1964) New tables for multiple comparisons with a control. Biometrics 20:482–491

Grisham JW, Charlton RK, Kaufman DG (1978) In vitro assay of cytotoxicity with cultured liver: accomplishments and possibilities. Environ Health Perspect 25:161–171

Hart A, Mattheyse FJ, Balinsky JB (1983) An organ culture of postnatal rat liver slices. In Vitro 19:841–852

Kissane JM, Robins E (1958) The fluorometric measurements of deoxyribonucleic acid in animal tissues with special reference to the central nervous system. J Biol Chem 233:184–188

Krebs HA, Cornell NW, Lund P, Hems R (1974) Isolated liver cells as experimental material. In: Lundquist F, Tygstrup N (eds) Regulation of hepatic metabolism. Munksgaard, Copenhagen, pp 726–750

Krumdieck CL, Dos Santos JE, Ho K (1983) A new instrument for the rapid preparation of tissue slices. Anal Biochem 104:118–123

Lowry OH, Rosebrough NJ, Farr AL, Randall RJ (1951) Protein measurement with the folin phenol reagent. J Biol Chem 193:265–275

Omura T, Sato R (1964) The carbon monoxide binding pigment of liver microsomes. J Biol Chem 239:2370–2378

Reid WD (1972) Mechanism of allyl alcohol-induced hepatic necrosis. Experientia 28:1058–1061

Smith PF, Gandolfi AJ, Krumdieck CL, Putnam CW, Zukoski CF, Davis WM, Brendel K (1985) Dynamic organ culture of precision liver slices for in vitro toxicology. Life Sci 36:1367–1375

Smith PF, Fisher R, Shubat PJ, Gandolfi AJ, Krumdieck CL, Brendel K (1986a) In vitro cytotoxicity of allyl alcohol and bromobenzene in a novel organ culture system Toxicol Appl Pharmacol (to be published)

Smith PF, Krack G, McKee R, Johnson DG, Gandolfi AJ, Hruby V, Krumdieck CL, Brendel K (1986b) Maintenance of adult rat liver slices in dynamic organ culture. In Vitro (to be published)

Steel RGD, Torrie JH (1960) Principles and practices of statistics. McGraw-Hill, New York

Wroblewski F, LaDue JS (1955) Lactic dehydrogenase activity in blood. Proc Soc Exp Biol Med 90:210–213

Mechanisms and Models in Toxicology
Arch. Toxicol., Suppl. 11, 34–38 (1987)
© by Springer-Verlag 1987

Some Aspects of Cell Defense Mechanisms of Glutathione and Vitamin E During Cell Injury

D. J. Reed, G. A. Pascoe, and K. Olafsdottir

Department of Biochemistry and Biophysics, and Environmental Health Sciences Center, Oregon State University, Corvallis, Oregon 97331, USA

Introduction

Glutathione (GSH) is well established as having important roles in the limiting of cell injury caused by a variety of chemicals and reduced species of molecular oxygen (Reed 1985). Less well understood is the possible interaction of glutathione and vitamin E in chemically induced cell injury, as well as the oxidation type of stress caused by incubation of cells in calcium-depleted medium. This laboratory has demonstrated that chemically induced injury, including alterations in calcium homeostasis, can be correlated with α-tocopherol (vitamin E) content of rat hepatocytes (Fariss et al. 1985a). Incubation of freshly isolated rat hepatocytes in the absence of extracellular calcium produces a "nonoxidant type" of oxidative stress, enhanced by the loss of cytoplasmic and mitochondrial GSH and stimulated lipid peroxidation (Fariss et al. 1984). These events appear to be "reversible" in the absence of chemical insult, but rapidly become irreversible in its presence (Fariss et al. 1984; Fariss et al. 1985a).

The following report describes the potential sparing effect of vitamin E on intracellular GSH and the effect of vitamin E supplementation on the GSH redox system and hepatocyte morphology during oxidative stress. The calcium ionophore A23187 has been used to alter calcium homeostasis of rat hepatocytes incubated in the presence and absence of extracellular calcium. This nonoxidant model of oxidative stress demonstrates the interdependence of GSH and vitamin E as protective agents during injurious events to the cell, and the susceptibility of protein thiols to oxidation-induced alterations.

Methods

Isolated Hepatocyte System: Freshly isolated hepatocytes were prepared and incubated in Fischer's medium, as previously described (Fariss et al. 1985b).

Experimental Protocol: Calcium (3.5 mM), α-tocopheryl succinate (25 μM), and the calcium ionophore A23187 (20 μM, Sigma Chemical Co., St. Louis, MO)

were supplemented to the incubation medium as indicated. Viable cells were separated from nonviable hepatocytes and analysed for glutathione contents (reduced and oxidized), intracellular K^+ content, lactate dehydrogenase (LDH) leakage (Fariss et al. 1985b), α-tocopherol content (Fariss et al. 1985a), and protein thiol content (Di Monte et al. 1984a).

Scanning Electron Microscopy: Viable hepatocytes were fixed in glutaraldehyde and sodium cacodylate, and a monolayer of cells was critical-point dried and coated with gold/palladium, as previously described (Fariss et al. 1985b). Cells were viewed with an AMRAY 1000 scanning electron microscope.

Results

Incubating rat hepatocytes in calcium-depleted medium reduced their calcium content to less than 10% of the cellular calcium content of control cells incubated with 3.5 mM calcium in the medium. In 5 h, endogenous α-tocopherol content of viable cells decreased from 0.1 to 0.01 nmol/10^6 cells compared with a 44% loss in control cells in the presence of extracellular calcium (Table 1). A 10-fold increase in production of thiobarbituric acid (TBA)-reactive substances was associated with this depletion (data not shown). α-Tocopherol depletion was followed by a 20% loss of intracellular K^+ with no detectable loss of LDH, as previously

Table 1. Changes in α-tocopherol content and loss of intracellular K^+ in isolated hepatocytes incubated with or without extracellular calcium (3.5 mM) in the presence or absence of α-tocopheryl succinate (25 μM). Values are mean ± SEM; $n=4$

Ca^{2+}	−	+	−	+
Vitamin E	−	−	+	+
α-Tocopherol content (nmol/10^6 cells) at:				
0 h	0.100 ± 0.020	0.125 ± 0.017	0.123 ± 0.019	0.122 ± 0.017
5 h	0.019 ± 0.005	0.060 ± 0.006	2.120 ± 0.520	0.646 ± 0.094
Intracellular K^+ (% of initial content) at:				
0 h			100	
5 h	67 ± 3	85 ± 4	84 ± 3	91 ± 3

Table 2. Changes in intracellular GSH and protein thiols in isolated hepatocytes incubated with or without extracellular calcium (3.5 mM) in the presence or absence of α-tocopheryl succinate (25 μM). Values are mean ± SEM, $n=4$–7)

Ca^{2+}	−	+	−	+
Vitamin E	−	−	+	+
Intracellular GSH (nmol/10^6 cells) at:				
0 h	20.3 ± 1.37	21.6 ± 1.20	19.9 ± 1.33	21.3 ± 2.89
5 h	9.53 ± 0.90	24.2 ± 1.81	18.7 ± 1.53	23.8 ± 1.86
Protein thiols (nmol/10^6 cells) at:				
0 h	96.6 ± 4.2	102.9 ± 6.7	106.7 ± 6.1	106.5 ± 9.0
5 h	32.8 ± 9.4	69.9 ± 4.3	89.2 ± 4.1	84.2 ± 3.1

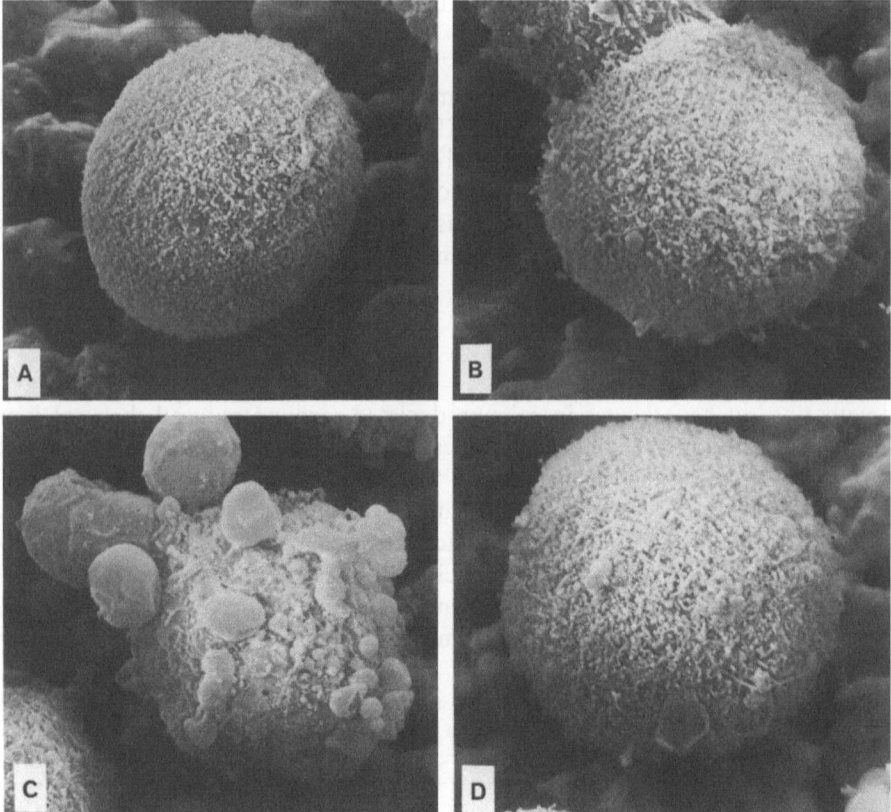

Fig. 1 A–D. Scanning electron micrographs of isolated hepatocytes freshly suspended as described in Methods (**A**), or resuspended and incubated for 5 h in calcium-supplemented medium (**B**), calcium-deficient medium (**C**), or calcium-deficient medium supplemented with α-tocopheryl succinate (25 μM; **D**). Magnification × 2500–3000

described (Fariss et al. 1984). Addition of α-tocopheryl succinate (25 μM) to calcium-depleted cells completely inhibited this loss of intracellular K^+.

Intracellular K^+ loss was preceded by a loss of intracellular GSH from calcium-depleted cells (Table 2). Vitamin E in the medium had no effect on GSH efflux, a normal function of these cells, whereas intracellular GSH was maintained at nearly control levels (Table 2). The loss in intracellular GSH from calcium-depleted cells was associated with a loss in protein thiols, which was similarly reversible upon supplementation with vitamin E (Table 2).

Peroxidation of membrane lipids following disturbance of calcium homeostasis resulted in massive blebbing of the plasma membrane of calcium-depleted cells (Fig. 1). The morphological alterations were preventable by vitamin E supplementation to these cells.

The presence of 20 μM A23187 in the medium resulted in 47% LDH leakage after 5 h incubation in the absence of calcium (Table 3). This toxicity was prevented by supplementation with vitamin E (Table 3), and was comparable to

Table 3. Influence of calcium ionophore A23187 (20 µM) on isolated hepatocytes incubated with or without extracellular calcium (3.5 mM) in the presence or absence of α-tocopheryl succinate (25 µM). Values are mean ± SEM; $n = 4-8$

Ca^{2+}	−	+	−	+
Vitamin E	−	−	+	+
LDH leakage (%) at:				
0 h	7.9 +0.5	7.6 + 0.6	6.9+0.4	6.5 +0.3
5 h	47.2 ±0.9	80.7 ± 0.9	25.5±2.1	71.0 ±5.6
Intracellular GSH (nmol/10^6 cells) at:				
0 h	27.3 ±0.36	28.4 ± 0.44	28.6±1.24	28.9 ±0.25
5 h	5.09±0.38	2.60± 1.65	12.6±1.05	3.12±1,82
Protein thiols (nmol/10^6 cells) at:				
0 h	120 ±5.9	128 ± 6.0	121 ±5.3	121 ±4.7
4 h	64.2 ±8.6	38.3 ±13	140 ±9.6	70.2 ±9.8

LDH leakage from control cells (data not shown). In contrast, in the presence of calcium, LDH leakage was almost total, and vitamin E had minimal effect on such leakage (Table 3).

Intracellular GSH was extensively depleted in the presence of calcium and A23187, and vitamin E had no effect on this loss (Table 3). In contrast, intracellular GSH was partially retained in the absence of calcium and maintained at double these levels with vitamin E supplementation. Changes in protein thiol levels, induced by the ionophore, paralleled the calcium- and vitamin E-induced changes in intracellular GSH levels, and directly correlated with the extent of cytotoxicity (Table 3).

Discussion

Hepatocytes incubated in calcium-free medium display a type of oxidative stress-induced injury that is characterized by a loss of intracellular K^+, in spite of an absence of LDH leakage. This is considered to be a reversible phenomenon and is preceded by stimulated lipid peroxidation and depletion of cellular vitamin E stores.

The present study presents evidence that the enhanced oxidative state of vitamin E-depleted cells depletes intracellular GSH with its resultant oxidation and efflux. GSH directly participates in the maintenance of both cytoplasmic and membrane protein thiol status as an intracellular reductant of disulfides (Kosower and Kosower 1983). The loss of protein thiol protection during GSH depletion resulted in the depletion of cellular protein thiols followed by extensive plasma membrane alterations and K^+ leakage.

Correlations between depletion of protein thiols and loss of cell viability during oxidative stress to hepatocytes have been repeatedly demonstrated (DiMonte et al. 1984a, b; Moore et al. 1985; Nicotera 1985; Ku and Billings 1986), with the suggestion that protein thiol status is directly linked to the balance between free cytosolic and membrane-bound calcium (Orrenius 1985). Based on the evidence presented herein, a novel role is suggested for vitamin E in preventing oxidation-induced injury via maintenance of cellular protein thiols, presumably secondary to the maintenance of intracellular GSH, regardless of the calcium status of the cells.

Calcium ionophore-induced perturbation of cellular calcium homeostasis was found to support the need for maintenance of intracellular GSH and protein thiols for cell viability. Influx of extracellular calcium, induced by A23187 and 3.5 mM calcium in the medium, as well as loss of intracellular calcium induced by A23187 and the absence of extracellular calcium, caused differing degrees of toxicity to the cells. The extent of toxicity was directly correlated with the extent of depletion of both GSH and protein thiols. Vitamin E maintenance of intracellular GSH above 20% of initial values ($-$ Ca + Vit E) was associated with maximal protein thiol content and minimal loss of cell viability. The strong correlations between these parameters support the hypotheses that intracellular GSH levels are related to vitamin E protection against oxidation-induced cell damage, and in concert with vitamin E, are critical for maintenance of protein thiols and cell viability.

References

Di Monte D, Ross D, Bellomo G, Eklöw L, Orrenius S (1984a) Alterations in intracellular thiol homeostasis during the metabolism of menadione by isolated rat hepatocytes. Arch Biochem Biophys 235:334–342

Di Monte D, Bellomo G, Thor H, Nicotera P, Orrenius S (1984b) Menadione-induced cytotoxicity is associated with protein thiol oxidation and alteration in intracellular Ca^{2+} homeostasis. Arch Biochem Biophys 235:343–350

Fariss MW, Olafsdottir K, Reed DJ (1984) Extracellular calcium protects isolated rat hepatocytes from injury. Biochem Biophys Res Commun 121:102–110

Fariss MW, Pascoe GA, Reed DJ (1985a) Vitamin E reversal of the effect of extracellular calcium on chemically-induced toxicity in hepatocytes. Science 227:751–754

Fariss MW, Brown MK, Schmitz JA, Reed DJ (1985b) Mechanism of chemical-induced toxicity. I. Use of rapid centrifugation technique for the separation of viable and nonviable hepatocytes. Toxicol Appl Pharmacol 79:283–295

Kosower NS, Kosower EM (1983) Glutathione and cell membrane thiol status. In: Larsson A et al. (eds) Functions of glutathione: biochemical, physiological, toxicological, and clinical aspects. Raven, New York, pp 307:315

Ku RH, Billings RE (1986) The role of the mitochondrial glutathione and cellular protein sulfhydryls in formaldehyde toxicity in glutathione-depleted rat hepatocytes. Arch Biochem Biophys 247:183–189

Moore M, Thor H, Moore G, Nelson S, Moldéus P, Orrenius S (1985) The toxicity of acetaminophen and N-acetyl-p-benzoquinone imine in isolated hepatocytes is associated with thiol depletion and increased cytosolic Ca^{2+}. J Biol Chem 260:13035–13040

Nicotera PL, Moore M, Mirabelli F, Bellomo G, Orrenius S (1985) Inhibition of hepatocyte plasma membrane Ca^{2+}-ATPase activity by menadione metabolism and its restoration by thiols. FEBS Lett 181:149–153

Orrenius S (1985) Biochemical mechanisms of cytotoxicity. Trends Pharmacol Sci, [Suppl]

Reed DJ (1985) Cellular defense mechanisms against reactive metabolites. In: Anders MW (ed) Bioactivation of foreign compounds. Academic, New York, pp 71–108

Mechanisms and Models in Toxicology
Arch. Toxicol., Suppl. 11, 39–41 (1987)

Structure Activity Requirements for Induction of Peroxisomal Enzyme Activities in Primary Rat Hepatocyte Cultures

D. F. V. Lewis[1], B. G. Lake[2], T. J. B. Gray[2], and S. D. Gangolli[2]

[1] Department of Biochemistry, University of Surrey, Guildford, Surrey, GU2 5XH, UK
[2] The British Industrial Biological Research Association,
   Woodmansterne Road, Carshalton, Surrey, SM5 4DS, UK

Introduction

A range of apparently structurally diverse compounds are known to produce liver enlargement and hepatic peroxisome proliferation in rodents (Reddy and Lalwani 1983). As the in vivo effects of peroxisome proliferators may be demonstrated in cell culture (Gray et al. 1983), the structure activity requirements for induction of peroxisomal enzyme activities by a series of 13 compounds in primary rat hepatocyte cultures has been studied.

Materials and Methods

Chemicals

2,4-Dichlorophenoxyacetic acid (I), 2,4,5-trichlorophenoxyacetic acid (II), 2-(2,4-dichlorophenoxy)propionic acid (III), 2-(2,4,5-trichlorophenoxy)propionic acid (IV), 4-(2,4-dichlorophenoxy)butyric acid (V), 4-chloro-o-tolyloxyacetic acid (VI), trichloroacetic acid (VII), acetylsalicylic acid (VIII), and clofibric acid [2-(4-chlorophenoxy)-2-methylpropionic acid, IX] were obtained from commercial sources. Mono-(2-ethylhexyl)phthalate (X) was synthesised (Gray et al. 1983). Methyl clofenapate {methyl-2-[4-(p-chlorophenyl)phenoxy]-2-methylpropionic acid; XI} and clobuzarit [2-(4-p-chlorophenylbenzyloxy)-2-methylpropionic acid; XII] were the generous gifts of ICI Pharmaceuticals Division, Cheshire, UK and ciprofibrate {2-[4-(2,2-dichlorocyclopropyl)phenoxy]-2-methylpropionic acid; XIII} was kindly donated by Sterling Winthrop, Alnwick, Northumberland, UK.

Hepatocyte Isolation and Culture

Hepatocytes were obtained from 6-week-old male Sprague-Dawley rats (180–220 g) by collagenase perfusion and maintained in culture as described previously (Gray et al. 1983). After 2 h in culture, treatment was commenced by replacing

the medium with either medium containing 0.4% (v/v) final concentration dimethyl sulphoxide (DMSO) or medium containing the test compounds dissolved
in DMSO. Subsequently the medium was changed and the cells redosed every
24 h. After 70 h the cells were harvested in 0.154 M KCl/50 mM Tris-HCl pH 7.4,
homogenised by sonication and assayed for enzyme activity.

Structure Activity Analysis

Electronic structural parameters were determined using molecular orbital
(MINDO/3) calculations (Bingham et al. 1975). Quantitative structure activity
relationships were generated by multiple linear regression analysis.

Results

The 13 peroxisome proliferators were cultured with rat hepatocytes for 70 h at
concentrations ranging from 0.005 to 6.0 mM depending on compound potency.

Table 1. Relative potencies for induction of palmitoyl-CoA oxidation in primary rat hepatocyte cultures
and results of molecular orbital calculations (MINDO/3 method) for a series of 13 peroxisome
proliferators

Com-pound[a]	Relative potency for induction of palmitoyl-CoA oxidation[b]	Electronic structural parameter				
		S_e	Q_t	$E(LEMO)$	Q_0	$Q_0(HOMO)$
I	0.258	4.5134	4.1176	−0.2119	−0.5684	0.0214
II	0.716	4.8977	4.3137	−0.4406	−0.5686	0.0144
III	1.33	4.9176	4.1368	−0.1533	−0.5816	0.0217
IV	2.59	5.3007	4.3524	−0.3794	−0.5795	0.0141
V	0.433	5.3126	4.5260	−0.0914	−0.5852	0.0039
VI	0.218	4.5179	3.9213	0.2328	−0.5725	0.0178
VII	0.074	2.6489	3.0808	−1.7624	−0.5131	0.2636
VIII	0.0060	4.3501	5.4142	0.2382	−0.6186	0.0280
IX	1.00	4.9074	3.8527	0.3690	−0.5922	0.0129
X	0.919	7.1571	4.6941	−0.2188	−0.5851	0.2672
XI	12.4	6.7694	4.3589	0.4950	−0.5926	0.0150
XII	4.01	7.2518	4.2242	0.4518	−0.5687	0.000001
XIII	20.3	6.5717	4.7390	−1.0132	−0.5903	0.0019

[a] The numeral identifies individual compounds listed in Materials and Methods. For purposes of
molecular orbital calculations, methyl clofenapate was considered as the free acid in XI.
[b] Cells were cultured for 70 h with various concentrations of the test compounds and the concentration
of each compound required for a three-fold induction of enzyme activity was determined. Relative
compound potencies were calculated as the ratio of potency of clofibric acid (μM) to potency of test
compound (μM).
S_e, sum of total electrophilic superdelocalizability; Q_t, sum of net atomic charges; $E(LEMO)$, energy of
lowest empty molecular orbital; Q_0, net atomic charge on the carboxyl group carbonyl oxygen atom;
$Q_0(HOMO)$, electron density on the carboxyl group carbonyl oxygen atom in the highest occupied
molecular orbital.

All compounds produced an induction of cyanide-insensitive palmitoyl-CoA oxidation. As a measure of potency, the concentrations of the compounds required to produce a three-fold increase (i.e. 300% of activity present in 70 h control cultures) in enzyme activity were calculated from linear portions of plots of enzyme activity against the logarithm of the compound concentration in the culture medium. However, in order to correct for variations between experiments all compound potencies (Table 1) were expressed relative to the potency of clofibric acid (compound IX) which was included in each experiment.

To determine whether there was a relationship between biological activity and chemical structure, the potency values (expressed as $\log_{10}A$) for induction of palmitoyl-CoA oxidation were compared with electronic structural parameters obtained by molecular orbital calculations. The best correlation observed ($r=0.979$) is described by the following equation:

$$\text{Log}_{10}A = 0.803S_e\ (\pm0.067) - 1.683Q_t\ (\pm0.303) - 1.039E(LEMO)\ (\pm0.188) - 24.717Q_O\ (\pm8.418) - 4.220Q_O(HOMO)\ (\pm0.946) - 11.445\ (\pm3.885)$$

where $\text{Log}_{10}A$ is the logarithm of compound potency relative to clofibric acid (see Table 1), and S_e, Q_t, $E(LEMO)$, Q_O, and $Q_O(HOMO)$ are the electronic structural parameters as defined in Table 1.

Discussion

These results demonstrate substantial quantitative differences in the effects of 13 compounds on enzymes of peroxisomal fatty acid β-oxidation in rat primary hepatocyte cultures. Despite the apparent structural diversity of the compounds used, a good correlation was obtained between biological activity and electronic structural parameters derived from molecular orbital calculations, suggesting that some critical features were common to all the compounds.

These results demonstrate the usefulness of primary hepatocyte cultures as a rapid and economical system for screening compounds for peroxisome proliferation and that such systems can be used to generate data for quantitative structure activity relationships (QSARs).

Acknowledgement. This work forms part of a research project sponsored by the United Kingdom Ministry of Agriculture, Fisheries and Food. The results of the research are the property of the Ministry of Agriculture, Fisheries and Food and are Crown Copyright.

References

Bingham RC, Dewar MJS, Lo DH (1975) Ground states of molecules. XXV. MINDO/3. An improved version of the MINDO semiempirical SCF-MO method. J Amer Chem Soc 97:1285–1293
Gray TJB, Lake BG, Beamand JA, Foster JR, Gangolli SD (1983) Peroxisome proliferation in primary cultures of rat hepatocytes. Toxicol Appl Pharmacol 67:15–25
Reddy JK, Lalwani ND (1983) Carcinogenesis by hepatic peroxisome proliferators: evaluation of the risk of hypolipidemic drugs and industrial plasticizers to humans. Crit Rev Toxicol 12:1–58

Mechanisms and Models in Toxicology
Arch. Toxicol., Suppl. 11, 42–44 (1987)
© by Springer-Verlag 1987

Oxidative and Reductive Biotransformation of Chloroform in Mouse Liver Microsomes

E. Testai, F. Gramenzi, S. Di Marzio, and L. Vittozzi

Department of Comparative Toxicology and Ecotoxicology, Istituto Superiore di Sanità, Viale Regina Elena, 299-00161 Rome, Italy

The carcinogenicity of chloroform seems species-, strain-, and sex-specific (see Davidson et al. 1982 for a review). Still further studies are in order, however, to assess its carcinogenic power in man, who may be exposed for long periods to $CHCl_3$ present in drinking water and the work environment. Thorough metabolic studies would be of particular importance to establish the dose dependency of the carcinogenic effect; indeed, a great deal of uncertainty is associated with the lower end of the dose-response curve due to differences between predicted tumors and tumors observed at the lower concentrations tested (Reitz et al. 1978). The reductive metabolism of chloroform by liver microsomes has been associated with the formation of reactive metabolites (Wolf et al. 1977; Tomasi et al. 1985), which have recently been shown to bind to cellular lipid and protein structures (Testai and Vittozzi 1986). It has also been suggested that $CHCl_3$ may occur in vivo (Testai and Vittozzi 1984). Therefore a study was undertaken to determine the effects of $CHCl_3$ on reductive and oxidative metabolism with particular emphasis on the relationship to $CHCl_3$ concentration. Male B6C3F1 mice, which have been reported (NCI 1976) to be sensitive to $CHCl_3$ hepatocarcinogenicity, were used.

Cytochrome P_{450} was determined according to Omura and Sato (1964); protein and lipid covalent binding was measured according to Ilett et al. (1973) and Uehleke (1973).

Data of protein and lipid covalent binding indicate that $CHCl_3$ metabolism produces reactive metabolites in aerobic and anaerobic incubations with both nonpretreated and induced mouse liver microsomes (Table 1). Covalent binding of $CHCl_3$ is induced by PB pretreatment only. The increase of total binding is accounted for by the lipid binding in the anaerobic incubations, whereas, aerobically, both lipid and protein fractions showed increased covalent binding. The level of anaerobic covalent binding ranges between a quarter and more than half the levels attained in the presence of oxygen. Addition of reduced glutathione (GSH) to microsomal incubations decreased the covalent binding of $CHCl_3$ metabolites (Table 2). In these conditions, the binding to the lipid fraction was com-

Table 1. In vitro covalent binding of $^{14}CHCl_3$ to liver microsomes of variously pretreated B6C3F1 mice

	Protein-bound $^{14}CHCl_3$ (nmol/mg protein)		Lipid-bound $^{14}CHCl_3$ (nmol/mg lipid)		Total bound ^{14}C (nmol/mg protein)	
	Anaerobiosis	Aerobiosis	Anaerobiosis	Aerobiosis	Anaerobiosis	Aerobiosis
Uninduced mice	12.2 (1.2)	23.0 (1.7)	10.0 (0.6)	14.0 (0.5)	20.9	35.2
PB-Pretreated mice	12.8 (1.0)	52.4 (3.0)	17.2 (1.0)	57.5 (4.2)	32.7	118.5
NF-Pretreated mice	7.7 (1.3)	19.7 (1.1)	9.2 (0.4)	18.0 (1.4)	15.7	35.4

$^{14}CHCl_3$ concentration was 5 mM. Figures represent differences from corresponding incubations without NADPH and are means of six experiments. Standard error is given in parentheses. A phospholipid content of 0.86 mg/mg microsomal protein was considered for the estimation of total (protein plus lipid) binding.

Table 2. Effect of GSH on in vitro covalent binding of $^{14}CHCl_3$ to protein and lipid of B6C3F1 mouse liver microsomes

$^{14}CHCl_3$ concentration	GSH (3 mM) addition	Anaerobiosis (nmol $^{14}CHCl_3$/mg)		Aerobiosis (nmol $^{14}CHCl_3$/mg)	
		Protein-bound	Lipid-bound	Protein-bound	Lipid-bound
5 mM	−	12.2 ± 1.2	10.0 ± 0.6	23.0 ± 1.7	14.0 ± 0.5
5 mM	+	0.46 ± 0.05	4.0 ± 0.7	1.1 ± 0.1	− 0.4 ± 0.6
1 mM	−	3.9 ± 0.4	−	13.7 ± 0.6	−
1 mM	+	0.33 ± 0.04	−	1.08 ± 0.1	−
0.1 mM	−	1.9 ± 0.2	−	10.8 ± 0.7	−
0.1 mM	+	0.27 ± 0.05	−	1.12 ± 0.17	−

Results are expressed as mean ± S.E. of six experiments.

pletely prevented aerobically, while being the highest after anaerobic incubations. The total (protein *plus* lipid) binding elicited by anaerobic conditions became about four times higher than that consequent to aerobic incubations. On decreasing CHCl$_3$ concentration the binding to microsomal protein was reduced although not proportionally, under either oxygen conditions; the level of protein binding occurring in the presence of GSH was not dependent on CHCl$_3$ concentration. The levels of cytochrome P_{450} were also affected by CHCl$_3$ metabolism (Fig. 1). At high CHCl$_3$ concentration anaerobic incubations produced a time-dependent loss of cytochrome P_{450} about twice higher than that measured after the aerobic metabolism, but at low concentrations a significant loss of cytochrome P_{450} occurred in anaerobiosis only. When NADPH was replaced by 1 mM NADH, cytochrome P_{450} loss was measured only after anaerobic incubations (19.4% ± 0.6%). These data indicate that CHCl$_3$ reactive metabolites produced without the use of O_2 as a cosubstrate give rise to biochemical alterations at least quantitatively similar to those successive to CHCl$_3$ oxidation. It is therefore possible that metabolites other than phosgene may be of relevance in the toxicity of CHCl$_3$. From this point of view, it is interesting to note that the CHCl$_3$ carcino-

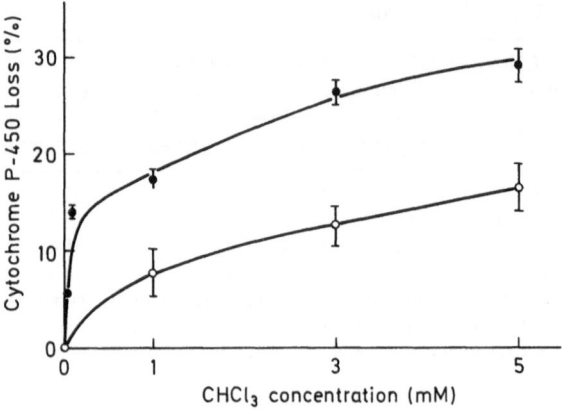

Fig. 1. Dependence of cytochrome P_{450} loss on chloroform concentration in anaerobic (●) or aerobic (○) incubations with B6C3F1 mouse liver microsomes in the presence of NADPH. Results are expressed as percentage decrease with reference to levels after blank incubations run in parallel (30 min, 37 °C). *Bars* represent SEM of determinations with at least three different microsomal preparations

genic potential is apparent in B6C3F1 mice but not in uninduced Sprague-Dawley rats, which are not able to anaerobically bioactivate chloroform (Testai and Vittozzi 1986).

Acknowledgement. This work has been partly supported by CNR, in the frame of the Target Project "Preventive and Rehabilitative Medicine," grant no. 85.00811.56.

References

Davidson IWF, Sumner DD, Parker JC (1982) Chloroform: a review of its metabolism, teratogenic, mutagenic, and carcinogenic potential. Drug Chem Toxicol 5(1):87

Ilett KF, Reid WD, Sipes IG, Krishna G (1973) Chloroform toxicity in mice: correlation of renal and hepatic necrosis with covalent binding of metabolites to tissue macromolecules. Exp Mol Pathol 19:215–229

NCI (1976) Report on carcinogenesis bioassay of chloroform. Natl Tech Inf Serv PB-264018. Springfield, Virginia

Omura T, Sato R (1964) The carbon monoxide binding pigment of liver microsomes. J Biol Chem 239:2370–2378

Reitz RH, Gehring PJ, Park CN (1978) Carcinogenic risk estimation for chloroform: an alternative to EPA's procedures. Fd Cosmet Toxicol 16:511–514

Testai E, Vittozzi L (1984) Different pathways of chloroform metabolism. Arch Toxicol [Suppl] 7:278–281

Testai E, Vittozzi L (1986) Biochemical alterations elicited in rat liver microsomes by oxidation and reduction products of chloroform metabolism. Chem Biol Interact 59:157–171

Tomasi A, Albano E, Biasi F, Slater TF, Vannini V, Dianzani MU (1985) Activation of chloroform and related trihalomethanes to free radical intermediates in isolated hepatocites and in the rat in vivo as detected by the ESR-spin trapping technique. Chem Biol Interact 55:303–316

Uehleke H (1973) The model system of microsomal drug activation and covalent binding to endoplasmic proteins. Proc Eur Soc Study Drug Toxic 15:119–129

Wolf CR, Mansuy D, Nastainczyk W, Deutschmann G, Ullrich V (1977) The reduction of polyhalogenated methanes by liver microsomal cytochrome P-450. Mol Pharmacol 13:698–705

Mechanisms and Models in Toxicology
Arch. Toxicol., Suppl. 11, 45–49 (1987)

Effects of Subchronic Low-Protein Diet on Some Tissue Glutathione – Related Enzyme Activities in the Rat

J.-M. Warnet[1], I. Bakar-Wesseling[2], M. Thevenin[1], J.J. Serrano[2], A. Jacqueson[1], M. Boucard[2], and J. R. Claude[1]

[1] Laboratoire de Toxicologie, Faculté de Pharmacie F-75006 Paris
and Laboratoire de la D.A.S.E.S., F-75017 Paris, France
[2] Laboratoire de Pharmacodynamie, Faculté de Pharmacie, F-34000 Montpellier, France

Introduction

Nutritional status influences the activity of drug metabolizing enzymes in the liver (Alvares et al. 1980; Basu and Dickerson 1974; Campbell and Hayes 1976; Magdalou et al. 1979). Deficiency of protein decreases the activity of the mixed-function oxidase system (cf. Hathcock 1985). Since glutathione (GS) and GS-related enzymes play an important role in the detoxification processes, the influence of subchronic low-protein diet (LPD) on GS content and GS-related enzyme activities was investigated in the liver, kidney, and gonads in the rat in order to develop an experimental system which may be used as a model to study the effect of drugs in protein-deficient animals.

Material and Methods

Animals and Experimental Procedure

Male (M) and female (F) Wistar rats, 3 week old, were fed with standard diet for 1 week. Then, 40 M and 40 F were fed with standard diet for 20 weeks (controls), 30 M and 30 F were fed for 12 weeks with an isocaloric diet containing only 5% casein (low-protein diet; LPD group), 10 M and 10 F were fed with LPD for 12 weeks and then fed with standard diet for 8 weeks (reverse group). From the control and LPD groups 10 M and 10 F were killed by carotid exsanguination after 4, 8, and 12 weeks. Remaining controls and reverse group were killed after 20 weeks. Liver, kidneys, and gonads were promptly excised and a 20% (w/v) solution of organ homogenates was prepared in 0.15 M KCl; cytosol was separated by differential sedimentation.

Analytical Methods

Total GS was determined in the cytosol using the enzymatic method of Tietze et al. (1969). The GS-related enzyme activities, peroxidase (GS Px), transferase

(GST), and reductase (GS Rd), were assayed using the method of Jaskott et al. (1983). Lipid peroxides were determined in the total homogenate by noting the thiobarbiturate reaction (Ohkawa et al. 1979).

All the results were expressed relative to the proteins as measured using a modified version of Lowry's method (Markwell 1978).

Statistical Analysis

All the results were statistically analyzed. The differences between the controls and the LPD rats were determined using Student's *t* test and a *P* value of 0.05 or less was considered significant.

Results and Discussion

Subchronic low-protein diet (LPD) produces a spectacular decrease in body weight which is more marked in males than females. This effect on the body weight leads to an involution of the liver, kidneys, testes, and ovaries. These changes are accompanied by variations in the GS levels/mg protein and the GS-related enzyme activities/mg protein in the different tissues examined, often at the early stages of the LPD. All these abnormalities proved reversible with return to normal protein diet (Tables 1–3).

The critical role of GS in detoxification reactions is well documented. Besides its direct antioxidant role, GS serves as a cosubstrate for GS peroxidases, which reduce hydrogen peroxide and/or organic peroxides, and for GS transferases which catalyze the reaction between the nucleophilic reduced GS and the electrophilic foreign substrate, forming a less toxic GS conjugate (cf. Kaplowitz 1980 and Stadtman 1980).

In the present work a distinction must be made between various investigated tissues. In the liver and gonads of both male and female LPD-fed rats, GS was decreased as early as the 4th week. At the same time, there was a significant decrease in GS Px activity in the male and female rat liver, whereas the decrease of GS Px in the gonads of both sexes was inconstant. GST activity was significantly decreased in the male rat liver, inconstant in the female rat liver, and remained unchanged in gonads.

In the kidney, by contrast, GS and GST were increased in male and female LPD-fed rats, whereas GS Px was not significantly changed. It seems that the increased GS levels and GST activities reflect in the kidney an adaptation to the consequences of the LPD intake.

It was observed that GS Rd activity was generally increased in the various tissues of male and female LPD-fed rats, except in the female kidney and testes. GS Rd catalyzes the reduction of oxidized GS by NADPH in order to replenish the level of reduced GS that has been oxidized by free radicals, peroxides, oxygen or enzymatic pathways such as GS Px (Staal et al. 1969). This increase in GS Rd seems related to the relative increase in dextrose caloric charge due to the LPD. This load could be responsible for an increase in NADPH needed by the enzyme activity.

Table 1. Effect of low protein diet (LPD) on glutathione (GS) and GS-related enzymes in male (M) and female (F) rat liver (mean ±SD)

Weeks	Total GS (µg/mg protein)		GS Transferase (GST)		GS Peroxidase (GS Px)		GS Reductase (GS Rd)	
	M	F	M	F	M	F	M	F
4 C	10.5±1.5	10.5±2.8	0.54±0.07	0.65±0.15	0.32±0.06	1.06±0.14	55.0±6.1	62.7±11.4
LPD	6.2±2.0 ***	6.3±1.9 ***	0.42±0.07 *	0.50±0.08	0.14±0.01 ***	0.19±0.02 ***	67.9±21.3	72.8±10.5
8 C	14.5±0.4	11.8±1.8	0.52±0.05	0.36±0.04	0.58±0.04	0.65±0.06	46.7±1.2	36.6±3.0
LPD	5.6±0.7 ***	7.1±1.1 ***	0.29±0.02 ***	0.47±0.02 ***	0.09±0.02 ***	0.14±0.01 ***	63.5±10.2 *	65.6±5.0 ***
12 C	14.2±1.4	11.6±1.6	0.63±0.08	0.62±0.03	0.54±0.05	0.60±0.04	63.0±5.4	52.8±2.8
LPD	6.2±0.6 ***	5.4±0.6 ***	0.53±0.02	0.64±0.07	0.09±0.01 ***	0.17±0.02 ***	88.6±5.9 ***	88.9±6.1 ***
20 C	13.7±1.5	14.5±0.7	0.66±0.04	0.53±0.03	0.58±0.03	0.76±0.07	50.5±3.1	48.4±4.5
R	14.0±1.4	14.9±0.6	0.69±0.04	0.55±0.04	0.55±0.05	0.79±0.05	59.4±3.7 **	52.5±8.9

C, controls; R, reverse group. GST data are µmol product formed/min/mg protein. GS Px and GS Rd data are µmol NADPH oxidized/min/mg protein. Significance of difference from controls: * $p < 0.05$; ** $p < 0.01$; *** $p < 0.001$.

Table 2. Effect of LPD on GS and GS-related enzymes in rat kidney (same legend as in Table 1)

Weeks	Total GS M	Total GS F	GST M	GST F	GS Px M	GS Px F	GS Rd M	GS Rd F
4 C	—	—	0.058 ± 0.002	0.042 ± 0.005	—	—	43.1 ± 3.8	50.2 ± 2.8
LPD	—	—	0.083 ± 0.002 ***	0.080 ± 0.005 ***	—	—	54.0 ± 3.0 ***	52.8 ± 3.7
8 C	0.40 ± 0.07	0.43 ± 0.02	0.055 ± 0.003	0.040 ± 0.003	0.027 ± 0.003	0.032 ± 0.002	36.7 ± 2.2	46.4 ± 2.6
LPD	1.04 ± 0.09 ***	0.91 ± 0.13 ***	0.081 ± 0.005 ***	0.083 ± 0.008 ***	0.038 ± 0.013	0.029 ± 0.001 *	44.2 ± 4.3 **	40.6 ± 3.1 *
12 C	0.29 ± 0.06	0.33 ± 0.05	0.054 ± 0.004	0.042 ± 0.005	0.025 ± 0.002	0.024 ± 0.001	35.2 ± 2.0	43.6 ± 2.8
LPD	0.86 ± 0.18 ***	1.71 ± 0.32 ***	0.069 ± 0.006 **	0.087 ± 0.008 ***	0.022 ± 0.002 *	0.024 ± 0.001	37.3 ± 2.1	42.4 ± 0.7
20 C	0.40 ± 0.08	0.45 ± 0.05	0.054 ± 0.006	0.045 ± 0.002	0.022 ± 0.001	0.029 ± 0.002	35.9 ± 1.5	46.0 ± 5.2
R	0.75 ± 0.19 ***	0.39 ± 0.08	0.059 ± 0.003	0.035 ± 0.004 **	0.021 ± 0.002	0.025 ± 0.002 *	37.4 ± 2.7	42.0 ± 1.7

Table 3. Effect of LPD on GS and GS-related enzymes in rat gonads (same legend as in Table 1)

Weeks	Total GS M	Total GS F	GST M	GST F	GS Px M	GS Px F	GS Rd M	GS Rd F
4 C	22.5 ± 1.4	4.78 ± 0.66	0.45 ± 0.04	0.085 ± 0.016	0.114 ± 0.006	—	3.7 ± 1.6	26.1 ± 7.5
LPD	19.2 ± 2.9	0.88 ± 0.57 **	0.54 ± 0.07	0.132 ± 0.050	0.057 ± 0.009 ***	—	7.8 ± 2.0 *	25.7 ± 8.8
8 C	19.7 ± 1.5	2.27 ± 0.27	0.72 ± 0.04	0.073 ± 0.008	0.110 ± 0.009	0.085 ± 0.008	12.1 ± 2.2	34.1 ± 2.9
LPD	15.7 ± 1.7 *	1.85 ± 0.42	0.68 ± 0.10	0.132 ± 0.017 **	0.096 ± 0.014	0.055 ± 0.016 *	12.3 ± 1.4	48.8 ± 7.1 *
12 C	20.3 ± 0.9	1.45 ± 1.40	0.83 ± 0.07	0.168 ± 0.113	0.105 ± 0.006	0.087 ± 0.009	15.3 ± 0.3	34.1 ± 2.1
LPD	14.8 ± 1.2 *	0.25 ± 0.05	0.77 ± 0.04	0.107 ± 0.015	0.088 ± 0.006 *	0.064 ± 0.011	13.6 ± 0.6	39.1 ± 5.2
20 C	18.1 ± 0.7	0.59 ± 0.09	0.79 ± 0.05	0.062 ± 0.004	0.094 ± 0.005	0.090 ± 0.009	14.5 ± 1.1	34.4 ± 1.6
R	20.0 ± 1.9	0.43 ± 0.27	0.86 ± 0.09	0.059 ± 0.007	0.098 ± 0.010	0.082 ± 0.002	14.6 ± 2.1	35.1 ± 0.8

From these results on LPD-fed rats, it can be inferred that a subchronic low protein diet intake in rats may reduce the defensive protection against xeno-biotics, particularly against their electrophilic metabolites. This is obvious for the liver, which is the major organ involved in the detoxification and the elimination of xenobiotics. However, this is not proof of a lipid peroxidation mechanism as a consequence of this reduction in protective mechanisms, since there were no marked variations in lipid peroxides. In contrast, the kidney appears to be able to partially compensate for the liver deficiency, although it can be considered a minor organ with respect to the liver.

Finally, all the variations observed in LPD-fed rats must be taken into account in the evaluation of drugs inducing protein absorption disorders or of drugs administered in protein-deficient patients.

References

Alvares AP, Anderson KE, Conney AH, Kappas A (1976) Interactions between nutritional factors and drug biotransformation in man. Proc Nat Acad Sci USA 73:2501–2504

Basu TK, Dickerson JWT (1974) Inter-relationships of nutrition and the metabolism of drugs. Chem Biol Interactions 8:193–206

Campbell TC, Hayes JR (1976) The effect of quantity and quality of dietary protein on drug metabolism. Fed Proc 35:2470–2474

Hathcock JN (1985) Metabolic mechanisms of drug-nutrient interactions. Fed Proc 44:124–129

Jaskott RH, Charlet EG, Grose EC, Grady MA (1983) An automated analysis of glutathione peroxidase, S-transferase and reductase activity in animal tissue. J Anal Toxicol 7:86–88

Kaplowitz N (1980) Physiologic significance of the glutathione S-transferases. Am J Physiol 239:439–444

Magdalou J, Steinmetz D, Batt AM, Poullain B, Siest G, Debry G (1979) The effect of dietary sulfur-containing amino acids on the activity of drug-metabolizing enzymes in rat-liver microsomes. J Nutr 109:864–871

Markwell MAK (1978) A modification of the Lowry procedure to simplify protein determination in membrane and lipoprotein samples. Anal Biochem 87:206–210

Ohkawa H, Ohishi N, Yagi K (1979) Assay for lipid peroxides in animal tissues by thiobarbituric acid reaction. Anal Biochem 95:351–358

Staal GEJ, Visser J, Veeger C (1969) Purification and properties of glutathione reductase of human erythrocytes. Biochim Biophys Acta (Amst) 185:39–48

Stadtman TC (1980) Selenium dependent enzymes. Annu Rev Biochem 49:93–110

Tietze F (1969) Enzymic method for quantitative determination of nanogram amounts of total and oxidized glutathione: applications to mammalian blood and other tissues. Anal Biochem 27:502–522

Mechanisms in Cancer Risk Assessment

Mechanisms and Models in Toxicology
Arch. Toxicol., Suppl. 11, 53–65 (1987)

Interorgan Shift of Nitrosamine Metabolism by Dietary Ethanol

O. D. Wiestler [1], A. von Deimling [1], E. von Hofe [2], I. Schmerold [2],
E. Wiestler [1], and P. Kleihues [2]

[1] Abteilung Neuropathologie, Pathologisches Institut, Universität Freiburg, 7800 Freiburg, FRG
[2] Abteilung Neuropathologie, Institut für Pathologie, Universität Zürich, 8091 Zürich, Switzerland

Introduction

Nitrosamines exceed most other classes of chemical carcinogens in their capacity to selectively induce tumors in a wide range of different tissues. Structure activity investigations have established that symmetric nitrosamines are often hepatocarcinogens, whereas most asymmetric nitrosamines selectively induce esophageal carcinomas. Furthermore, dibutylnitrosamine and related long-chain nitrosamines cause the development of bladder tumors while the nervous system is frequently the target for alkylnitrosoureas (Druckrey et al. 1967; Preussmann and Stewart 1984). For many nitroso compounds the origin and location of tumors varies with species, route of administration, and age or developmental stage. The biological basis of organ and species specificity has only been elucidated for a limited number of agents and a few selected target tissues (Langenbach et al. 1983; Kleihues and Wiestler 1986). From these studies it appears that the extent of DNA alkylation in target tissues as well as the capacity for enzymic repair of DNA modifications constitute key determinants. Additional factors influencing the location of tumors are cell division and tumor promoters.

Since the half-life of proximate and ultimate carcinogens is usually too short to allow for extensive systemic distribution, the carcinogenicity of nitroso compounds is in most cases restricted to those tissues possessing the P_{450} isozymes required for their bioactivation. If different organs compete for the same substrate, the extent of interaction with cellular DNA can be extensively modified by pharmacokinetic factors. In addition, several drugs and diets (e.g., protein deficiency) have been identified which, by inhibition of nitrosamine metabolism in liver, lead to an increased exposure of extrahepatic tissues. This is often paralleled by an acceleration of tumorigenesis or malignant transformation in organs which are not normally target tissues. A marked interorgan shift of nitrosamine metabolism can be caused by ethanol (Swann 1984). In this report the effects of dietary ethanol on the metabolism and reaction with DNA of four nitrosamines known to induce tumors in rat liver (N-nitrosodimethylamine, NDMA; N-nitrosomethylethylamine, NMEA; and N-nitrosodiethylamine, NDEA), esophagus

(*N*-nitrosomethylbenzylamine, NMBzA; and NDEA), and kidney (NDMA) are compared. With all compounds an inhibition of hepatic nitrosamine metabolism was observed, but changes in the extent of DNA alkylation in the target tissues varied considerably. Evidence is also provided that the observed modulation of carcinogen metabolism could be mediated by acetaldehyde, i.e., the major metabolite of ethanol.

Materials and Methods

Animals

Male inbred Lewis rats and male Wistar rats were obtained from Ivanovas (Kisslegg, FRG). Male F344 rats were from Charles River Wiga (Sulzfeld, FRG) and female Han:Wist rats were from Zentralinstitut für Versuchstiere (Hannover, FRG). The animals were fed a standard laboratory diet (Altromin) and were given water ad libitum.

Chemicals

N-Nitroso[^{14}C]dimethylamine ([^{14}C]NDMA) was synthesized by Dr. P.F. Swann (Courtauld Institute of Biochemistry, University of London) at a specific radioactivity of 58 mCi/mmol or was purchased from New England Nuclear (Dreieich, FRG; specific activity 54 mCi/mmol). The radiochemical purity was checked using HPLC and proved to be greater than 98%. Unlabeled NDMA (Schuchardt, München, FRG) was added to lower the specific activity.

   N-Nitroso[^{14}C]methylbenzylamine ([^{14}C]NMBzA, specific activity 58 mCi/ mmol) and *N*-nitrosodi[1-^{14}C]ethylamine ([1-^{14}C]NDEA, specific activity 57 mCi/mmol) were obtained from Amersham International (Buckinghamshire, England). The radiochemical purity was checked using HPLC and proved to be greater than 96%. Unlabeled NMBzA, synthesized by Dr. M. Wiessler (Deutsches Krebsforschungszentrum, Heidelberg, FRG), and unlabeled NDEA (Schuchardt, München, FRG), were added to lower the specific radioactivity. Details are given in table and figure legends. Ethanol (ethyl alcohol, anhydrous, p.a.) was purchased from Roth (Karlsruhe, FRG) and acetaldehyde was obtained from Merck (Darmstadt, FRG). Sephasorb HP Ultrafine was from Deutsche Pharmacia (Freiburg, FRG); Lumagel scintillation cocktail was from LKB (Karlsruhe, FRG).

Metabolic Cage Experiments

After deprivation of water overnight, rats received a single oral dose of the ^{14}C-labeled nitrosamine (for details see figure and table legends) and were placed in a metabolic cage (Jencons Metabowl, Hemel Hempstead, UK). The carcinogens were dissolved in approximately 5 ml tap water or in 5 ml tap water containing 5% (v/v) ethanol. This volume was readily imbibed within 20 min. Alternatively, nitrosamines were dissolved in 10% (v/v) acetaldehyde. Of this solution 1 ml per

100 g body weight was administered by stomach tube. Exhaled $^{14}CO_2$ was adsorbed in two serially connected Nilox columns, each containing 600 ml 1 N NaOH. Samples (0.5 ml) were diluted with distilled water (1:4) and mixed with 8 ml Lumagel. The counting efficiency was 86%.

DNA Alkylation In Vivo

Nitrosamines and ethanol were administered as described above (for details see figure and table legends). Following 5–7 h survival, animals were killed by exsanguination in ether anesthesia. Organs were rapidly removed, frozen in liquid N_2 and stored at -70 °C. DNA was isolated from the pooled organs of seven to eight rats by phenolic extraction, as described elsewhere (Margison and Kleihues 1975), hydrolized in 0.1 N HCl (20 h, 37 °C), neutralized and separated on a Sephasorb HP column (1 × 50 cm) using 10 mM NaH$_2$PO$_4$ (pH 5.5) as mobile phase (flow rate, 1.5 ml/min; fraction volume, 3.7 ml). The absorbance at 260 nm was measured in a Perkin Elmer spectrophotometer and radioactivity was determined after addition of 8 ml Lumagel to each fraction (counting efficiency, 85%). The amounts of methylated DNA purines were expressed as fractions of the parent base (guanine), assuming that the specific activity of the methyl adducts was the same as that of the administered [^{14}C]NMBzA and half of that of [^{14}C]NDMA.

Autoradiographic Studies

Tissues were fixed in buffered formaldehyde (5%, pH 7.2), dehydrated in 20%–100% ethanol and xylene, embedded in paraffin and cut into 5 μm sections. The slides were exposed for 14–21 days in X-ray cassettes using LKB 3H-Ultrofilm. Autoradiographs were developed in Kodak D-19 developer and fixed in Kodak Unifix. Some slides were counterstained with hematoxylin and eosin for anatomical localization of labeled areas.

Results

In a series of experiments involving ^{14}C-labeled NDMA, NDEA, and NMBzA, the time course of $^{14}CO_2$ expiration in rats was determined in a metabolic cage. Following a single oral dose (16.5 μmol/kg) exhalation of $^{14}CO_2$ was completed after 5–7 h as indicated by a plateauing of the cumulative radioactivity curves (Fig. 1). At this time, 40%–60% of the total radioactivity administered had been converted to $^{14}CO_2$. Simultaneous administration of ethanol caused a marked retardation in the rate of metabolism, with a two- to three-fold increase in the $t_{1/2\,max}$ i.e., the time at which 50% of the plateau value had been reached (Table 2). When NDMA and NMBzA were administered with acetaldehyde, a similar retardation of nitrosamine metabolism was noted (Fig. 2), although the increase in the $t_{1/2\,max}$ was somewhat less than with ethanol (Table 1).

The effects of dietary ethanol on DNA alkylation in target and nontarget tissues are shown in Table 2. Following a single oral dose of [^{14}C]NDMA, 7-methylguanine concentrations were highest in DNA from the liver, followed by lung

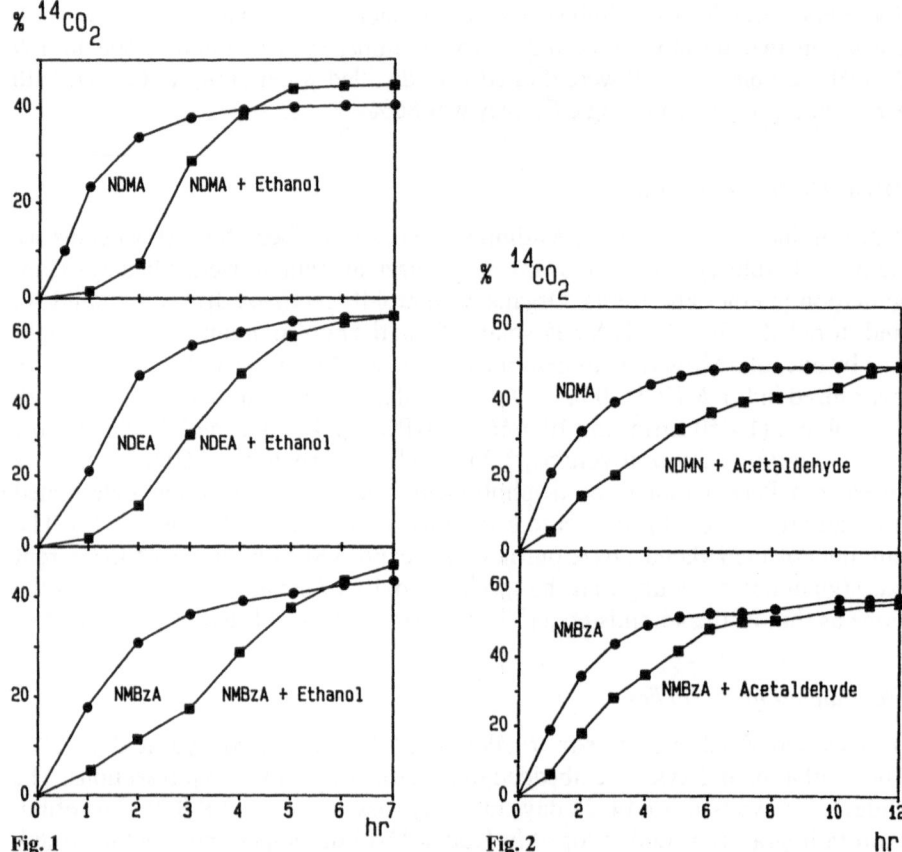

Fig. 1. Effect of ethanol on the time course of $^{14}CO_2$ exhalation following administration of ^{14}C-labeled nitrosamines. The data are plotted as cumulative percentages of the total ^{14}C-radioactivity administered. Male Lewis rats received a single oral dose of [^{14}C]NDMA (1.22 mg/kg; 1 mCi/mmol) or [^{14}C-methyl]NMBzA (2.5 mg/kg; 2.06 mCi/mmol) in 5 ml tap water (●) or in 5 ml tap water containing 5% ethanol (v/v) (■). Male Wistar rats were similarly given a single oral dose of [1-^{14}C]NDEA (1.68 mg/kg; 1 mCi/mmol) in 5 ml tap water or in 5 ml tap water containing 5% ethanol

Fig. 2. Effect of acetaldehyde on the time course of $^{14}CO_2$ exhalation following administration of ^{14}C-labeled nitrosamines. The data are presented as cumulative percentages of the total ^{14}C-radioactivity administered. Male Wistar rats received a single oral dose of 0.1 mg/kg [^{14}C]NDMA (10.65 mCi/mmol) in 1 ml tap water or tap water plus 10% acetaldehyde (v/v) per 100 g body weight. Female Han:Wist rats received 0.19 mg/kg [^{14}C]NMBzA (24.5 mCi/mmol) in tap water or tap water plus acetaldehyde as described above

and esophagus. Concurrent administration of ethanol did not alter the extent of methylation in liver or lung. However, methylation of kidney DNA showed a 150% increase and in esophageal DNA, 7-methylguanine was only detectable if animals received [^{14}C]NDMA with ethanol. Autoradiographic visualization of the ^{14}C-labeled reaction products with cellular macromolecules showed a characteristic centrilobular distribution in rat liver. In the lung, labeling by [^{14}C]NDMA

Table 1. Retardation of nitrosamine metabolism in rats by ethanol or acetaldehyde

Treatment	Nitrosamine dose		$t_{1/2\,max}$ [d] (h)
	(mg/kg)	(μmol/kg)	
NDMA[a]	1.22	16.5	0.9
NDMA + 5% ethanol	1.22	16.5	2.7 (300%)
NDEA[a]	1.68	16.5	1.4
NDEA + 5% ethanol	1.68	16.5	3.0 (214%)
NMBzA[a]	2.5	16.6	1.3
NMBzA + 5% ethanol	2.5	16.6	3.4 (261%)
NDMA[b]	0.1	1.4	1.4
NDMA + 10% acetaldehyde	0.1	1.4	4.0 (286%)
NMBzA[b]	0.18	1.2	1.8
NMBzA + 10% acetaldehyde	0.18	1.2	3.2 (178%)
NMBzA[c]	2.5	16.6	1.8
NMBzA + 10% acetaldehyde	2.5	16.6	2.8 (156%)

[a] Experimental conditions as described in Fig. 1.
[b] Experimental conditions as described in Fig. 2.
[c] Male Wistar rats received a single oral dose of 2.5 mg/kg [^{14}C]-NMBzA (1 mCi/mmol) in 1 ml tap water per 100 g body weight or tap water plus 10% acetaldehyde (v/v).
[d] Time at which one-half the maximal amount of radioactivity was exhaled; the numbers in parenthesis refer to the percent retardation of metabolism.

was uniformly diffuse, whereas [^{14}C]NDEA (Fig. 3) and [^{14}C]NMBzA (Fig. 5) showed a preferential reaction with the bronchiolar epithelium.

Following a single oral dose of [^{14}C]NMBzA, DNA methylation was highest in the target tissue, i.e., the esophagus, followed by liver, lung, and kidney. Simultaneous administration of ethanol caused a substantial reduction (52%) in hepatic DNA alkylation and a concurrent increase in esophageal (250%) and lung (503%) DNA. Representative radiochromatographs are shown in Fig. 4. With the specific radioactivity of [^{14}C]NMBzA available (13.7 mCi/mmol), O^6-methyl-guanine values were close to the limit of quantitative detection. An increase by ethanol of approximately 300% was calculated. This marked interorgan shift in DNA alkylation was also evident from autoradiographic analysis (Fig. 5). Ethanol caused a decrease of labeling in the liver and a marked increased in esophagus and lung without changing the basic pattern of tissue labeling. This figure also demonstrates that in rat esophagus, the metabolism of NMBzA is restricted to the mucosa proper.

Discussion

A common finding in all nitrosamines investigated was a marked ethanol-induced retardation of $^{14}CO_2$ exhalation (Fig. 1). It should, however, be noted that the time course of $^{14}CO_2$ expiration does not directly reflect the rate of metabolism.

Table 2. Effect of ethanol on DNA alkylation by nitrosamines. Adult rats received an oral dose of [14C]-NDMA (1.22 mg/kg; 11.6 mCi/mmol), [14C]-NMEA (4.4 mg/kg; 4.5 mCi/mmol), or [14C]-NMBzA (2.5 mg/kg; 13.7 mCi/mmol) in 5 ml tap water or water containing 5% ethanol (v/v); [2-3H]-NDEA (20 µg/kg; 3.15 Ci/mmol) was given as a single oral dose in 1 ml water or 5% ethanol in water

Organ	7-Methylguanine[a]		7-Ethylguanine[b]		7-Methylguanine[a]		7-Methylguanine[a]	
	NDMA	NDMA+EtOH	NDEA	NDEA+EtOH	NMEA	NMEA+EtOH	NMBzA	NMBzA+EtOH
Liver	406	417 (103%)	87	92 (106%)	910	791 (87%)	135	70 (52%)
Esophagus	n.d.	5	14	25 (179%)	9.1	15 (16%)	213	532 (250%)
Lung	17	16 (94%)	n.a.	n.a.	4.0	4.6 (115%)	40	201 (503%)
Kidney	10	15 (150%)	3.6	1.9 (53%)	57	30 (53%)	4	n.d.

[a] Expressed as µmol/mol guanine; n.d., not detected.
[b] Expressed as nmol/mol guanine; n.a., not available.
Data for NDEA from Swann et al. (1984); NMEA data from von Hofe et al (1986).

This radioactivity is derived from [14C]formaldehyde of [14C]acetaldehyde that is produced subsequent to enzymic α-C hydroxylation of NDMA, NMEA, and NDEA, respectively. In addition, methyl and ethyl diazonium ion, i.e., the ultimate carcinogens, react with water to form methanol and ethanol, and these, too, will enter the C1 pool and ultimately form $^{14}CO_2$. A retardation of $^{14}CO_2$ exhalation can be due to either an inhibition of nitrosamine metabolism or any factors interfering with the processing of formaldehyde in the C1 pool. However, numerous studies have shown that the latter is not rate limiting and that the time course of $^{14}CO_2$ production closely parallels the overall metabolism of ^{14}C-labeled nitroso compounds (Swann 1969; Fiume et al. 1970; Hodgson et al. 1980; Wiestler et al. 1985). The results shown in Fig. 1 do not allow the conclusion that the metabolism of these nitrosamines is generally inhibited by ethanol. The available evidence suggests rather that this retardation mainly reflects an inhibition of hepatic bioactivation since the liver is the predominant nitrosamine-metabolizing organ and amounts to approximately 5% of the total body mass.

DNA alkylation as a biological endpoint of nitrosamine metabolism is, in the view of the authors, the most relevant parameter in assessing the extent of interorgan shift and the potential effects of ethanol on the incidence and location of tumors induced. The data shown in Table 2 clearly indicate that the response to ethanol is not uniform amont the nitrosamines and tissues investigated. Following a single oral dose of NDMA, DNA methylation was by far the highest in liver, i.e., the principal target tissue, followed by lung and kidney. Simultaneous adminis-

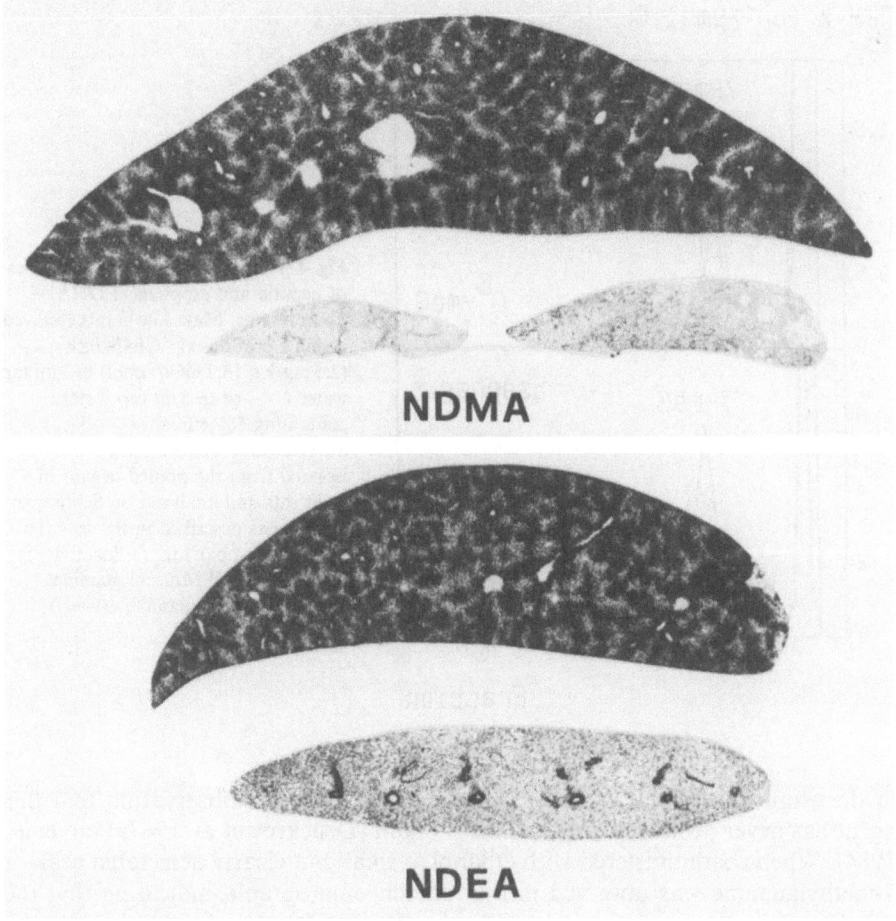

Fig. 3. Autoradiographs from the liver and lung of male Lewis rats which received a single oral dose of [^{14}C]NDMA (1 mg/kg; 51 mCi/mmol) and of male F344 rats which were given an i.p. injection of [1-^{14}C]NDEA (6.91 mg/kg; 17.07 mCi/mmol). Survival time was 4–5 h. Tissue sections were exposed for 14 days in X-ray cassettes using LKB 3H-Ultrofilm

tration of ethanol did not affect hepatic DNA methylation, but caused a 150% increase in renal 7-methylguanine concentrations. Ethanol is a competitive inhibitor of NDMA metabolism in rat liver (Schwarz et al. 1980; Peng et al. 1982), and has been shown to abolish the hepatic first-pass clearance observed after oral administration of NDMA at doses below approximately 30 µg/kg (Diaz-Gomez et al. 1977; Pegg 1980; Swann et al. 1984). This effect is similar to that observed in rats kept on a protein deficient diet (Swann and McLean 1971). This dietary regimen decreases the activity of hepatic microsomes to a greater extent than those of kidney, thereby causing a higher level of renal DNA alkylation and a marked increase in the incidence of tumors in this organ by a single dose of NDMA (Swann 1982). NDMA alone did not produce detectable levels of methylpurines

DPM x 10^{-3}/µmol G

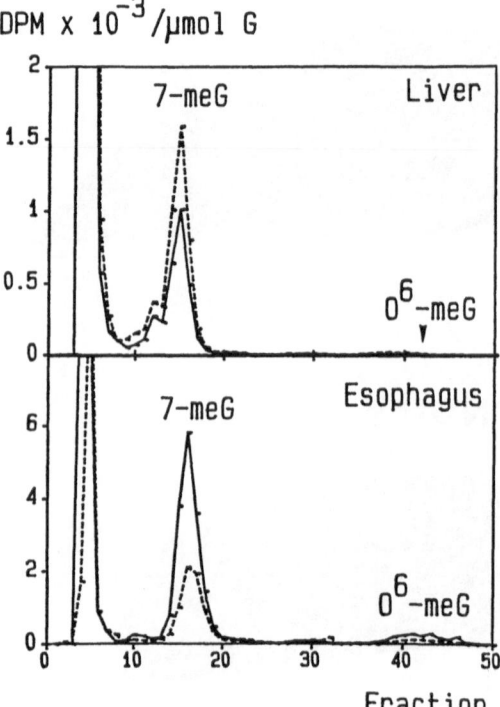

Fig. 4. Radiochromatographic profiles of hepatic and esophageal DNA hydrolysates. Male Lewis rats received a single oral dose [^{14}C]NMBzA (2.5 mg/kg; 13.7 mCi/mmol) in 5 ml tap water (---) or in 5 ml tap water containing 5% ethanol (–––). Survival time was 7 h. DNA was isolated from the pooled organs of eight rats and analyzed on Sephasorb columns as described in the text. To facilitate comparison, radioactivity is expressed as DPM/µmol guanine. *7-meG*, 7-methylguanine; *O^6-meG*, O^6-methylguanine

in the esophagus (Table 2) and this corresponds with the observation that this agent has never produced tumors in this organ (Druckrey et al. 1967; Peto et al. 1984). When coadministered with ethanol, a small but clearly detectable peak of 7-methylguanine was observed in the radiochromatograph, indicating that the esophagus may possess a very small amount of NDMA demethylase activity. Chronic bioassay studies on the simultaneous administration of NDMA and ethanol in rats have not been reported, but in mice this treatment causes, in addition to hepatic carcinomas, a high incidence of tumors of the nasal cavity (Griciute et al. 1981). The finding that ethanol does not reduce hepatic DNA alkylation is probably due to the small amount metabolized in the kidney. Ethanol retards hepatic NDMA metabolism and the reaction with cellular macromolecules, but since the parent carcinogen is not excreted via the urine, the overall extent of hepatic DNA alkylation remains unaffected.

In contrast to its methyl analog, NDEA also induces a high incidence of esophageal carcinomas (Druckrey et al. 1967). Concurrent administration of NDEA and ethanol greatly increased esophageal DNA alkylation. This corresponds to the observation by Gibel (1967) of a three-fold increase in the incidence of esophageal tumors in rats given NDEA in 30% ethanol instead of water. In other chronic bioassay studies, no such effect was observed (Habs and Schmähl 1981), probably because ethanol and NDEA were administered subsequently rather than simultaneously. It is noteworthy that ethanol decreased the ethylation of kidney DNA (Table 2). The reason for this is not clear, but the most likely expla-

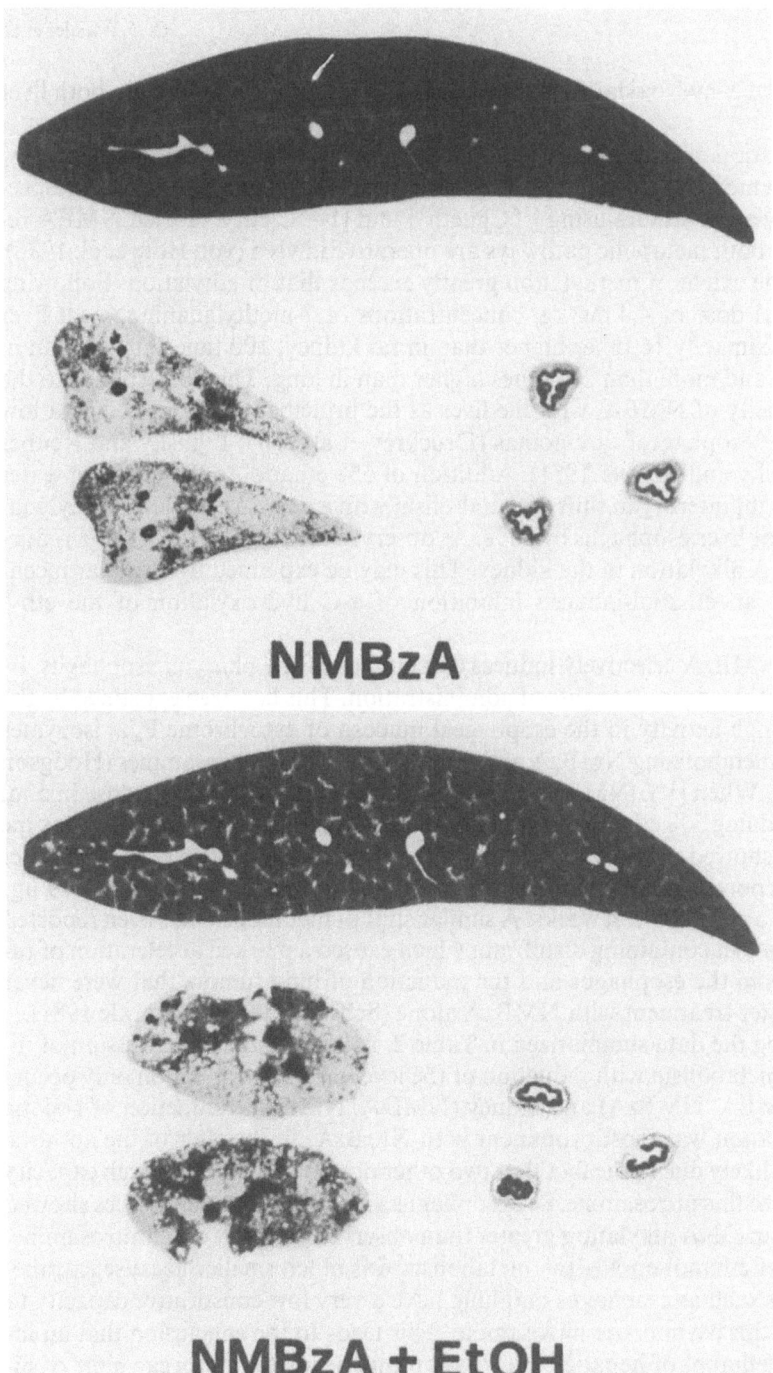

Fig. 5. Effect of alcohol on macromolecular binding of [^{14}C]NMBzA in liver, lung, and esophagus. Male Lewis rats received a single oral dose of [^{14}C]NMBzA (2.5 mg/kg; 13.7 mCi/mmol) in 5 ml tap water or in 5 ml tap water containing 5% ethanol. Following 7 h survival, organs were removed, fixed in buffered formaldehyde (5%; pH 7.2), embedded in paraffin, and cut in 2-μm sections. All slices were exposed for 14 days in X-ray cassettes using LKB 3H-Ultrofilm

nation is that α-hydroxylation at one of the ethyl groups is inhibited in both liver and kidney.

Bioactivation of NMEA can be initiated by hydroxylation of either the methyl or the ethyl moiety, leading to an ethylating or methylating intermediate, respectively. Alkylation studies using [^{14}C]methyl and [1-^{14}C]ethyl labeled NMEA revealed that both metabolic pathways are operative in vivo (von Hofe et al. 1986), although the extent of methylation greatly exceeds that of ethylation. Following a single oral dose of 4.4 mg/kg, concentrations of 7-methylguanine in rat liver were approximately 16 times higher than in rat kidney, 100 times higher than in esophagus, and more than 200 times higher than in lung. This corresponds to the carcinogenicity of NMEA, with the liver as the principal target tissue and a low incidence of esophageal carcinomas (Druckrey et al. 1967; Lijinsky and Reuber 1980; Lijinsky and Reuber 1981). Addition of 5% ethanol to the drinking water caused a slight interorgan shift of metabolism with a decrease in the 7-methylguanine ratio for liver:esophagus by 50%. As observed for NDEA, there was a reduction of DNA alkylation in the kidney. This may be explained by a similar mechanism, i.e., an ethanol-induced inhibition of α-C hydroxylation of the ethyl group.

In rats, NMBzA selectively induces carcinomas of the pharynx/esophagus, irrespective of the dose and route of administration. This has been explained by the unusually high activity in the esophageal mucosa of cytochrome P_{450} isozymes capable of metabolizing NMBzA and related asymmetric nitrosamines (Hodgson et al. 1980). When [^{14}C]NMBzA was administered orally as a single dose in 5 ml water containing 5% ethanol, hepatic DNA alkylation was decreased, whereas the esophagus showed a 2.5-fold and lung a five-fold increase (Table 2). Kouros et al. (1983) reported an analogous effect in rats pretreated with alcohol (45–69 µg/kg/day) for a period of 3–4 weeks. A similar shift of metabolism has been reported for rats on a diet containing disulfiram which caused a marked acceleration of tumorigenesis in the esophagus and the induction of lung tumors that were never observed after treatment with NMBzA alone (Schweinsberg and Bürkle 1981).

Reviewing the data summarized in Table 2, it emerges that a depression of nitrosamine metabolism with reduction of the level of DNA alkylation only occurs in liver (NMEA, NMBzA) and kidney (NMDA, NMEA). Reduction of hepatic DNA alkylation was most prominent with NMBzA. In the view of the authors, this is most likely due to the fact that two other organs show a fairly high capacity to metabolize this nitrosamine, i.e., esophagus and lung. The latter tissues showed an increase in DNA alkylation greater than observed with any other nitrosamine. The effect of ethanol on NMEA metabolism was much smaller because extrahepatic tissues such as esophagus and lung have a very low constitutive capacity to bioactivate this asymmetric nitrosamine. This leads to the conclusion that an inhibition by ethanol of hepatic bioactivation only leads to interorgan shift of nitrosamine metabolism if extrahepatic tissues are able to gain from the increased exposure. Only in this case will the retardation of hepatic metabolism and the increased exposure of extrahepatic tissues via the systemic circulation change the relative extent of DNA alkylation among the potential target tissues.

The depression of renal DNA alkylation observed with NDEA and NMEA shows that the inhibitory effect of ethanol is not always restricted to rat liver.

DNA ethylation by NDEA and DNA methylation by NMEA both require α-C hydroxylation of an ethyl moiety. In contrast, the metabolism of NDMA is initiated by α-hydroxylation of a methyl group and with this agent, ethanol caused an increase in renal DNA alkylation. This strongly suggests that α-C hydroxylation of methyl and ethyl groups is mediated by isozymes of the microsomal cytochrome P_{450} system (Peng et al. 1982) differing in their susceptibility to inhibition by ethanol.

With all nitrosamines investigated, simultaneous administration of ethanol led to a marked increase of esophageal DNA alkylation, indicating that bioactivation in this tissue is not depressed by ethanol at doses employed in the present experiments. Epidemiological studies show that in Western countries a high incidence of tumors of the oropharynx and esophagus is associated with increased alcohol consumption. This is particularly true for heavy smokers: exposure to tobacco smoke and to ethanol seem to act synergistically in the production of esophageal neoplasms (Tuyns 1978; Doll and Peto 1981; Seitz and Kommerell 1985). Several mechanisms have been proposed to explain this effect, including an ethanol-mediated induction of cytochrome P_{450}. The experiments reviewed here and pharmacokinetic studies on N-nitrosopyrrolidine, N-nitrosodipropylamine, and N-nitrosonornicotine suggest that the interorgan shift of carcinogen metabolism constitutes an important pathogenic mechanism which may also be applicable to other classes of chemical carcinogens (Swann 1984). The experiments carried out with acetaldehyde (Fig. 2) indicate that this metabolite rather than the ethanol itself might be responsible for the retardation of nitrosamine metabolism. In this context, it is noteworthy that alcoholics maintain increased blood acetaldehyde levels, while nonalcoholics do not (Korsten et al. 1975).

Determination of adducts in DNA isolated from whole tissues (Table 2) would not reveal ethanol-induced changes in specific target-cell populations. Autoradiographic studies on the distribution of [^{14}C]labeled reaction products with cellular macromolecules reveal that, in rat liver, nitrosamines are predominantly metabolized in the centrilobular areas (Figs. 3 and 5). In the esophagus, bioactivation of NMBzA is restricted to the mucosa. In rat lung, we found that NDEA (Fig. 3), NMEA, and NMBzA (Fig. 5) are preferentially metabolized in the bronchiolar epithelium, whereas [^{14}C]NDMA leads to a diffuse labeling of the lung parenchyma (Fig. 3). Coadministration of ethanol caused changes in the extent of labeling, similar to those determined biochemically (Table 2 and Fig. 5). There was no indication that ethanol caused an intraorgan shift in target-cell population.

Summary and Conclusions

The effect of dietary ethanol on the metabolism and reaction with DNA of four nitrosamines was investigated in rats. ^{14}C-Labelled N-nitrosodimethylamine (NDMA), N-nitrosodiethylamine (NDEA), N-nitrosomethylethylamine (NMEA) and N-nitrosomethylbenzylamine (NMBzA) were given as a single oral dose (1.2 to 16.5 μmol/kg) with or without the addition of 5% ethanol. Co-administration of ethanol caused a marked inhibition of nitrosamine metabolism, as determined by a retardation of ^{14}CO$_2$ expiration, the $t_{\frac{1}{2}max}$ being increased by a factor of 1.3 to 3. This effect was also observed when nitrosamines were co-administered with acetaldehyde, i.e. the major metabolite of ethanol. DNA alkylation studies revealed that the ethanol-induced depression of nitrosamine metabolism occurred mainly in liver, leading to an increased exposure of extrahepatic tissues. In all experiments, ethanol caused an increased level of DNA alkylation in the esophagus and this was most extensive in the case of NMBzA, for which the esophageal mucosa has a high constitutive bioactivating activity. Similarly, NMBzA was also subject to the most extensive shift in metabolism from liver to lung (5-fold increase in pulmonary DNA alkylation). NDMA produced detectable levels of 7-methylguanine in esophagus only after simultaneous administration of ethanol. With this agent, ethanol caused a 50% increase in kidney DNA alkylation whereas with NDEA and NMEA, the concentrations of 7-methylguanine in renal DNA were reduced by approximately 50%. DNA ethylation by NDEA and DNA methylation by NMEA both require α-C hydroxylation of an ethyl moiety, whereas the metabolism of NDMA is initiated by α-C hydroxylation of a methyl group. This suggests that α-C hydroxylation of methyl and ethyl groups is mediated by isozymes of the microsomal cytochrome P_{450} system differing in their susceptibility to inhibition by ethanol. Autoradiographic studies with [^{14}C-methyl]NMBzA identified the esophageal mucosa, bronchial epithelium and centrilobular areas of the liver as the principal target cell populations and this pattern was not changed by ethanol. The biological consequences of interorgan shift in nitrosamine metabolism by ethanol have been discussed, in particular the potential acceleration of tumorigenesis in extrahepatic organs which are not usually target tissues. The common finding of an ethanol-induced shift in metabolism from liver to esophagus may explain epidemiological observations of an increased risk for esophageal cancer in individuals with high alcohol consumption.

Acknowledgement. This work was supported by the Deutsche Forschungsgemeinschaft (SFB 31) and the Schweizerischer Nationalfonds zur Förderung der wissenschaftlichen Forschung.

References

Diaz-Gomez MI, Swann PF, Magee PN (1977) The absorbtion and metabolism in rats of small oral doses of dimethylnitrosamine. Biochem J 164:497–500

Doll R, Peto R (1981) The causes of cancer. J Natl Cancer Inst 66:1191–1308

Druckrey H, Preussmann R, Ivankovic S, Schmähl D (1967) Organotrope carcinogene Wirkungen bei 65 verschiedenen N-Nitroso-Verbindungen an BD-Ratten. Z Krebsforsch 69:103–201

Fiume L, Campadelli-Fiume G, Magee PN, Holsman J (1970) Cellular injury and carcinogenesis. Inhibition of metabolism of dimethylnitrosamine by acetonitrile. Biochem J 120:601–606

Gibel W (1967) Experimentelle Untersuchungen zur Synkarzinogese beim Ösophaguskarzinom. Arch Geschwulstforsch 30:181–189

Griciute L, Castegnaro M, Bereziat J-C (1981) Influence of ethyl alcohol on carcinogenesis with N-nitrosodimethylamine. Cancer Lett 13:345–352

Habs M, Schmähl D (1981) Inhibition of the hepatocarcinogenic acitivity of diethylnitrosamine (DENA) by ethanol in rats. Hepatogastroenterology 28:242–244

Hodgson RM, Wiessler M, Kleihues P (1980) Preferential methylation of target organ DNA by the oesophageal carcinogen N-nitrosomethylbenzylamine. Carcinogenesis 1:861–866

Kleihues P, Wiestler OD (1986) Structural DNA modifications and DNA repair in organ-specific tumor induction. In: Cohen GM (ed) Target Organ Toxicity, Vol. II, pp 159–180, CRC Press, Boca Raton, Florida

Korsten MA, Matsuzaki S, Feinman L, Lieber CS (1975) High blood acetaldehyde levels after ethanol administration. Difference between alcoholic and nonalcoholic subjects. N Engl J Med 292:386–389

Kouros M, Mönch W, Reiffer FJ, Dehnen W (1983) The influence of various factors on the methylation of DNA by the oesophageal carcinogen N-nitrosomethylbenzylamine. I. The importance of alcohol. Carcinogenesis 4:1081–1084

Langenbach R, Nesnow S, Rice JM (eds) (1983) Organ and species specificity in chemical carcinogenesis. Plenum, New York

Lijinsky W, Reuber MD (1980) Carcinogenicity in rats of nitrosomethylethylamines labeled with deuterium in several positions. Cancer Res 40:19–21

Lijinsky W, Reuber MD (1981) Comparative carcinogenesis by some aliphatic nitrosamines in Fischer rats. Cancer Lett 14:297–302

Margison GP, Kleihues P (1975) Chemical carcinogenesis in the nervous system. Preferential accumulation of O^6-methylguanine in rat brain deoxyribonucleic acid during repetitive administration of N-methyl-N-nitrosourea. Biochem J 148:521–525

Pegg AE (1980) Formation and subsequent repair of alkylation lesions in tissues of rodents treated with nitrosamines. Arch Toxicol [Suppl] 3:55–68

Peng R, Young Tu Y, Yang CS (1982) The induction and competitive inhibition of a high affinity microsomal nitrosodimethylamine demethylase by ethanol. Carcinogenesis 3:1457–1461

Peto R, Gray R, Brantom P, Grasso P (1984) Nitrosamine carcinogenesis in 5120 rodents: chronic administration of sixteen different concentrations of NDEA, NDMA, NPYR, NPIP in the water of 4440 inbred rats, with parallel studies on NDEA alone of the effect of age of starting (3, 6 or 20 weeks) and of species (rats, mice or hamsters). In: O'Neill IK, von Borstel RC, Miller CT, Bartsch H (eds) N-Nitroso compounds: occurrence, biological effects and relevance to human cancer. IARC Sci Publ 57:627–665

Preussmann R, Stewart BW (1984) N-Nitroso carcinogens. In: Searle CE (ed) Chemical carcinogens, vol 2, 2nd edn. American Chemical Society, Washington, pp 643–828 (ACS monograph 182)

Schwarz M, Appel KE, Schrenk D, Kunz W (1980) Effect of ethanol on microsomal metabolism of dimethylnitrosamine. J Cancer Res Clin Oncol 97:233–240

Schweinsberg F, Bürkle V (1981) Wirkung von Disulfiram auf die Toxizität und Carcinogenität von N-Methyl-N-nitrosobenzylamin bei Ratten. J Cancer Res Clin Oncol 102:43–47

Seitz HK, Kommerell B (eds) (1985) Alcohol related diseases in gastroenterology. Springer, Berlin Heidelberg New York

Swann PF (1969) The rate of breakdown of methyl methanesulphonate, dimethyl sulphate and N-methyl-N-nitrosourea in the rat. Biochem J 110:49–52

Swann PF (1982) Metabolism of nitrosamines: observations on the effect of alcohol on nitrosamine metabolism and on human cancer. In: Magee PN (ed) Nitrosamines and human cancer. Cold Spring Harbor Laboratory, New York, pp 53–68 (Banbury report 12)

Swann PF (1984) Effect of ethanol on nitrosamine metabolism and distribution. Implications for the role of nitrosamines in human cancer and for the influence of alcohol consumption on cancer incidence. In: O'Neill IK, von Borstel RC, Miller CT, Long J, Bartsch H (eds) N-Nitroso compounds: occurrence, biological effects and relevance to human cancer. IARC Sci Publ 57:501–512

Swann PF, McLean AEM (1971) Cellular injury and carcinogenesis: the effect of a protein-free high-carbohydrate diet on the metabolism of dimethylnitrosamine in the rat. Biochem J 124:283–288

Swann PF, Coe AM, Mace R (1984) Ethanol and dimethylnitrosamine and diethylnitrosamine metabolism and disposition in the rat. Possible relevance to the influence of ethanol on human cancer incidence. Carcinogenesis 5:1337–1343

Tuyns AJ (1978) Alcohol and cancer. Alcohol Health Res World 2:20–31

von Hofe E, Grahmann F, Keefer LK, Lijinsky W, Nelson V, Kleihues P (1986) Methylation versus ethylation of DNA in target and nontarget tissues of Fischer 344 rats treated with N-nitrosomethylethylamine. Cancer Res 46:1038–1042

Wiestler OD, Schmerold I, Fringes B, Volk B, Kleihues P (1985) Nafenopin-induced rat liver peroxisome proliferation reduces DNA methylation by N-nitrosodimethylamine in vivo. Carcinogenesis 6:1309–1313

Mechanisms and Models in Toxicology
Arch. Toxicol., Suppl. 11, 66–74 (1987)

Quantitative Evaluation of DNA-Binding Data In Vivo for Low-Dose Extrapolations

W. K. Lutz

Institute of Toxicology, ETH and University of Zurich, CH-8603 Schwerzenbach, Switzerland

Introduction

The risk of tumor formation from exposure to a chemical carcinogen is dependent on the exposure, the potency of the carcinogen, and the individual host reaction. Humans are exposed to chemical carcinogens at dose levels which are orders of magnitude below the levels used in animal studies on carcinogenicity. The latter experiments provide significant data only at high-dose levels which lead to tumor incidences on the order of percent (Fig. 1). For humans, tolerable exposures producing not more than one additional tumor in one million lives should be defined. The extrapolation range therefore covers four to five orders of magnitude. Instead of using purely mathematical models for the extrapolation, it would be desirable to have a biologically relevant indicator which could be investigated in the dose range to be bridged.

A large group of chemical carcinogens is known to bind covalently to DNA in the target cell. Under appropriate conditions, this primary DNA lesion can be expressed as a mutation finally leading to cancer. The primary interaction of the carcinogen with DNA can be investigated with appropriate techniques (radiolabeled test compound, phosphorylation with ^{32}P, or immunological methods) at low dose levels which would not give rise to a detectable increase in tumor yield with a limited number of animals treated. It is therefore possible to investigate the shape of the dose-response curve in the region of interest.

Methods

With radiolabeled test compound, the limit of detection is dependent on the specific activity, on the binding potency (covalent binding index, CBI; Lutz 1979), on the amount of DNA analyzed, and on the radioactivity in a vial considered significant. Under optimal conditions met, for instance, with tritiated aflatoxin B_1 of 8 Ci/mmol and a CBI of 10000, a single dose of 1 ng/kg rat was the observed limit of detection for liver DNA binding (10 dpm net radioactivity in 6 mg DNA).

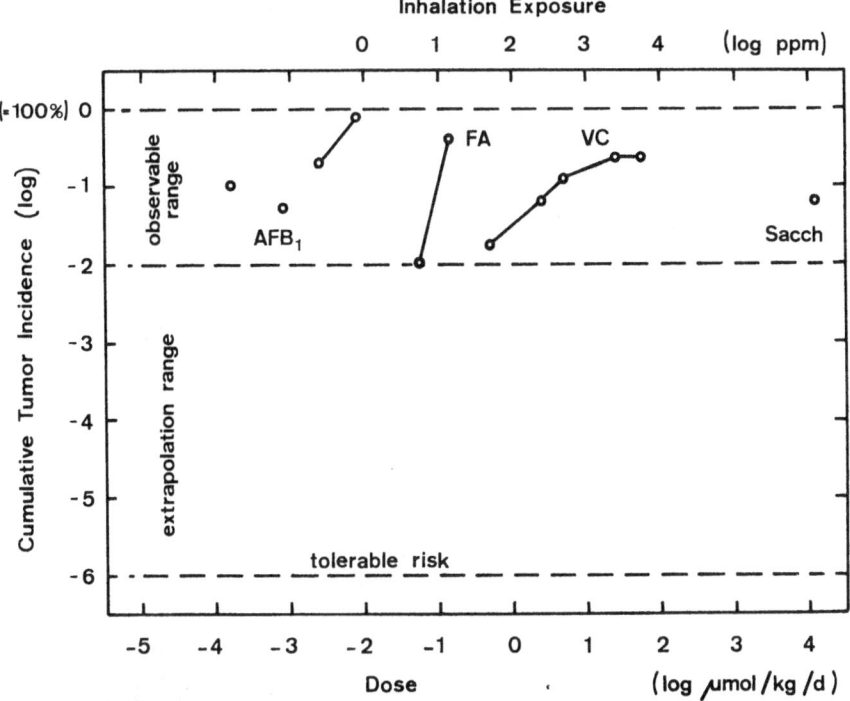

Fig. 1. Cumulative tumor incidence in rats as a function of the level of exposure. For aflatoxin B_1 (*AFB*$_1$) and saccharin (*Sacch*) the compound was admixed to the diet; the bottom dose scale applies. For formaldehyde (*FA*) and vinyl chloride (*VC*) exposure was by inhalation, 6 h/day, 5 days/week, for 2 years; the top dose scale applies. The two scales were combined on the assumption of a respiratory minute volume of 750 ml air/kg and an absorption of 20%

This corresponded to 3 adducts per 10^{11} nucleotides, i.e., less than 1 adduct per liver cell genome. With ^{14}C-labeled compounds of 10 mCi/mmol, the limit of detection would have been about 500 times higher, i.e., 1 adduct in 10^8 nucleotides.

A model calculation for the postlabeling technique using HPLC methods gives the following results: With $[\gamma\text{-}^{32}\text{P}]$ATP of a specific activity of 1000 Ci/mmol, an assumed limit of detection of 20 dpm would correspond to 0.01 fmol adduct, i.e., a level of 3 in 10^9 nucleotides in a 1-µg DNA sample.

With antibodies and the slot-blot technique (Rajewsky, personal communication), 0.1 fmol adduct can be detected in 3 µg DNA. This corresponds to an adduct level of 1 in 10^8 nucleotides.

A comparison of the three methods therefore shows that for the testing of new compounds, and where only small amounts of DNA are available from a specific tissue, the postlabeling technique seems most versatile.

Theoretical Considerations of the Shape of the Dose-Response Curve for DNA Binding

Many of the DNA-binding carcinogens require metabolic activation to form electrophilic, reactive, so-called ultimate carcinogens. DNA binding therefore involves enzymatic processes, diffusion processes, and electrophilic substitution reactions. In principle, the rate of all these steps is proportional to the concentration in the low range, so that a linear dose-DNA binding relationship would be postulated. The rate of DNA repair has been found to be proportional to the level of the DNA adducts in the case of O^6-methylguanine (Lutz 1982). If this first order kinetics for DNA repair holds also for other adducts, a linear dose-DNA binding relationship would hold not only for the time of maximum binding, but also at later times of DNA analysis.

Experimental Findings on the Dose-DNA Binding Relationship

A number of compounds have been studied in this respect. The dose range investigated is shown in Fig. 2. A small arrow indicates for each compound the TD_{50}

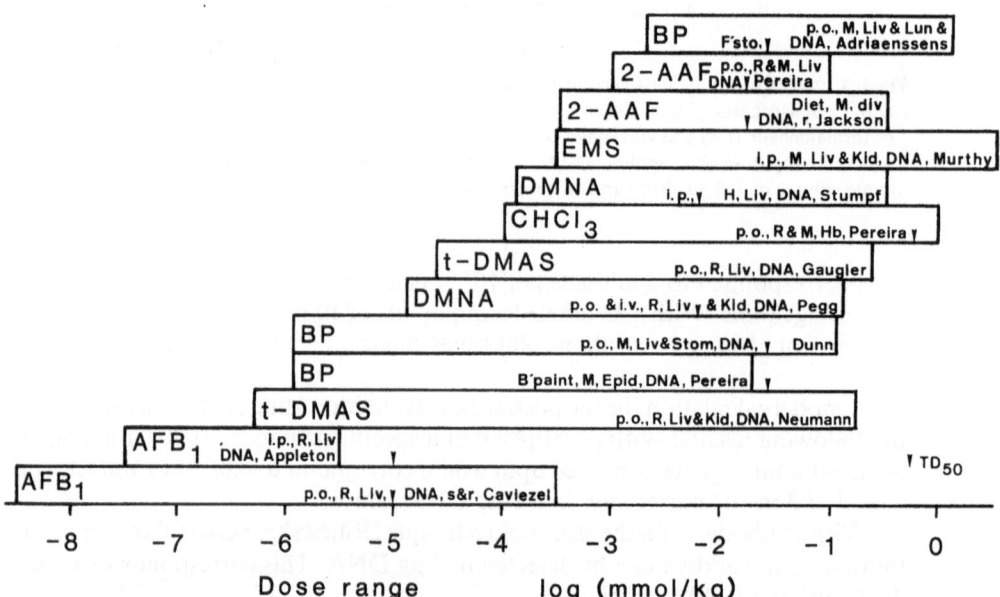

Fig. 2. Range of doses investigated with various carcinogens for macromolecular binding in vivo. The *small arrows* indicate the TD_{50} value (Gold et al. 1984), i.e., a measure for carcinogenic potency. Abbreviations of substances from left to right: *AFB₁*, aflatoxin B₁; *t-DMAS*, *trans*-4-dimethylaminostilbene; *BP*, benzo[a]pyrene; *DMNA*, dimethylnitrosamine; *EMS*, ethyl methanesulfonate; *2-AAF*, 2-acetylaminofluorene. Other abbreviations indicate the route of exposure, the animal species, the organ of interest, the type of macromolecule, and a specification of single (*s*) or repeated (*r*) administration: *R*, rat; *M*, mouse; *H*, hamster; *Liv*, liver; *kid*, kidney; *Epid*, epidermis; *Stom*, stomach; *Lun*, lung; *F'sto*, forestomach; *div*, diverse organs; *Hb*, hemoglobin. The respective reference is listed under the first author's name. (From P. Buss, Ph.D. thesis, ETH Zurich, in preparation)

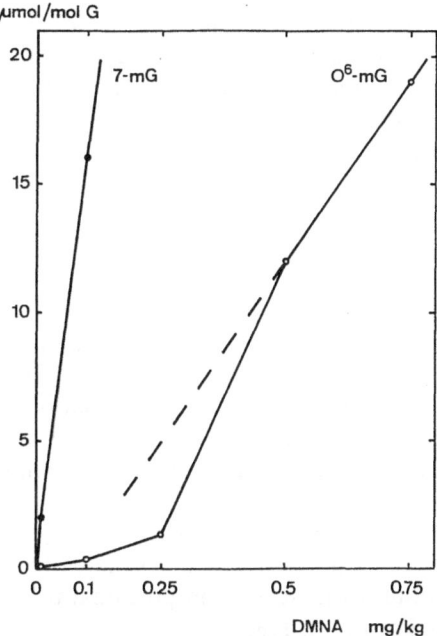

μmol/mol G

Fig. 3. Dose-response curve for the determination of 7-methylguanine (*7-mG*) and *O⁶*-methylguanine (O^6-*mG*) in liver DNA isolated from male Syrian golden hamsters, 5 h after i.p. injection of radiolabeled dimethylnitrosamine (DMNA). (Original data from Stumpf et al. 1979)

value (Gold et al. 1984), i.e., the approximate daily dose required to induce a tumor in 50% of the animals treated. With respect to the problem of extrapolation of tumor-inducing doses to lower exposures, those studies are the most relevant which cover three or more orders of magnitude below the TD_{50}. Studies which did not extend beyond one order of magnitude below the TD_{50} were not included in the list. All studies except those investigating specific methylated DNA bases showed a linear dose-response curve. The lowest dose used was 1 ng/kg with aflatoxin B_1 (Caviezel 1984). The theoretical prediction of proportionality could therefore be verified experimentally.

The only situation showing a nonlinearity is exemplified in Fig. 3. The formation of 7-methylguanine increased linearly with the DMNA dose, whereas the level of O^6-methylguanine was proportional to the dose only above 0.5 mg/kg. Below that dose, the level of O^6-methylguanine was lower than extrapolated from the high dose levels. This phenomenon was indicative of a fast-acting repair process which was exhausted at higher levels of O^6-methylguanine (Lutz 1982). For this adduct it could also mean that a linear extrapolation of the tumor incidence data to lower doses might be too conservative because a small DNA damage might be more quickly repaired than a large one. A nonlinear dose-response relationship results. Since DNA methylation so far is the only DNA damage leading to this type of dose response it is possible that this constitutive, fast repair of erroneous DNA methylations has evolved in nature in order to control errors in the formation of 5-methylcytidine by the endogenous methyl donor *S*-adenosylmethionine.

It is becoming evident that DNA binding is nonrandom with respect both to sequence and arrangement of the DNA. This does interfere with the quantitative relationship of total DNA binding to the number of critical mutations, but it should not affect the analysis of the dose-response relationship because it can be assumed that the fraction of critical adducts will be proportional to the total number of adducts.

Single Vs Repetitive Exposure

In a standard carcinogenicity bioassay, the test compound is given continuously. The level of DNA adducts therefore is a result of a constant daily increase from new exposure and the removal by repair, cell death, or cell division. What is decisive for the tumorigenicity of DNA adducts in the steady-state level. Only two studies have been dealing with the low dose-response relationship for DNA binding after repetitive exposure.

1. Various concentrations of 2-acetylaminofluorene (2-AAF) were admixed to the diet fed for 2 weeks to mice of different strains. DNA was isolated from different organs. The level of DNA adducts was strictly proportional to the concentration of 2-AAF in the diet (Jackson et al. 1980).

2. In this laboratory, tritiated aflatoxin B_1 was administered p.o. to F344 rats on 10 consecutive days (Caviezel 1984). Liver DNA was isolated 24 h after the last dose and the level of DNA damage was determined. Again, a linear dose-response relationship was found over 4 orders of magnitude (Fig. 4). The damage set by the highest dose was no longer proportional to the dose, probably because of a saturation of the activating enzyme systems. This phenomenon was also observed with DNA adducts induced by trans-4-dimethylaminostilbene (t-DMAS; Neumann 1980) and vinyl chloride (Watanabe et al. 1978) and is reflected in carcinogenicity studies by a flattening out of the dose-response curve at the highest exposure levels (see Fig. 1 vinyl chloride, VC).

Conclusions on DNA-Binding in Exposed Individuals

The data summarized above indicate that the level of genotoxicity is proportional to the dose in the low dose range after both single and repetitive administration of a DNA-binding compound. In the high dose range, a flattening out of the curve can be seen if the metabolic activation is becoming saturated.

The lowest dose used so far for a DNA-binding study was 1 ng aflatoxin B_1 administered per kg rat. This corresponds to about 60 ng per man, i.e., a dose which is taken up daily in certain areas of tropical Africa and Asia. The lowest point shown in Fig. 4 therefore represents a dose to which humans can be exposed.

For risk extrapolation of DNA-binding carcinogens it therefore seems most appropriate to underline the idea that the primary lesion is strictly proportional to the dose. The nonlinearity seen with O^6-methylguanine is one exception to the rule and probably cannot be used for other types of adducts.

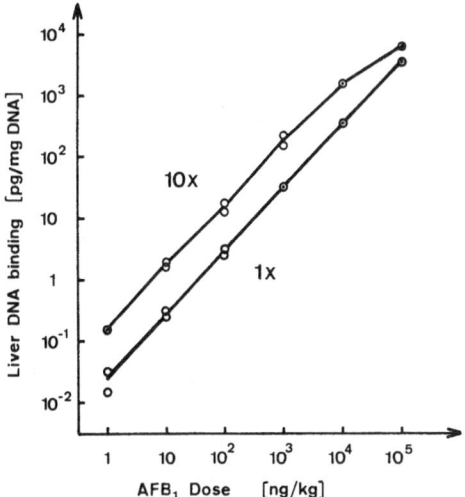

Fig. 4. Binding of tritiated aflatoxin B$_1$ (*AFB$_1$*) to liver DNA of male F344 rats, 24 h after one single (*1x*) or the last of ten daily oral doses (*10x*), as a function of the dose

Low-Dose Extrapolations in Populations

Both theoretical analysis and experimental data indicate that, for the primary lesion in chemical carcinogenesis by DNA-binding compounds, a linear extrapolation is appropriate. This proportionality cannot, however, be extended to the question of the dose-response relationship for the appearance of tumors in a population without additional considerations. In general toxicology it is very often seen that the distribution of individuals giving a predetermined response (yes or no criterion) to an agent is gaussian (normal) if the doses are scaled logarithmically. This log-normal distribution can be derived exactly from the reasonable pharmacological assumption that the effect will become observable if the concentration of the toxic principle is above a certain limit during a critical period of time. If it is further accepted that the individuals in the population differ according to a normal distribution with respect to either the critical time period necessary or the rate of detoxication, the values of a minimal effective concentration will be log-normally distributed (Koch 1966).

An element of time is therefore required for the logarithm to enter into the dose-response relationship. Time is also of predominant importance in the process of chemical carcinogenesis, but here it is not a matter of an all or none response, but rather of a stochastic succession of stages where the probability is dependent on the period of time available. For instance, a heritable mutation can only be derived from a DNA adduct if the DNA is replicating to produce a genetic alteration in a daughter cell. The fixation of the primary lesion is therefore dependent on the relative rates of DNA repair and DNA replication. A reduction of the time available for the mutational expression of the DNA adduct will therefore reduce the probability of a mutation.

Many mathematical risk models take into account that carcinogenesis is a multistage process with several hits being required with or without specific sequence assumptions. The observed tumor incidences are used to determine best-fit values of the parameters of the underlying function. If such functions are used for low-dose extrapolations, an unresolvable problem arises from the assumption that the host reaction to the high dose levels also determines the shape of the dose-response curve at lower dose levels (FDA 1971).

Dose-Response Relationship for Combination Mechanisms of Carcinogenic Action

DNA binding is only one out of a number of activities resulting in increased tumor formation (Lutz 1986). Cell division seems to be an absolute requirement in carcinogenesis, and agents or processes which stimulate the rate of DNA synthesis are often found to increase the tumor incidence. Some compounds most probably produce DNA adducts and stimulate cell division: hexachlorocyclohexane isomers could be named (Sagelsdorff et al. 1983) and formaldehyde might also be an example (Swenberg et al. 1983). In both cases it is considered that the DNA-binding activity is low so that it would not alone be sufficient to lead to a significant increase in tumor formation in a standard bioassay (Fig. 5, dashed line). Only together with sufficient promotion would an effect become observable. With formaldehyde, this promoting activity – in a mechanistic sense – could be due to cytotoxicity and tissue regeneration. Since cell death is an "all or nothing" phenomenon, discussed above, as the basis of a log-normal dose-response relationship, a nonlinear curve could result. A combination of DNA binding with stimulation of cell division would still be nonlinear (Fig. 5). The steep slope observed for the tumor incidence from formaldehyde inhalation exposure to 5.6 and 14.3 ppm (Fig. 1) could therefore be explained by a combination of direct genotoxicity and tissue irritation.

The slope shown for aflatoxin B_1 and vinyl chloride (low dose part only) is approximately one in the double-log plot. The proportionality of dose and DNA

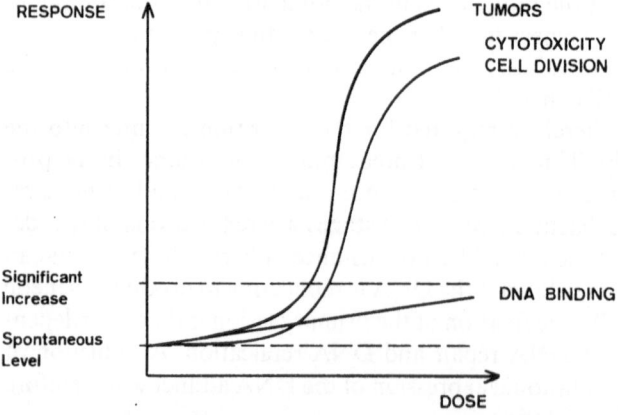

Fig. 5. Potential dose-response relationship for a chemical carcinogen exhibiting more than one biological activity related to tumor induction. Cytotoxicity with regenerative cell division is given as one possible example for a promoting type activity

binding as discussed above therefore seems to determine the dose-response relationship for the tumor incidence. This could mean that DNA binding is the predominant factor in chemical carcinogenesis by AFB_1 and VC. DNA binding is only one mechanism of genotoxicity. Stimulation of cell division is only one aspect in tumor promotion. The present analysis of the available data shows that these two aspects might explain tumor formation by a large number of chemicals. Nevertheless, other types of activities might be involved in the process of carcinogenesis. Such critical biochemical processes should be searched for.

The present discussion has shown that the assessment of the risk of exposure to a tumor-inducing agent at low dose levels could be improved if mechanisms of action were taken into account. Low-dose extrapolations should therefore be based more often on biological models. Neither standard carcinogenicity bioassays nor mathematical models provide such information.

Acknowledgement. We thank the Swiss League Against Cancer for financial support (FOR 267 AK 84/5).

References

Adriaenssens PI, White CM, Anderson MW (1983) Dose-response relationships for the binding of benzo[a]pyrene metabolites to DNA and protein in lung, liver, and forestomach of control and butylated hydroxyanisole-treated mice. Cancer Res 43:3712–3719

Appleton BS, Goetchius MP, Campbell TC (1982) Linear dose-response curve for the hepatic macromolecular binding of aflatoxin B_1 in rats at very low exposure. Cancer Res 42:3659–3662

Caviezel M (1984) Untersuchungen zur kovalenten Bindung an DNS und Protein in vivo durch die Steroide Cholesterin-5,6-epoxid, Oestron, Oestradiol und Trenbolon, sowie durch Aflatoxin B_1. Ph.D. Thesis, ADAG Zürich, Diss. ETH Nr. 7564

Dunn BP (1983) Wide-range linear dose-response curve for DNA binding of orally administered benzo[a]pyrene in mice. Cancer Res 43:2654–2658

FDA (1971) Food and drug administration advisory committee on protocols for safety evaluation: panel on carcinogenesis report on cancer testing in the safety evaluation of food additives and pesticides. Toxicol Appl Pharmacol 20:419–438

Gaugler BJM, Neumann HG (1979) The binding of metabolites formed from aminostilbene derivatives to nucleic acids in the liver of rats. Chem-Biol Interact 24:355–372

Gold LS, Sawyer CB, Magaw R, Backman GM, de Veciana M, Levinson R, Hooper NK, Havender WR, Bernstein L, Peto R, Pike MC, Ames BN (1984) A carcinogenic potency database of the standardized results of animal bioassays. Environ Health Perspect 58:9–319

Jackson CD, Weis C, Shellenberger TE (1980) Tissue binding of 2-acetylaminofluorene in BALB/c and C57Bl/6 mice during chronic oral administration. Chem-Biol Interact 32:63–81

Koch AL (1966) The logarithm in biology: 1. Mechanisms generating the log-normal distribution exactly. J Theor Biol 12:276–290

Lutz WK (1979) In vivo covalent binding of organic chemicals to DNA as a quantitative indicator in the process of chemical carcinogenesis. Mutat Res 65:289–356

Lutz WK (1982) Inducible repair of DNA methylated by carcinogens. Trends Pharmacol Sci 3:398–399

Lutz WK (1986) Quantitative evaluation of DNA binding data for risk estimation and for classification of direct and indirect carcinogens. J Cancer Res Clin Oncol 112:85–91

Murthy MSS, Calleman CJ, Osterman-Golkar S, Segerbäck D, Svensson K (1984) Relationship between ethylation of hemoglobin, ethylation of DNA and administered amount of ethyl methanesulfonate in the mouse. Mutat Res 127:1–8

Neumann HG (1980) Dose-response relationship in the primary lesion of strong electrophilic carcinogens. Arch Toxicol [Suppl] 3:69–77

Pegg AE, Perry W (1981) Alkylation of nucleic acids and metabolism of small doses of dimethylnitrosamine in the rat. Cancer Res 41:3128–3132

Pereira MA, Burns FJ, Albert RE (1979) Dose response for benzo[a]pyrene adducts in mouse epidermal DNA. Cancer Res 39:2556–2559

Pereira MA, Lin LHC, Chang LW (1981) Dose-dependency of 2-acetylaminofluorene binding to liver DNA and hemoglobin in mice and rats. Toxicol Appl Pharmacol 60:472–478

Pereira MA, Chang LW (1982) Binding of chloroform to mouse and rat hemoglobin. Chem-Biol Interact 39:89–99

Sagelsdorff P, Lutz WK, Schlatter C (1983) The relevance of covalent binding to mouse liver DNA for the carcinogenic action of hexachlorocyclohexane isomers. Carcinogenesis 4:1267–1273

Stumpf R, Margison GP, Montesano R, Pegg AE (1979) Formation and loss of alkylated purines from DNA of hamster liver after administration of dimethylnitrosamine. Cancer Res 39:50–54

Swenberg JA, Barrow CS, Boreiko CJ, Heck HA, Levine RJ, Morgan KT, Starr TB (1983) Non-linear biological responses to formaldehyde and their implications for carcinogenic risk assessment. Carcinogenesis 4:945–952

Watanabe PG, Zempel JA, Pegg DG, Gehring PJ (1978) Hepatic macromolecular binding following exposure to vinyl chloride. Toxicol Appl Pharmacol 44:571–579

Mechanisms and Models in Toxicology
Arch. Toxicol., Suppl. 11, 75–83 (1987)

Persistent Organ Damage and Cancer Production in Rats and Mice

P. Grasso

131, Old Lodge Lane, Purley, Sussey, UK

Introduction

The reparative processes that take place in response to tissue injury are indubitably of great importance in restoring the integrity of a damaged organ, but they are not usually thought of as a mechanism.

Since "Mechanism in Carcinogen Risk Assessment" is the theme of this symposium it is worthwhile to see whether the term "mechanism" is applicable to repair processes that follow a single or repeated injury to a particular organ.

Strictly speaking, the word "mechanism" is an engineering term and is used to designate any appliance which is made up of a number of parts, so arranged as to work in harmony together. An easily understood example is the mechanical watch, and, in fact, when a famous engineer analysed the workings of the mechanical watch, he called his treatise "The Mechanism of the Watch" (Swinburne 1950).

In biology, the term mechanism is usually reserved for the study of molecular mechanisms, but in fact biological mechanisms occur at various levels – cellular, or organelle level as well as molecular. From carcinogenicity studies in rodents an attempt will be made to illustrate the way in which biological mechanisms involved in tissue damage and repair at the cellular level may be employed in the assessment of risk for man.

Subcutaneous Sarcoma – A Doubtful Index of Carcinogenic Hazard

Historically, Oppenheimer (1953) was one of the earliest investigators to study such mechanisms in experimental carcinogenesis and his studies were so successful that at one time the mode of cancer development described by him was widely known as the "Oppenheimer Effect". Oppenheimer was a physician and was interested in treating hypertension. He developed a simple technique for making a hypertensive rat model to test new ideas and drugs in antihypertensive therapy. The technique consisted of wrapping the kidneys of rats in cellophane film which caused some degree of cortical ischaemia and this in turn resulted in the production of hypertension in the rat (Bischoff et al. 1964).

Whether by chance or design, Oppenheimer preserved some of his rat models for several months and one day he discovered that some of them had developed sarcoma around the cellophane film (Bischoff et al. 1964). His inquisitive nature led him to investigate this phenomenon further. His findings, and those of others who became interested in the "Oppenheimer Effect" can be summarized as follows:

Pieces of solid material about 2 cm × 2 cm (or 2 cm in diameter) induced a high incidence of tumours. Smaller pieces induced less tumours, while the same amount of material by weight implanted as a powder or in the shredded form did not produce any tumours at all. These observations were first established with cellophane implants and then with many other solids, including plastics material, gold, silver, glass and other solid substances which were biologically inert (Bischoff et al. 1964).

Three sets of observations demonstrated that the tissue reaction was the determining factor in the production of the sarcomas. First, a marked granulomatous reaction developed around the large solid implant, but very little reaction was found around the shredded material. Secondly, if the reaction was allowed to continue for at least 4 months, then removal of the solid foreign body did not prevent the onset of tumours. Thirdly, if pieces of the granulomatous tissue or of the film were re-implanted in appropriate recipient rats, then tumours developed in the recipients. Obviously transformed cells had developed within the tissue reaction (Bischoff et al. 1964; Grasso et al. 1966; Brandt et al. 1976).

When this mechanism became established, many questions were asked about its relevance for man. It is not certain whether the final answer has been found to these questions, but so far there has been no substantial evidence that sarcoma develops around large pieces of solid material embedded for several years in humans – such as shell fragments or bone prostheses (Grasso et al. 1966). Obviously, this is only part of the story of solid-state carcinogenesis, since asbestos is a well-known carcinogen in man and experimental animals, but the physical state of asbestos is very different from that of the metallic and polymeric foreign bodies which have just been referred to and is, therefore, a separate issue.

The significance of sarcoma arising at the site of injection in rats and mice was an off-shoot of the debate that took place during the study of the "Oppenheimer Effect." From the point of view of mechanisms relevant to man, the sarcomas induced by repeated injection of Fe-dextran can provide some interesting clues on how to approach problems of risk assessment. Fe-dextran was at one time an extremely popular remedy for iron-deficiency anaemias, real or imaginary, in humans and was given therapeutically by subcutaneous injection. When tested in animals by this route, it produced sarcomas at the site of injection in both rats and mice. Investigations into the mechanism of tumour production revealed that two major events occurred in the rodent following repeated injection of Fe-dextran.

First, there was a rapid overloading of the test animal with Fe. Secondly, when this point was reached, no further absorption of Fe occurred from the injection site so that it accumulated locally in macrophages as haemosiderin, forming a large granuloma. This lesion underwent progressive increase in fibrous tissue and after several weeks foci of cells without haemosiderin appeared which heralded the development of local sarcomas (Golberg 1963). There was a strong resemblance in the evolution of this lesion to that found around plastic films, but this was not enough to allay concern about the possible effects on man. To provide information on this point data were collected from patients who had been treated with Fe-dextran and two observations have been made. It was found that under conditions of therapeutic use no iron overloading occurred in man since the amount of Fe given to man on a mg/kg basis was much smaller than that administered to the rat or mouse; no massive local accumulation of the type observed in animals occurred in man (Golberg 1963). Second, up to the present day (i.e., 30 years or so from the time the problem was recognised), no convincing evidence of sarcoma at the site of injection of Fe-dextran has been established in man.

This episode led to a searching reappraisal of the significance of this route of administration in terms of human hazard. A search of the literature revealed that glucose and common salt and even distilled water, when injected repeatedly and in large doses into experimental rodents, induced sarcomas (Grasso et al. 1966). The concentrations at which these substances were administered were strongly hypertonic and dose/volumes of 4–5 ml per injection appeared to be the norm. Someone suggested (Boyland 1958) that these tumours were due to "osmotic shock" although it was not made clear who it was that suffered from shock, whether it was the rat when it had the injection or the experimentalist when he saw tumours developing!

Many experimentalists, at that time, had shocks of this kind when they used this route for testing compounds for carcinogenicity and none more so than the food industry which then used a large range of food colours in processed food; it was found that a high proportion of these induced sarcomas when tested by repeated subcutaneous injection (Grasso et al. 1966).

Some work was done at the British Industrial Biological Research Association (BIBRA) to throw more light on this problem. It was quickly realized that some of the triphenylmethane, xanthene or azo-colourings which induced sarcoma were closely related in structure to those which did not do so. Careful study of the tissue reaction produced at the site of repeated injection revealed that those substances which did not induce sarcoma produced a self-limiting reaction, while

Table 1. Surface activity and sarcoma (from Gangolli et al. 1967)

Food colour	Surface activity	Amphipathy	Sarcoma
Blue VRS	+		+
Brilliant blue FCF	+		+
Patent blue V Na	+		+
Patent blue V CA			−
Amaranth		−	−
Eosine G	−	+	+
Rhodamine B	−	+	+

Table 2. Relationship between surface tension, type of reaction and
sarcoma production in rats (Grasso et al. 1971)

Lowering of surface tension (%)	Concentration[a] in water (%)	Dose (ml)	Type of reaction	Sarcoma[b] (%)
0	0		Mild	0
10	0.5		ND	ND
15	1.0	1.5	Mild	0
30	1.5		ND	ND
50	2.0	1.0	Severe and progressive	56
50	3.0	0.5	Severe and progressive	61

[a] Patent blue V sodium.
[b] Groups of 20 rats.

those that did induce sarcoma produced a progressive reaction in which sometimes macrophages predominated.

The pathology induced locally not only correlated with the production of tumours, but also with the surface activity or amphipathy of the compound
(Table 1; Gangolli et al. 1967). It was subsequently demonstrated that, when a
surface active food colouring (Patent Blue V), was administered in three concentrations and the dose/volume adjusted to keep the amount by weight constant,
sarcomas only developed at those concentrations which exhibited, a high surface
activity (Table 2; Grasso et al. 1971).

These results indicate that great care has to be exercised in interpreting results
of sarcoma production at the site of repeated injection, since compounds which
are without any activity when given by some other route may well produce positive results by this route if given in concentrated solutions. Such results bear little
relevance for substances that normally would be ingested or inhaled by man.

Urothelial Hyperplasia and Cancer

The examples given so far were derived from studies of connective tissue tumours,
but examples of pathological mechanisms involving hyperplasia and tumour formation exist in epithelial tissues as well. The first evidence of the existence of this
mechanism came from a study by Weil et al. (1965) following the finding of bladder tumours in rats treated with diethylene glycol – a most unexpected event.
Along with the transitional cell carcinomas there were several bladder stones.
Weil showed that if the stones were washed and cleaned and then implanted in
young rats, urothelial carcinomas developed in the recipient rats. This experiment
was followed by studies from other authors which showed that foreign bodies implanted in the bladder of rats and mice developed urothelial carcinoma (Table 3;
Clayson 1974), but the best illustration of the importance of hyperplasia in tumour production is afforded by the experiment of Flaks et al. (1973) with 4-eth-

Table 3. Tumour induction in mouse blader by foreign bodies

Substance	Tumour incidence (%)	
	Papilloma	Carcinoma
Paraffin wax[a]	5.4	3.6
Paraffin wax[b]	1.2	3.6
Cholesterol[b]	1.8	9.1
Palmitic acid		14.0
Hexamethylbenzene[b]		11.0
Arachid acid[b]		15.0
Glass beads	1.5	1.5
Calcium oxalate stone[c]		3.0

From Clayson (1974):
[a] Pellets after heating to 80° C.
[b] Powdered and compressed in tablet machine.
From Weil et al. (1959).
[c] Formed during dietary treatment with diethylene glycol rat experiment.

Table 4. Bladder carcinoma in mice

Treatment	Concentration (%)	Bladder pathology		
		Tumours	Stones	Epithelial hyperplasia
ENS	0.01	7	13	18[a]
NHCl	1.0	–	–	–
ENS + NHCl	–	–	–	22[b]
None	–	–	–	–

Groups of 26 female mice. ENS, 4-Ethylsulphonylnaphthalene-1-sulphonamide.
[a] Marked.
[b] Mild.

ylsulphonylnaphthalene-1 sulphonamide. This compound produced a high incidence of bladder tumours when it was first used as an experimental model and was hailed as a model compound for the study of human bladder cancer. But it was noticed that the rats voided a copious amount of an alkaline urine which contained a considerable number of crystals. Stone formation was also noted in the bladder. Acidification of the urine caused crystals, stones and tumours to disappear (Table 4).

These results have a number of implications in attempting to assess hazard for man, but the principal message is that chronic bladder pathology involving prolonged episodes of hyperplasia is an important confounding factor in assessing the carcinogenic potential of a chemical and care should be taken to understand the extent to which it has contributed to the development of the vesical tumours before coming to any conclusion on risk for man.

Considerations of this sort may well have saved a considerable amount of unnecessary anxiety to those who are constrained to take saccharin which for a time was suspected to carry a substantial carcinogenic risk for man (Grasso 1984).

Induction of tumours in the liver or in endocrine glands are two other areas where a consideration of pathological findings might assist in assessing hazard to man.

Liver Growth and Cancer Development

Episodes of cell necrosis in the liver lead first to nodular hyperplasia and then to cancer. This process is exemplified by CC14 and CH3Cl, but no doubt it applies to other compounds as well (ECETOC 1982).

However, there are numerous compounds which produce liver tumours without any of the classical signs of pathological damage observed histologically in conventionally stained sections. This class of compounds possesses two main characteristics – they are nongenotoxic (as the term is interpreted generally) and they produce liver growth (Schulte-Hermann 1974). The relationship of liver growth to the development of tumours has not been investigated in depth, but there are two pieces of evidence which suggest that some link may exist between liver growth and hepatocellular carcinoma. In a carcinogenicity study with four isomers of benzenehexachloride, only the isomer which produced the greatest degree of liver enlargement led to the induction of liver tumours (Table 5), the degree of enzyme induction did not appear to have the same significance. Secondly, as Table 6 shows, the minimum dose that produces tumours is much greater than the threshold dose for liver growth, suggesting that when substanial liver growth occurs the risk for developing hepatic tumours is very high indeed.

There is, at the moment, no clear relationship between the severity of liver enlargement and tumour development, but in general it would seem that when the liver weight is approximately 50% higher than the control values the probability of cancer development in the liver is considerable.

Many of the compounds that induce liver enlargement also induce profound biochemical and ultrastructural changes in this organ. They involve changes in

Table 5. Liver enlargement, enzyme induction and liver cancer in rats treated with hexachlorocyclohexane (HCH) isomers

Isomer	% of controls		
	LE	AP demethylase[a]	Cancer[b]
B-HCH	40	30	– ve
d-HCH	30	30	NT
a-HCH	100	30	+ ve
g-HCH	20	100	– ve

[a] Aminopyrene demethylase, from Schulte-Hermann (1974).
[b] From IARC (1979).

Table 6. Liver enlargement and cancer production

Compound	Species	Threshold dose[a] for LE[c]	Lowest effective dose for cancer production
Phenobarbital	Mouse	30 mg/kg/bw	70 mg/kg/bw[b]
a-HCH	Rat	10 ppm	1500 ppm[c]
DDT	Rat	128 ppm	?800 ppm[d]
BHT	Rat	75 mg/kg/bw	250 mg/kg/bw[e]

LE, liver enlargement.
[a] Oral; from Schulte Hermann (1974).
[b] IARC (1977).
[c] IARC (1979).
[d] IARC (1974).
[e] Olsen et al. (1985).

the activity of a variety of enzymes as well as an increase in lysosomes, mitochondria, smooth and rough ER, and peroxisomes. But perhaps the most important cellular changes in the hepatocytes are an increased mitotic activity and an increase in ploidy (Schulte-Hermann 1974; ECETOC 1982). Although mitosis is usually confined to the early stage of liver enlargement (3–4 days), the increase in ploidy appears to be gradual and continuous so long as the compound is administered. It is now seemingly generally accepted that an increase in cell ploidy is the equivalent of hyperplasia (Brodsky and Uryvaeva 1977), so that in liver enlargement there would appear to be a prolonged process of hyperplasia analogous perhaps to that observed in the subcutaneous tissue and the bladder. Here again the mechanism of cancer induction would appear to involve a pathological process involving DNA replication at a higher rate than the normal one.

Endocrine Overactivity and Tumours

The other area which deserves to be mentioned because it illustrates so clearly the importance of pathological changes developing through a disturbance of the homoeostatic mechanism is tumour production by hormonal imbalance. The role of hormones in tumour production has been suspected for several years in human pathology and has been extensively investigated in animals in order to understand better the human disease. Several years ago Lacassagne (1956) showed that natural or synthetic oestrogens increased the natural incidence of mammary tumours in mice when administered at very high doses. It is known that when serum prolactin is increased either by drugs or secondary to a neoplastic disease of the pituitary, the incidence of these tumours in both mice and rats increases considerably (Welsch et al. 1977). Studies of the mammary tissue in both rats and mice revealed that long before tumours appear, the mammary glands undergo hyperplasia which gradually progresses until tumours appear (Foulds 1975). Other endocrine organs are also affected by drugs. The best-known example of these are the thyroid tumours which result from the administration of thiourea and

Table 7. Fatty acids and stomach tumours in rats

Acid	Number of C atoms	Pappilomatous Growths	Hyperplasia	Carcinoma
Propionic	3	+	+	+[a]
Butyric	4	+	+	
Valeric	5	+	+	
Capronic	6	−	−	
Capric	11	−	−	
Lauric	12	−	−	
Palmitic	16	−	−	

Mixed with diet up to 10%; fed for 150 days (Mori 1953).
[a] Mixed with diet up to 4%; fed for 2 years (Griem 1986).

thiouracil (Purves et al. 1947). These chemicals suppress thyroxine production. The resulting absence of feedback on the pituitary increases the level of circulating TSH. In turn this results in thyroid hyperplasia and eventually tumours.

Other examples exist which appear to support the observation that repeated tissue damage may lead to tumours. The most recent of these is the production of forestomach tumours in the rat, with the unexpected production of such tumours by butylated hydroxyanisole (BHA; Ito et al. 1983) and the subsequent demonstration of a marked hyperplastic reaction when the compound was given in the feed for a few days. But this is not the only compound that has given rise to tumours of this sort. Propionic acid was recently reported to produce similar tumours when given in the feed to rats (Griem 1985). As Table 7 indicates, propionic acid is known to produce hyperplasia in the rat stomach and apparently is not the only compound of this sort to produce this kind of change (Mori 1953). Judging from the data so far, butyric and valeric acid will also produce tumours if administered in the same way as propionic acid, since they also produce marked hyperplasia.

Thus, there would appear to be substantial evidence that prolonged tissue damage could be a major component in the induction of tumours of both the connective and epithelial tissues. Whether initiated cells are a prerequisite for tumours to appear in the presence of such tissue damage is not known for certain and it is a concept which certainly cannot be dismissed. But perhaps these cells would never have had the chance to develop into tumours if they were not involved in the reactive response to injury.

One does not wish to dismiss the mechanism of chronic injury in the production of cancer as irrelevant for man since chronic injury may lead to tumour production in man as it does in animals. For example, the lesions of lupus vulgaris, lupus erythematosus and chronic ulcers (varicose or tropical) are known to be associated with a high risk for the development of squamous cell carcinoma, while cirrhosis has long been associated with the development of hepatocellular carcinoma. Nevertheless, it is perhaps possible to arrive at some rational assessment of a safe level of use for those nongenotoxic compounds in which hyperplasia due to chronic injury can be demonstrably shown to be a major factor in the production of cancer. At a dose level which does not produce a reactive lesion, no tumours are likely to develop. Such an assessment at the moment is not possible for genotoxic carcinogens.

References

Bischoff F, Bryson G (1964) Carcinogenesis through solid state surfaces. Prog Exp Tumot Res 5:85

Boyland E (1958) The biological examination of carcinogenic substances. Br Med Bull 14:93–96

Brand KG, Johnson KH, Buoen LC (1976) Foreign body tumorigenesis. CRC Crit Rev Toxicol 4:353–394

Brodsky WY, Uryvaeva IV (1977) Cell polyploidy: its relation to tissue growth and function. Int Rev Cytol 50:275–332

Clayson DB (1974) Bladder carcinogenesis in rats and mice. Possibility of artefact. JNCI 52:1685–1689

ECETOC (1982) Hepatocarcinogenesis in laboratory rodents: relevance for man. European Chemical Industry Ecology and Toxicology Centre, p 21

Flaks A, Hamilton JM, Clayson DB (1973) Effect of ammonium chloride on incidence of bladder tumours induced by 4-ethylsulphonylnaphthalene-1-sulfonamide. JNCI 51:2007–2008

Foulds L (1975) Neoplastic development vol 2. Academic, London, chap 9

Gangolli SD, Grasso P, Golberg L (1976) Physical factors determining the early local tissue rections produced by food colourings and other compounds injected subcutaneously. Fd Cosmet Toxicol 5:601–621

Golberg L (1963) Die Wirkung von Eiseninjektionen im Tierversuch. Arzneimittelforsch 13:939–947

Grasso P (1984) Carcinogens in food. In: Serle CE (ed) Chemical carcinogens, vol 2, 2nd edn. American Chemical Society, Washington, p 1205 (ACS monograph 182)

Grasso P, Gangolli SD, Golberg L, Hooson J (1971) Physicochemical and other factors determining local sarcoma production by food additives. Fd Cosmet Toxicol 9:463–475

Grasso P, Golberg L (1966) Subcutaneous sarcoma as an index of carcinogenic potency. Fd Cosmet Toxicol 4:297–320

Griem W von (1985) Tumorigene Wirkung von Propionsäure an der Vormagenschleimhaut von Ratten im Fütterungsversuch. Bundesgesundheitsblatt 28:322–327

IARC (1974) Some organochlorine pesticides.IARC Monogr Eval Carcinog Risk Chem Hum 5:83–124

IARC (1977) Some miscellaneous pharmaceutical substances. IARC Monogr Eval Carcinog Risk Chem Hum 13:157–183

IARC (1979) Some halogenated hydrocarbons. IARC Monogr Eval Carcinog Risk Chem Hum 20:195–239

Ito N, Fukushima S, Hagiwara H, Shibata M, Ogiso T (1983) Carcinogenicity of butylated hydroxyanisole in F344 rats. JNCI 70:343–352

Lacassagne A (1936) A comparative study of the carcinogenic action of certain estrogenic hormones. Am J Cancer 28:735–740

Mori K (1953) Production of gastric lesions in the rat by the diet containing fatty acids. Gann 44:421–426

Olsen P, Bille N, Meyer O (1983) Hepatocellular neoplasms in rats induced by butylated hydroxytoluene. Acta Pharmacol Toxicol 53:433–434

Oppenheimer BS, Oppenheimer ET, Stout AP (1953) Carcinogenic effect of imbedding various plastic films in rat and mice. Surg Forum 4:672–678

Purves HD, Griesbach WE (1947) Studies on experimental goitre. VIII. Thyroid tumours in rats treated with thiourea. Br J Exp Path 28:46–53

Schulte-Hermann R (1974) Induction of liver growth by xenobiotic and other stimuli. CRC Crit Rev Toxicol 3:97 158

Swinburne J (1950) The mechanism of the watch. NAG Press, London

Weil CS, Carpenter CP, Smyth HF (1965) Urinary bladder response to diethylene glycol. Calculi and tumours following repeated feeding and implants. Arch Environ Health 11:569–581

Welsch CW, Nagasawa H (1977) Prolactin and murine mammary tumorigenesis: a review. Cancer Res 37:951–963

Mechanisms and Models in Toxicology
Arch. Toxicol., Suppl. 11, 84–88 (1987)
© by Springer-Verlag 1987

Sensitivity of DNA and Nucleotides to Oxidation by Permanganate and Hydrogen Peroxide

P. Sagelsdorff and W. K. Lutz

Institute of Toxicology, ETH and University of Zürich, CH-8603 Schwerzenbach, Switzerland

Introduction

For a number of cytotoxic and tumorigenic agents, active oxygen species such as hydroxyl radical are postulated to be responsible for indirect DNA damage (Cerutti 1981). Besides the formation of strand breaks, hydroxylation of DNA bases is assumed to occur, as shown earlier with ionizing radiation. It was the aim of this work to determine in vitro the DNA-damaging potency of hydrogen peroxide (H_2O_2), and to compare that with the potency of the strong oxidant permanganate ion.

Materials and Methods

Chemicals

Chemicals were obtained from Merck (Darmstadt, FRG) or Fluka (Buchs, Switzerland) and were of analytical grade. Nucleotides and calf thymus DNA were from Sigma (St. Louis, Mo., USA); [^{14}C]thymidine from the Radiochemical Center (Amersham, Buckinghamshire, GB).

Oxidation of Nucleotides and DNA

Oxidation with $KMnO_4$ was performed at 0 °C as described by Frenkel et al. (1981). The H_2O_2 reaction was carried out in 0.2 M sodium phosphate, pH 7.8, at 37 °C with 25 µM $FeCl_3$. Single-stranded DNA was obtained by heat denaturation of double-stranded calf thymus DNA followed by rapid cooling at -30 °C. The concentration of the oxidant is given in Table 1 and Figs. 1 and 2.

Isolation of Oxidized DNA

The reaction mixture was dialysed; DNA was precipitated with ethanol and stored at -20 °C overnight. The DNA was centrifuged for 20 min at 1000 g,

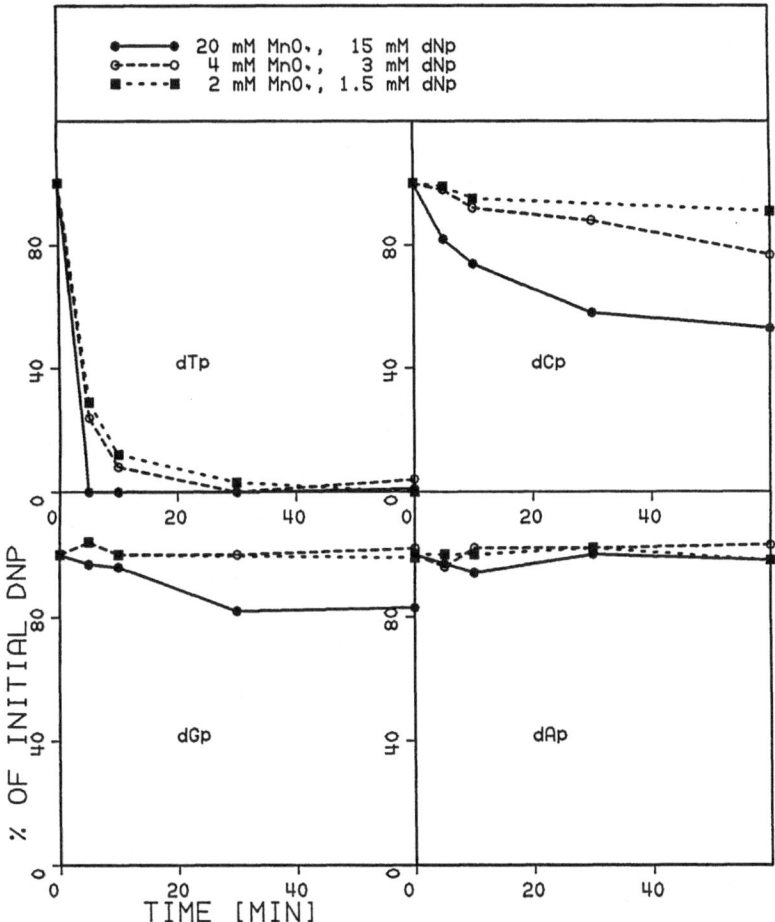

Fig. 1. Sensitivity of deoxyribonucleotides towards oxidation with $KMnO_4$ at 0 °C for various periods of time. *dTp*, thymidine monophosphate; *dCp*, deoxycytidine monophosphate; *dGp*, deoxyguanosine monophosphate; *dAp*, deoxyadenosine monophosphate

Table 1. Molar fraction and relative amount of nucleotides after oxidation for 48 h at 37° C of double-stranded DNA with H_2O_2. The least sensitive nucleotide dAp, was set to 100%. Oxidation of dAp cannot be excluded on the basis of these results.

dNp	Control		$1\,M\,H_2O_2$	
	Molar fraction	Relative amount (%)	Molar fraction	Relative amount (%)
dTp	0.22	100	0.24	62
dCp	0.28	100	0.14	46
dGp	0.28	100	0.24	78
dAp	0.22	100	0.39	100

dTp, thymidine monophosphate; dCp, deoxycytidine monophosphate; dGp, deoxyguanosine monophosphate; dAp, deoxyadenosine monophosphate

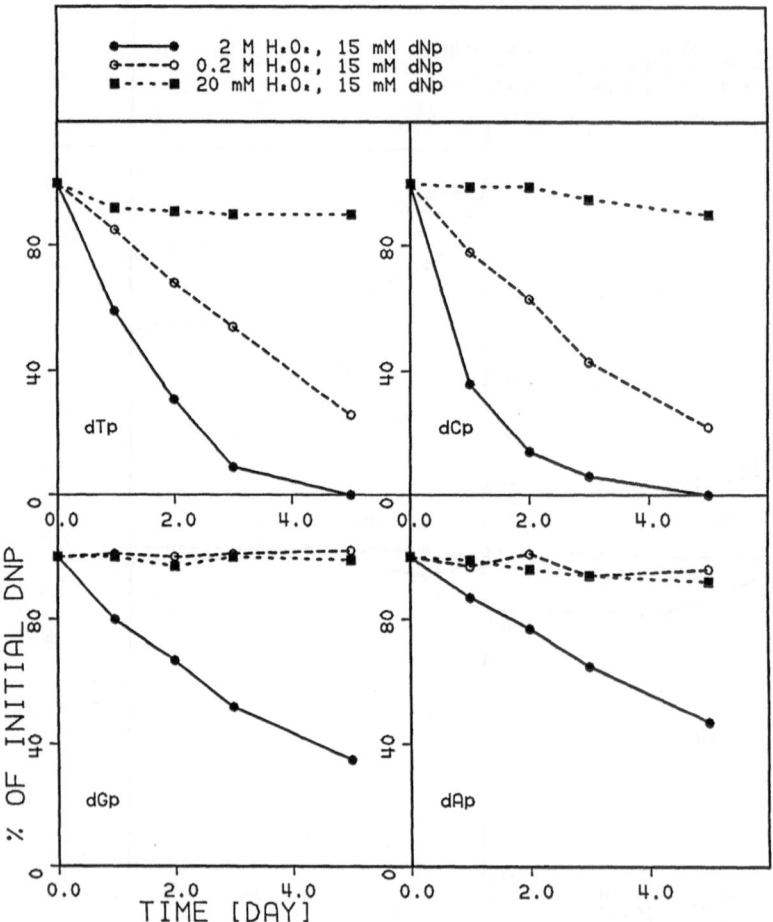

Fig. 2. Sensitivity of deoxyribonucleotides towards oxidation with H_2O_2 plus 25 µM Fe^{3+} at 37 °C for various periods of time. *dTp*, thymidine monophosphate; *dCp*, deoxycytidine monophosphate; *dGp*, deoxyguanosine monophosphate; *dAp*, deoxyadenosine monophosphate

dried in vacuo, and dissolved in 8 mM $CaCl_2$ and 20 mM sodium succinate, pH 6.0. Digestion to nucleotides was performed with 2.5 U micrococcal endonuclease (EC 3.1.31.1, Sigma) and 0.05 U spleen exonuclease (EC 3.1.16.1, Boehringer Mannheim, FRG; Rotkreuz, Switzerland) for 16 h at 37 °C.

Separation of Oxidation Products

The nucleotides were separated by HPLC on a Lichrosorb RP18 (7 µm) column (4.2 mm × 250 mm), eluting at a flow of 1.5 ml/min with 50 mM sodium phosphate buffer, pH 5.8, containing 3% methanol for 5 min, followed by a linear gradient to 20% methanol in 10 min.

Isolation of Thymidine Glycol

The reaction products of the oxidation of [^{14}C]thymidine were separated on a Lichrosorb RP18 (7 μm) column (4.2 mm × 250 mm), eluting at a flow of 0.75 ml/min with 1% aqueous methanol for 15 min, followed by a linear gradient to 100% methanol in 5 min.

GC/MS Analysis

The reaction products were silylated in 0.2 ml pyridine with 0.5 ml N,O-bis-(trimethylsilyl)trifluoroacetamide for 30 min at 150 °C. Pyridine was blown off with nitrogen and the residue dissolved in hexane; 1 μl was injected on a capillary column (19 m × 0.32 mm), coated with SE-54 (film thickness, 0.10 μm). Elution was at 60 kPa He, at a temperature of 60 °C for 2 min, followed by a gradient of 10 °C/min.

Results

Sensitivity of Nucleotides

Figs. 1 and 2 show that the pyrimidines (top) were more sensitive than the purines (bottom), both with $KMnO_4$ (Fig. 1) and H_2O_2 (Fig. 2). After 20 min incubation with 20 mM $KMnO_4$, a reduction of the optical density to 10% and 80% was observed for thymidine monophosphate and cytidine monophosphate, respectively, whereas no reduction was detectable for the purines. With 20 mM H_2O_2, no effect was detectable at all. Only after 2 days of incubation with 0.2 M H_2O_2 was a reduction to 70% and 60% observed for thymidine monophosphate and cytidine monophosphate, respectively. No oxidation of the purines was detectable at this H_2O_2 concentration.

Oxidation Products of Thymidine

Oxidation of [^{14}C]thymidine with 20 mM $KMnO_4$ yielded only one product, which was identified by mass spectrometry as thymidine glycol. With 2 M H_2O_2, at least three different products could be detected. Thymidine-5,6-glycol represented about 30% of the products. Fragmentation by mass spectrometry of another product was compatible with 5-hydroxy-5-methyl-hydantoin deoxyriboside. This compound has been postulated by Teoule and Cadet (1971) as a possible product of thymidine irradiation.

Sensitivity of DNA

Single-stranded (ss) and double-stranded (ds) DNA was oxidized with H_2O_2 and the loss of optical density at 254 nm was taken as a measure of the damage. It was shown that single-stranded DNA was more sensitive to oxidation than double-stranded DNA. Incubation with 2 M H_2O_2 resulted in a time-dependent decrease of optical density. After 2 days with 2 M H_2O_2, the optical density was reduced to 30% and 70% for ssDNA and dsDNA, respectively. The sensitivity of the four nucleotides in intact DNA was dCp > dTp > dGp > dAp, i.e., the same ranking as found with isolated nucleotides (Table 1). The yield of high-molecular, oxidized DNA decreased with increasing concentration of H_2O_2. Under the present incubation conditions, only 30% of the DNA could be retained during dialysis. The loss is thought to be due to strand breaks.

Discussion

Thymine was not the most sensitive target base for an oxidation by hydroxyl radical in this in vitro system. A quantification of thymidine glycol must therefore lead to an underestimation of the DNA damage mediated by the hydroxyl radical. H_2O_2 was found to be an astonishingly mild DNA oxidizing agent in vitro and it is questionable whether, in vivo, base hydroxylations occur to a relevant extent. The hypothesis of an oxidative stress as one possible genotoxic process in carcinogenesis must be carefully examined and the relative importance of strand breaks and DNA hydroxylations has to be assessed in vivo.

Acknowledgement. This work was supported by the Swiss National Science Foundation (SNF Grant no. 3.626-0.84).

References

Cerutti PA (1981) Measurement of thymidine damage induced by oxygen radical species. In: Friedberg EC, Hanawalt PC (eds) DNA repair. Decker, New York, pp 57–68
Frenkel K, Goldstein MS, Duker NJ, Teebor GW (1981) Identification of the *cis*-thymine glycol moiety in oxidized deoxyribonucleic acid. Photochem Photobiol 4:963–969
Teoule R, Cadet J (1971) Radiolysis of thymidine in aerated aqueous solution. J Chem Soc Chem Commun 1971:1269–1270

Mechanisms and Models in Toxicology
Arch. Toxicol., Suppl. 11, 89–92 (1987)
© by Springer-Verlag 1987

A Postlabelling Assay for N^7-(2-Oxoethyl)Guanine, the Principal Vinyl Chloride-DNA Adduct

W. P. Watson, A. E. Crane, R. Davis, R. J. Smith, and A. S. Wright

Shell Research Ltd., Sittingbourne Research Centre, Sittingbourne, Kent, ME9 8AG, UK

Introduction

Human exposures to high concentrations of vinyl chloride (VC) have been associated with the occurrence of angiosarcoma of the liver (Maltoni et al. 1982; Creech and Johnson 1974; Spirtas and Kaminski 1978). A programme of studies in this laboratory is investigating the relationships between exposure to VC, the dose at critical cellular targets, e.g. DNA, and the carcinogenic response in experimental species, e.g. rat. A key aspect of this work has been the development of highly sensitive quantitative methods for measuring the DNA dose of vinyl chloride in target tissues.

Vinyl chloride is a precursor genotoxic agent which undergoes biotransformation in mammals to chlorooxirane, which rearranges to chloroacetaldehyde (Hopkins 1979; Gwinner et al. 1983). The products of reactions of these metabolites with DNA are believed to constitute the primary lesions responsible for the mutagenic and carcinogenic actions of vinyl chloride (Laib et al. 1981). The principal adduct occurring in the DNA of rats exposed to vinyl chloride is N^7-(2-oxoethyl)guanine (N^7-OEG; Laib et al. 1981).

The use of radiolabelled genotoxic agents greatly facilitates the determination of DNA adducts in experimental species. However 'cold' analytical procedures are also required in certain situations, e.g. in conventional carcinogenicity studies or human biomedical monitoring programmes. One possible approach for quantitating VC-DNA adducts is based on postradiolabelling techniques. This approach has been employed in the current study and the aim was to develop a quantitative assay for N^7-OEG with a sensitivity of 1 molecule of adduct per 10^7 nucleotide units: equivalent to the detection of about 1 picomole of adduct in a 5-mg sample of DNA.

Materials and Methods

[U-^{14}C]Guanosine and [1-^{14}C]acetic anhydride were obtained from Amersham International (UK). N^7-(2-Oxoethyl)[^{14}C]guanine was prepared from the reaction of [^{14}C]guanosine with 2,3-epoxy-1-propanol followed by acid hydrolysis, then periodate cleavage (Scherer et al. 1981; Roe et al. 1973; Piper et al. 1980). All solvents were of at least Analar grade.

DNA samples were spiked with a known trace amount of N^7-(2-oxoethyl)[^{14}C]-guanine (1.0 pmol, 555 dpm, specific radioactivity 250 mCi/mmol). The spiked DNA was then treated in aqueous solution with a large excess of sodium borohydride for 1 h at room temperature. The resulting mixture was neutralized with aqueous sodium dihydrogen phosphate and heated at 100 °C for 1 h to release N^7-(2-hydroxyethyl)guanine. The adducted base was purified by ultrafiltration through a 1000 dalton cut-off membrane filter (Amicon YM2) followed by HPLC. The purified product was then converted to its N-,O-diacetate by treatment (2 h at 110 °C) with a large excess of [^{14}C]acetic anhydride (specific radioactivity 120 mCi/mmol) in dry DMF. After purification to radiochemical purity using column-switching HPLC (1, Waters Sep-Pak ODS precolumn eluted with water; 2, Ultrasphere ODS eluted with methanol-water gradients; 3, Aquagel eluted with 50% methanol-water) the product was treated with n-propylamine for 8 h at 60 °C. N-Acetylpropylamine and N^7-(2-hydroxyethyl)guanine were then separated by HPLC (Ultrasphere ODS). Radioactivity in the N-acetylpropylamine fraction gave a measure of the total N^7-(2-oxyethyl)guanine in the sample

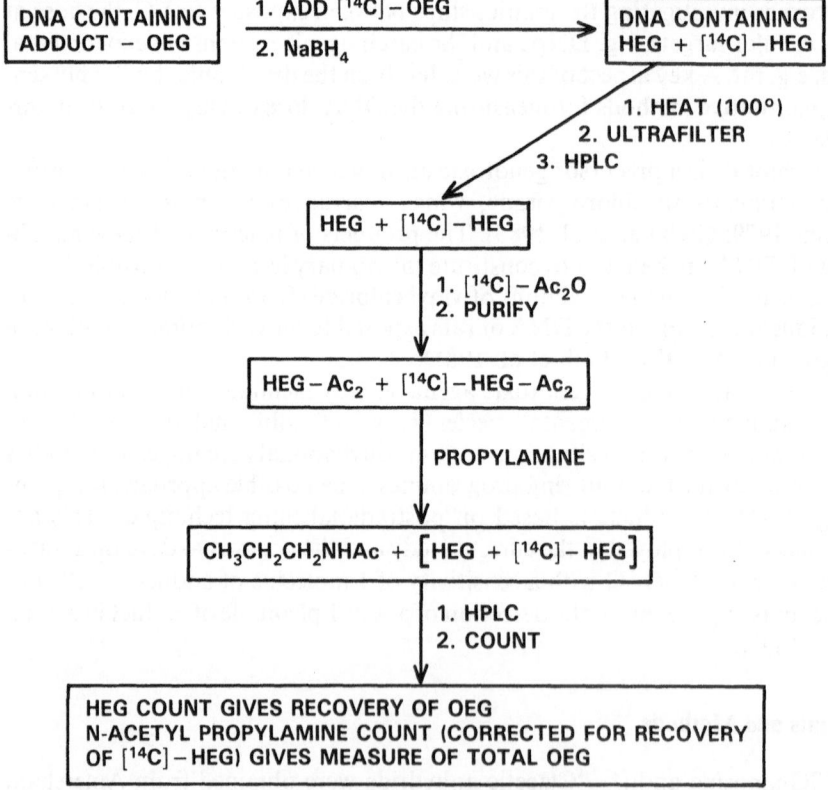

Fig. 1. Dual carbon-14 label approach for assay of N^7-(2-oxoethyl)guanine

and radioactivity in the N^7-(2-hydroxyethyl)guanine permitted correction for losses.

Results and Discussion

This strategy employing a radiolabel to quantitate unlabelled adducts and a radiolabelled 'spike' of the required adduct to determine recoveries offers a general approach for the quantitation of DNA adducts. Attempts to label N^7-(2-oxoethyl)guanine by reduction with sodium borotritiide gave variable results due to difficulties associated with tritium exchange and led to a design shown in Fig. 1, based on dual carbon-14 labels. The release of N^7-(2-oxoethyl)guanine from DNA by heating resulted in degradation and poor yields. The 2-oxoethyl group was, therefore, first reduced with sodium borohydride since the reduction product could be easily released from DNA by heating. The reduction proceeded in an essentially quantitative conversion. After purification by ultrafiltration and HPLC,

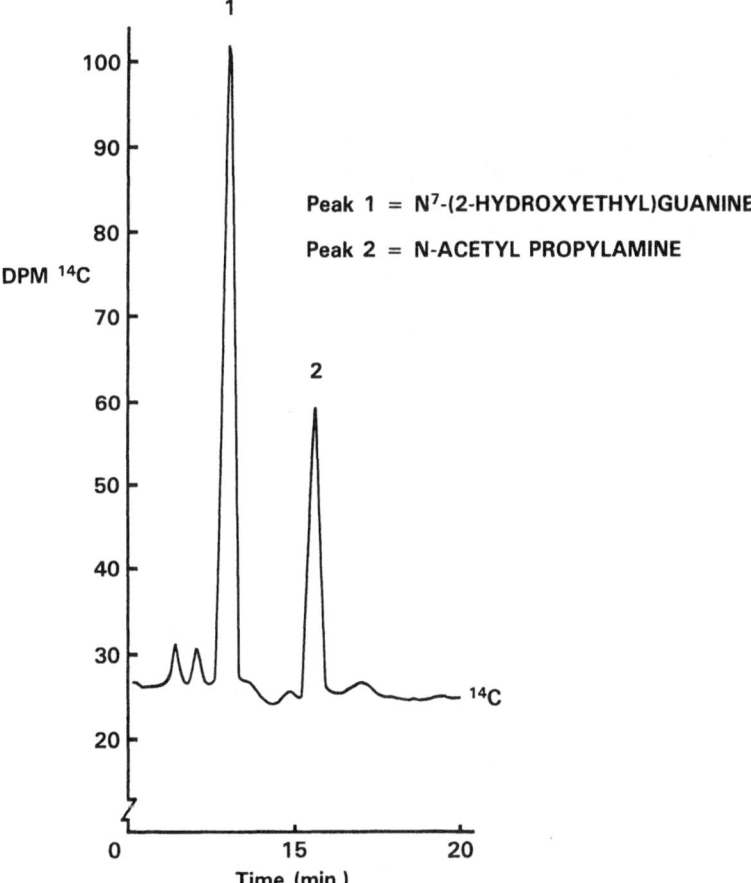

Fig. 2. HPLC (Ultrasphere ODS) separation of products from reaction of the diacetate of N^7-(2-hydroxyethyl)guanine with n-propylamine

Table 1. Postradiolabelling of standard samples of N^7-(2-hydroxyethyl)guanine

		1	2
Starting materials:			
N^7-(2-Hydroxyethyl)[^{14}C]guanine	pmol	2.86	2.0
	mCi/mmol	250	250
	dpm	1589	1110
[^{14}C]Ac$_2$O	μmol	3.3	2.2
	mCi/mmol	114	114
Products:			
N^7-(2-Hydroxyethyl)[^{14}C]guanine	dpm	119.4	142.8
[^{14}C]N-Ac. propylamine	dpm	59.9	73.8
Result:			
Calculated			
N^7-(2-Hydroxyethyl)[^{14}C]guanine		3.15	2.26

N^7(2-hydroxyethyl)guanine at the 2 pmol level could be converted to its N-,O-[^{14}C]diacetate in about 20% conversion using a large (10^6 molar) excess of [^{14}C]acetic anhydride. This derivitisation step and subsequent purification of the diacetate to radiochemical purity are both critical to the success of the assay. After purification of the product by column-switching HPLC, the labelled acetate groups were quantitatively removed by reaction with n-propylamine and the products separated by HPLC (Fig. 2). The ratio of radioactivity occurring in N^7-(2-hydroxyethyl)guanine and N-acetyl propylamine provided a measure of N^7-(2-oxoethyl)guanine in samples of DNA. Results for measurements on reference samples of N^7-(2-hydroxyethyl)guanine are shown in Table 1.

References

Creech JL, Johnson MN (1974) Angiosarcoma of liver in the manufacture of polyvinylchloride. J Occupational Med 16:150–151

Gwinner LM, Laib RJ, Filser JG, Bolt HM (1983) Evidence of chloroethylene oxide being the reactive metabolite of vinyl chloride towards DNA: comparative studies with 2,2'-dichlorodiethyl ether. Carcinogenesis 4:1483–1486

Hopkins J (1979) Vinyl chloride – Part 1: Metabolism. Fd Cosmet Toxicol 17:403–412

Laib RJ, Gwinner LM, Bolt HM (1981) DNA alkylation by vinyl chloride metabolites: etheno derivatives or 7-alkylation of guanine? Chem-Biol Interact 37:219–231

Maltoni C, Lefemine G, Ciliberti A, Cotti G, Caretti D (1982) Vinyl chloride: a model carcinogen for risk assessment. Environ Sci Research 25:329–344

Piper JR, Laseter AG, Montgomery JA (1980) Synthesis of potential inhibitors of hypoxanthine-guanine phosphoribosyltransferase for testing as antiprotozoal agents. 1. 7-Substituted 6-oxopurines. J Med Chem 23:357–364

Scherer E, Van Der Laken CJ, Gwinner LM, Laib RJ, Emmelot P (1981) Modification of deoxyguanosine by chloroethylene oxide. Carcinogenesis 2:671–677

Spirtas R, Kaminski R (1978) Angiosarcoma of the liver in vinyl chloride/polyvinylchloride workers. J Occup Med 20:427–429

Roe R, Paul JS, Montgomery PO'B (1973) Synthesis and PMR Spectra of 7-hydroxyalkylguanosinium acetates. J Heterocycl Chem 10:849–857

Mechanisms and Models in Toxicology
Arch. Toxicol., Suppl. 11, 93–98 (1987)
© by Springer-Verlag 1987

Comparison of Hydrocarbon – DNA Adducts Formed in Mouse and Human Skin Following Treatment with Benzo [A] Pyrene

W. P. Watson, R. J. Smith, K. R. Huckle, and A. S. Wright

Shell Research Ltd., Sittingbourne Research Centre, Sittingbourne, Kent, ME9 8AG, UK

Introduction

The assessment of human risk associated with exposure to carcinogens is often based on the use of experimental model systems. However, possible qualitative differences may exist between the bioactivation of carcinogens in man and experimental species employed as prospective risk models (Gori 1980; Wright 1980, 1981, 1983). By studying the interactions between DNA and metabolites of precursor carcinogens, the investigation of qualitative and, possibly, quantitative species differences in the metabolism of such genotoxic agents is possible. Valid comparisons of metabolism in risk models and man are particularly important where alternative bioactivation pathways are possible, e.g. polycyclic aromatic hydrocarbons. In certain instances there are difficulties in discriminating between genotoxic and nongenotoxic metabolites. Qualitative analyses of chromatographic profiles of DNA adducts formed by reaction of the ultimate genotoxic metabolites with DNA provide an approach to this problem. This approach effectively dispenses with aspects of metabolism that have no bearing on genotoxicity and therefore provides a selective procedure for the detection of qualitative differences between species and strains in the metabolic activation of precursor genotoxic agents. Direct comparative procedures may be readily applied in experimental species. With man, however, model in vitro preparations must be developed to qualitatively mimic human metabolism in vivo. The validation of such human systems is clearly not amenable to direct experimentation. However, validation may be indirectly accomplished by demonstrating that the profiles of DNA adducts generated using analogous preparations of tissues from experimental species are qualitatively identical with those generated in these species in vivo.

Materials and Methods

[G-^{3}H]Benzo(a)pyrene (BP; specific radioactivity 20 Ci/mmol) and [7,10-^{14}C]-benzo[a]pyrene (specific radioactivity 58.5 mCi/mmol) were purchased from

Amersham International (UK). Tritiated BP was diluted with nonradioactive BP (Sigma Chemical) to a specific radioactivity of 1.26 Ci/mmol; ^{14}C-labelled BP was used directly. Female CD1 mice aged 8–9 weeks were bred at Shell Research, in Sittingbourne.

Mice (10 per group) received an initiating dose of [^{14}C]- or [^{3}H]-benzo[a]pyrene (17 µg/cm^2) in acetone. Animals were killed after 24 h and the skin DNA (epidermal and dermal) was isolated and purified. Explants of freshly excised mouse dorsal skin were prepared and maintained in short-term organ culture, as described previously (Huckle et al. 1986). Analogous explants of human skin were prepared from a mastectomy patient. Skin explants were treated with [^{3}H]-BP in acetone, then incubated at 37 °C. Removal of the epidermis from skin samples was performed as described by Mars and Voorhees (1971). DNA was isolated and purified by phenol extraction followed by hydroxylapatite chromatography (Adriaenssens et al. 1982). The modified DNA was enzymically hydrolysed to nucleosides (Baird and Brookes 1973) and adducts were then bulk separated on Sephadex LH20 followed by analysis on reverse-phase HPLC (5 µm, 25 × 0.46 cm, Ultrasphere ODS) using methanol-water gradients (three-step programme: 0.7 ml/min, linear gradient 40%–50% methanol over 60 min; isocratic for 30 min followed by linear gradient to 75% methanol over 25 min). The assignments for BP-DNA adducts were based on cochromatography with authentic standards and comparison with literature data (see Huckle et al. 1986 and references therein).

Results and Discussion

The profiles of DNA adducts obtained after treatment of mouse skin in vivo, mouse skin explants in vitro or human skin explants in vitro were all qualitatively very similar. A reference profile of BP-DNA adducts from mice treated in vivo with [^{14}C]-BP is shown in Fig. 1. In each case the principal adduct was the N^2-deoxyguanosine adduct derived from (+)-7R,8S-dihydroxy-9R,10R-epoxy-7,8,9,10-tetrahydrobenzo[a]pyrene [anti-BPDE]. The ratios of different adducts in the in vivo and in vitro situation also showed a close similarly. In particular, the ratios of products derived from anti and syn isomers of BPDE, peaks D and E (Fig. 2), respectively, were similar in both the in vivo and in vitro experiments. Moreover, on a quantitative basis, the formation of BP-DNA in mouse skin in culture was approximately 50% of that occurring in vivo. The short-term mouse skin culture system is thus an acceptable model for BP metabolism in vivo. This suggests that the human explant system also provides an accurate model for BP metabolism in vivo.

Qualitative and quantitative comparisons of BP-DNA adducts from mice treated in vivo with either [^{14}C]- or [^{3}H]-BP showed excellent agreement, thus providing a sound reference for the in vivo situation. In the mouse studies the amount of radioactivity incorporated into DNA adducts was between five and ten times higher in the epidermis than the dermis. However, the qualitative profile of adducts was the same in mouse epidermis and dermis.

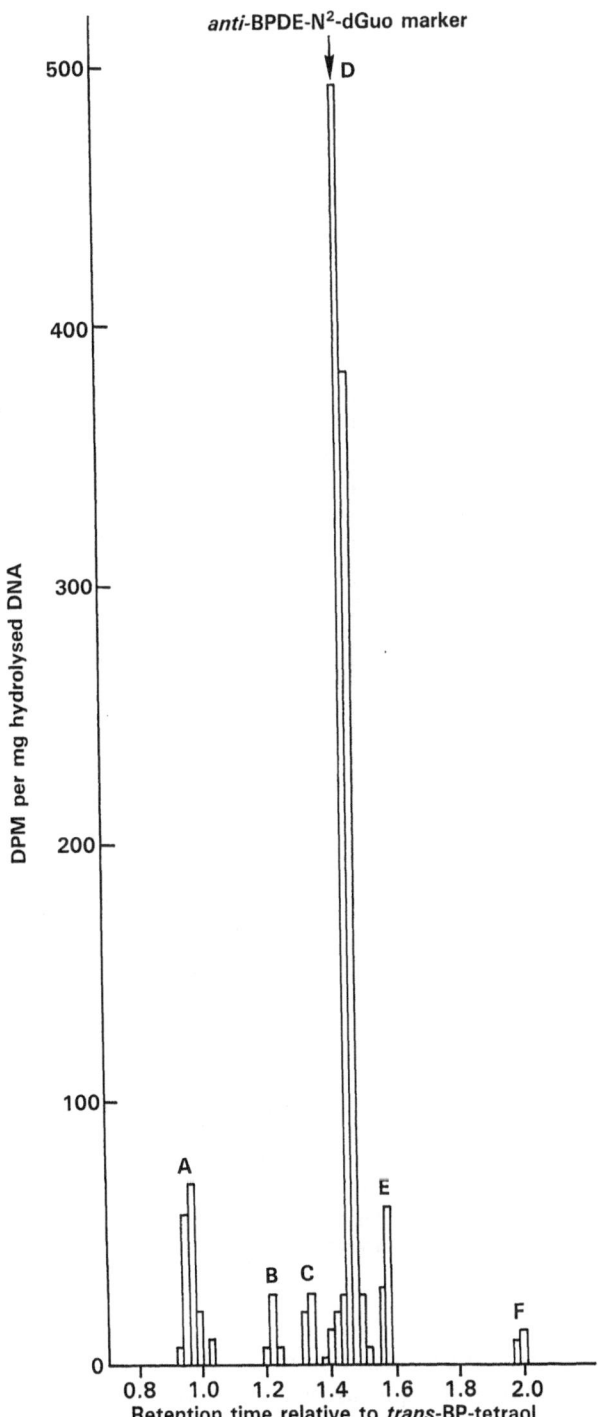

Fig. 1. Profile of [^{14}C]-BP-deoxyribunucleoside adducts obtained from epidermis of CD1 mice treated in vivo with [^{14}C]-BP

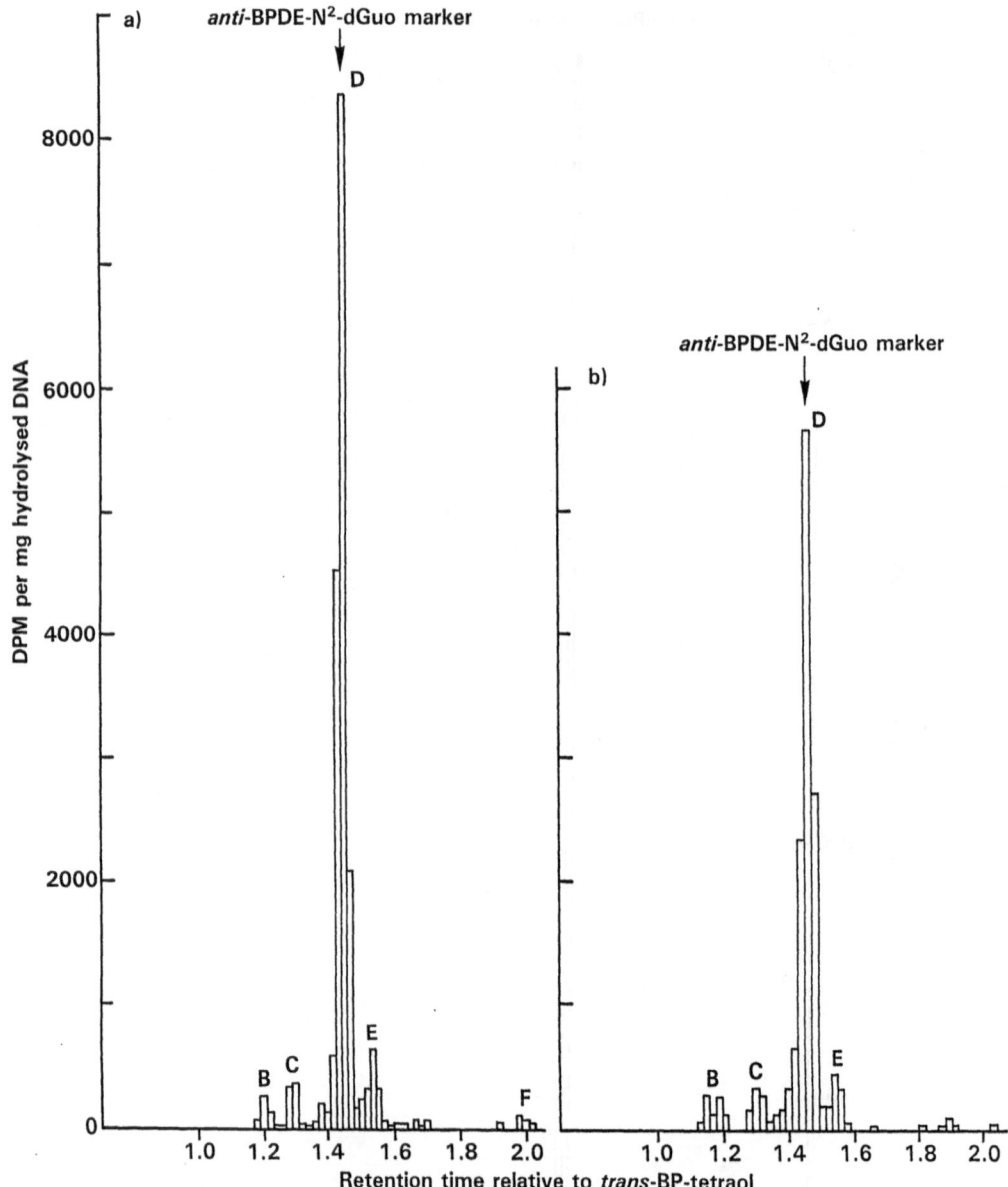

Fig. 2. Profile of [³H]-BP-deoxyribonucleoside adducts obtained from epidermal DNA of (**a**) CD1 mice treated in vivo (**b**) CD1 mouse skin explant treated in vitro

Concluding Remarks

This study has shown that with careful consideration of conditions for maintenance of explanted skin, organ culture techniques are valid models for in vivo metabolism. These techniques have been readily transferred to human skin (Fig. 3) and provide a valid model for the determination of the metabolism of carcinogens in human tissue in vivo.

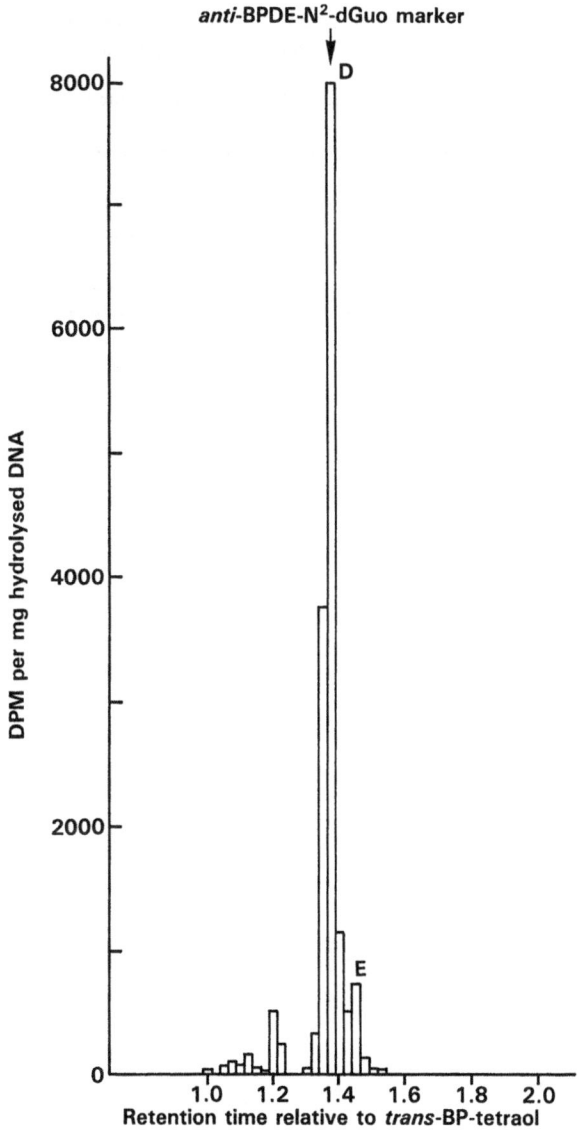

Fig. 3. Profile of [^{3}H]-BP deoxyribonucleoside adducts obtained from epidermal DNA of human skin explant treated in vitro with [^{3}H]-BP

References

Adriaenssens PI, Bixler CJ, Anderson MW (1982) Isolation and quantitation of DNA-bound benzo[a] pyrene metabolites: comparison of hydroxylapatite and precipitation procedures. Anal Biochem 123:162–169

Baird MW, Brookes P (1973) Isolation of the hydrocarbon-deoxyribonucleoside products from the DNA of mouse embryo cells treated in culture with 7-methylbenzo[a]anthracene-^{3}H. Cancer Res 33:2378–2385

Gori GB (1980) The regulation of carcinogenic hazards. Science 208:256–261

Huckle KR, Smith RJ, Watson WP, Wright AS (1986) Comparison of hydrocarbon-DNA adducts formed in mouse skin in vivo and in organ culture after treatment with benzo[a]pyrene. Carcinogenesis 7:965–970

Marrs JM, Voorhees JJ (1971) A method for bioassay of an epidermal chalone-like inhibitor. J Invest Dermatol 56:174–181

Wright AS (1980) The role of metabolism in chemical mutagenesis and chemical carcinogenesis. Mutat Res 75:215–241

Wright AS (1981) New strategies in biochemical studies for pesticide toxicity. In: Bandal SK, Marco GJ, Golberg L, Leng L (eds) The pesticide chemist and modern toxicology. American Chemical Society, Washington, p 285 (ACS Symposium No. 160)

Wright AS (1983) Molecular dosimetry techniques in human risk assessment: an industrial perspective. In: Hayes AW, Schnell RC, Miya TS (eds) Developments in the science and practice of toxicology. Elsevier, Amsterdam, p 311

Mechanisms and Models in Toxicology
Arch. Toxicol., Suppl. 11, 99–101 (1987)

Combined Radiolabelling Distribution and Covalent DNA-Binding Studies to Discriminate Between a Carcinogen/Noncarcinogen Pair of Monoazo Dyes Related to the Hepatocarcinogen Butter Yellow (DAB)

R. H. Dashwood [1], R. D. Combes [1] and J. Ashby [2]

[1] Department of Biological Sciences, Portsmouth Polytechnic, Portsmouth, Hants, UK
[2] ICI Central Toxicology Laboratory, Macclesfield, Cheshire, UK

Introduction

6BT 6-(p-dimethylaminophenylazo)benzothiazole and 5I 5-(p-dimethylamino-phenylazo)indazole) are a pair of mutagenic monoazo dyes related to the hepato-carcinogen butter yellow (DAB). 6BT is an exceptionally potent hepatocarci-nogen (Elliott et al. 1983) and initiates unscheduled DNA synthesis (UDS) in rat liver in vivo (Ashby et al. 1985), while 5I is weakly active in the latter and is a reported noncarcinogen, although only under suboptimal conditions of bioassay (Brown and Fisher 1969). However, the major difference between 6BT and 5I re-garding carcinogenic/genotoxic potency is well established, as is the potent muta-genicity of *both* compounds in vitro (Ashby et al. 1982). In view of the aforemen-tioned database, DNA-binding studies in vitro and in vivo were suggested, to in-clude assays employing isolated intact hepatocytes.

Materials and Methods

Chemicals

^{14}C-Labelled 6BT and 5I were as described elsewhere (Dashwood et al. 1986). Collagenase (Type 1), calf thymus DNA (Type I), and NADPH were from Sigma; DNA grade hydroxylapatite (HAP) from BioRad; scintillation fluid (Op-tiphase MP) from Fisons; aroclor from ICI. All other chemicals (purest grade) were from BDH.

Isolation of Hepatocytes and Microsomes

Hepatocytes (91%–96% viability, $> 250 \times 10^6$ viable cells from the liver of a 200 g rat) were isolated using a two-step in situ perfusion technique, as described by Mitchell et al. (1984). Aroclor-induced rat liver microsomes were prepared as de-scribed in Walters and Combes (1983).

Incubations

In vitro concentrations of 6BT and 5I were chosen to reflect those levels detected in the liver after oral dosing. Thus, an in vivo equivalent dose was derived as follows: $\cong 2\%$ of the ^{14}C-label administered p.o. to rats (both compounds) was detected in the entire livers from which DNA was extracted (12 h and 24 h after dosing; Dashwood et al. 1986); this is equivalent to 10 µg 6BT or 5I per g liver. Converting this to 10 µg/ml liver yields $\cong 35$ µM (both compounds). This concentration was used in subsequent in vitro studies.

Results

From Table 1 it is seen that at the in vivo equivalent dose (a) the carcinogen is always covalently bound to DNA more effectively, and (b) a trend is evident from metabolism by liver cells in situ, through intact hepatocytes in vitro, to liver microsomes in vitro, since the binding ratios 6BT : 5I correspondingly decrease.

Discussion

In a recent publication, in vivo covalent DNA binding was presented in the form of covalent binding index (CBI; Dashwood et al. 1986). Since CBI is defined as a function of dose administered/kg animal (Lutz 1979), orally administered compounds, even of similar chemical structure, may be taken up from the gut to different extents and reach target organ(s) in significantly different concentrations. This is likely to affect the resulting CBI values. Concomitant observations of DNA binding and gross organ/tissue concentrations of chemical could improve the relationship between DNA binding and carcinogenicity for orally administered chemicals. The detection of similar levels of both 6BT and 5I in the liver facilitated comparison of DNA binding (Dashwood et al. 1986) and pointed to the importance of similar compound concentrations in DNA studies ex vivo. The in

Table 1. The covalent DNA binding of 6BT and 5I in various assay systems at the in vivo equivalent dose

	In vivo		In vitro		
	12 h	24 h	Hepatocyte DNA	Calf thymus DNA	
				Hepatocytes[b]	Microsomes[c]
6BT[a]	212 ±4.7	169 ±8.8	169±19.3	134±29.9	153
5I	3.2±0.6	8.1±4.9	33±14.0	10± 2.2	87
6BT:5I	66.3	20.9	5.1	13.4	1.8

[a] Compound bound in nmol/g DNA; mean±SD from ≥ 3 separate determinations, except for microsomes which were extrapolated from dose-response curves (data not presented). In vivo data are derived from covalent binding indices (CBIs) presented previously (Dashwood et al. 1986).
[b, c] Activation systems in calf thymus DNA studies.

vitro/in vivo divergence of 6BT and 5I is reflected in the DNA binding data. Thus, the ratio 6BT:5I is some 37-fold greater in vivo than occurs in vitro with microsomal activation. Since the carcinogen consistently binds to DNA more effectively at the in vivo equivalent dose, it would be predicted that, at the same dose as in the Ames test, 6BT would be the more mutagenic of the pair. The fact that this is not so (see below) raises the question of the correlation between DNA binding to *Salmonella* and expression of that binding as mutagenicity.

In recent studies it was found that, at the in vivo equivalent dose ($\cong 4$ µg/plate), 6BT bound at 69.2 ± 14.9 nmol/g DNA and gave 154 ± 2.5 revertants/plate, whereas 5I bound at 87.7 ± 21.6 nmol/g DNA and gave 336 ± 13.5 revertants/ plate (mean $\pm$ SD; three separate experiments). Expressed as per unit 5I/6BT bound/unit DNA, 5I is therefore 1.72 times more mutagenic at the in vivo equivalent dose. Thus, for this particular pair of compounds the correlation between DNA binding and mutagenicity in the Ames test is not good. This has significant implications for the efficacy of the *Salmonella* data for these compounds with respect to predicted carcinogenicity.

References

Ashby J, Lefevre PA, Styles J, Charlesworth J, Paton D (1982) Comparisons between carcinogenic potency and mutagenic potency to Salmonella in series of derivatives of 4-dimethylaminoazobenzene (DAB). Mutat Res 93:67–81

Ashby J, Lefevre PA, Burlinson B, Penman MG (1985) An assessment of the in vivo rat hepatocyte DNA-repair assay. Mutat Res 156:1–18

Brown EV, Fisher WM (1969) Carcinogenic activities of analogues of *p*-dimethylaminoazobenzene. IX. Activity of quinoxaline and indazole analogues. J Med Chem 12:1113–1114

Dashwood RH, Combes RD, Ashby J (1986) The disposition and in vivo covalent binding to liver DNA of the monoazo dyes 6-(*p*-dimethylaminophenylazo)benzothiazole (6BT) and 5-(*p*-dimethylaminophenylazo)indazole (5I) after administration to the rat. Carcinogenesis 7:1029–1033

Elliott BM, Robinson M, Ashby J (1983) 6-(*p*-dimethylaminophenylazo)benzothiazole (6BT); a potent hepatocarcinogen in the rat. Cancer Res 21:69–76

Lutz WK (1979) In vivo covalent DNA binding as a quantitative indicator in the process of chemical carcinogenesis. Mutat Res 65:289–356

Mitchell AM, Bridges JW, Elcombe CR (1984) Factors influencing peroxisome proliferation in cultured rat hepatocytes. Arch Toxicol 55:239–246

Walters JM, Combes RD (1983) Evaluation of a methodology for the use of rat small intestine in the Salmonella/microsome assay. Mutat Res 113:393–402

Mechanisms and Models of Teratogenesis

Mechanisms and Models in Toxicology
Arch. Toxicol., Suppl. 11, 105–114 (1987)

Teratogenicity Testing in Vitro:
Status of Validation Studies

N. A. Brown

MRC Experimental Embryology and Teratology Unit, Medical Research Council Laboratories, Woodmansterne Road, Carshalton, Surrey, SM5 4EF, UK

Introduction

Alternatives to the standard method of using pregnant mammals to test for teratogenicity have been the subject of extensive review and comment in recent years (see, for example, Shepard et al. 1983; Johnson 1984; Sadler and Warner 1984; Brown and Freeman 1984; Neubert et al. 1985). There has been much debate on the uses and limitations of alternative tests, although no consensus has yet emerged. Regardless of these considerations, several test systems are commercially available and being used for the initial estimation of teratogenicity (variously termed "screening" or "prescreening"). The purpose of this study was to examine the current status of validation studies of the various model systems which have been proposed as potential tests. There are many other aspects of this field which will not be considered here: for example, the practicality of tests and the scientific basis of test design. The above reviews can be consulted for further discussion of these topics. It is appropriate, however, to make clear the limitations of any in vitro test for teratogenicity. (Strictly speaking, several of the models proposed as tests are not "in vitro" systems, but the terms "alternative test" and "in vitro test" are used synonymously in this paper.)

A standard teratogenicity test in vivo is only one segment of reproductive toxicity screening. It provides no information on the potential of a chemical to interfere with most aspects of the reproductive cycle. This must also be true of alternative teratogenicity tests. At best, an alternative test for teratogenicity will indicate the potential of a chemical or mixture to interfere with a limited portion of the reproductive process. There are four manifestations of developmental (or prenatal) toxicity: embryo or fetal death; malformation; retardation; and functional (including behavioural) impairment. A standard "teratogenicity" test can detect the first three of these. There is no current agreement on nomenclature in this field. It may be appropriate to name these tests developmental, or prenatal, toxicity tests and to reserve the terms "teratogenicity" and "teratogen" for description of structural malformations only. However, it is currently common practice to use these terms in a broader sense to encompass all adverse effects of prenatal insult, and this practice is generally followed here.

Many of the alternative tests proposed monitor specific cell processes which are important in development, e.g. cell adhesion or proliferation. It is not known what the manifestation of interference with such processes would be in vivo, and these tests should therefore be considered indicators of potential developmental toxicity, not specifically of the induction of structural malformation. This is not a barrier to the use of these tests in screening; the point is that the same chemical insult may induce different manifestations of developmental toxicity in different species in vivo, so a positive result in a test in vivo or in vitro should be considered only as a warning of potential to induce some kind of developmental toxicity.

Although biochemical mechanisms of developmental toxicity are poorly understood, it is clear that chemicals can act initially on the embryo, the placenta or the maternal system. Actions on the embryo can be intracellular or at the level of cell–cell interaction, extracellular matrix function or fluid and haemodynamic balance. It follows that as test systems are reduced in complexity, from the pregnant animal down to the isolated cell, then more and more potential teratogens will be "missed". This has to be accepted as an unavoidable consequence of simplifying test systems. Just how many teratogens will be missed with each step of simplification is not currently known, but will become clearer as more teratogens of known mechanism are screened in different tests.

In common with other in vitro systems, most alternative teratogenicity tests have no pharmacokinetic component. They are usually static closed systems in which exposure is to a constant concentration for an extended period. Clearly, the maternal physiological disposition of a chemical, and also maternal toxicity, will often prevent the conceptus from ever being exposed to the kinds of dosage that can be generated in vitro. Because induction of malformation is usually observed to be a threshold phenomenon in vivo, many agents will induce responses in vitro but would be effectively inactive in a pregnant animal. These factors must be considered for each individual test compound and cannot be evaluated without pharmacokinetic information.

Validation is the process of selecting a number of compounds which have well characterized mammalian teratogenic potential in vivo, testing them in the model system, and comparing the results with the known mammalian data. There have been three general approaches. The simplest, and by far the most common, is based upon the dichotomous classification of test compounds as "teratogens" and "non-teratogens" and test results as "positive" or "negative". Evaluation of performance is then based on a contingency table analysis. The second approach is to correlate measured potency in the test system with teratogenic doses in vivo. The third possibility is to compare "developmental hazard" estimates from in vivo and in vitro testing.

The concept of "developmental hazard" is critical in designing a teratogenicity test. All substances are toxic in vivo and an LD_{50} value can be determined for virtually any compound. Similarly, all substances must be potentially developmentally toxic, that is, they could induce some form of embryo-fetal toxicity if they could be delivered to the conceptus at a high enough dosage. The purpose of teratogenicity testing is to identify substances that are toxic to development with exposures that are not toxic to the adult. Such substances are "developmental hazards", and the degree of hazard can be quantified by some ratio of adult toxic to developmentally toxic doses (Johnson 1980, 1981, 1984; Fabro et al. 1982). Validation studies using each of the above three approaches have been analysed.

Methods

From literature searches which were completed in October, 1985, 14 tests were identified for which some kind of systematic validation study had been performed (Table 1). There is published information on another 12 potential test systems but these are not included because few chemicals have been tested and no systematic validation data are available. The data which were analysed were taken from the references listed in Table 1, plus unpublished information provided by Dr. S. Keller on the Pox Virus system and Dr. R. Jelinek on CHEST. The data on the FE-TAX system is incomplete, being available in abstract form only (Dumont and Epler 1984).

In the computerized analysis, two attempts were made to reduce the problems of comparing performance across tests which have utilized widely different groups of chemicals, many of which are not well accepted as "teratogens" or "non-teratogens". Firstly, a group of 81 compounds were identified which had been tested in three or more different systems. These compounds are listed in

Table 1. Model systems for which validation data were analysed

System	Abbreviation	References
Mammalian		
Rodent whole embryo culture	WEC	Schmid et al. (1983)
Non-Mammalian		
Chick embryotoxicity screening test	CHEST	Jelinek (unpublished)
Frog embryo teratogenesis assay: Xenopus	FETAX	Dumont and Epler (1984)
Hydra regeneration	Hydra	Johnson and Gabel (1983)
Primary cell cultures		
Micromass Mouse embryo limb mesenchyme	MM M L	Guntakatta et al. (1984)
Rat embryo CNS/limb	MM R C/L	Flint and Orton (1984)
Rat embryo, in vivo dosed, CNS/limb	MM RV C/L	Flint et al. (1984)
Chick embryo limb mesenchyme	MM CH L	Wilk et al. (1980); Hassel and Horigan (1982)
Chick embryo neural crest	CH NCC	Wilk et al. (1980); Greenburg (1982)
Drosophila embryo	DEC	Bournais-Vardiabasis et al. (1982)
Established cell lines		
Mouse ovarian tumor – attachment	MOT	Braun et al. (1979, 1982)
Human embryonal palatal mesenchyme – proliferation	HEPM	Pratt and Willis (1985)
Neuroblastoma – differentiation	NBLA	Mummery et al. (1984)
Pox virus infected cells – pox virus replication	Pox virus	Keller and Smith (1982); Keller (unpublished)

Table 2. Chemicals tested in three or more model systems

Teratogens		Non-teratogens
5-Fluorouracil[a]	EDTA	Amaranth[a]
6-Aminonicotinamide	Ethanol[a]	Aminopyrine
6-Mercaptopurine	Griseofulvin	Ammonium chloride
Acetazolamide[a]	Hydrocortisone	Ascorbic acid
Actinomycin D	Hydroxyurea[a]	Bendectin
Allopurinol	Indomethacin	Butylated hydroxyanisole
Aminopterin	Insulin	Cyclamate[a]
Aspirin[a]	Isoproteranol	Cysteine
Atropine	L-Dopa	Glutamate
Azathioprine	Lithium	Glutethimide
BAPN	Meclizine	Heparin
Benzo[A]pyrene	Methotrexate[a]	Isoniazid[a]
Bromodeoxyuridine	Mitomycin C	Lysine
Busulfan	Nicotine	Ouabain
Cadmium chloride	Nicotinic acid	Penicillin[a]
Caffeine[a]	Pentobarbital	Phenol
Chloramphenicol	Phenobarbital	Pyridoxine hydrochloride
Chlorcyclizine	Phenylbutazone	Quinine
Colchiceine	Progesterone	Saccharin[a]
Cortisone	Reserpine	Streptomycin
Cycloheximide	Retinoic acid[a]	Thiamine
Cyclophosphamide[a]	Salicylic acid	Tween
Cytosine arabinoside	Sucrose	
Dexamethasone[a]	Testosterone[a]	
Diazepam[a]	Thalidomide[a]	
Diethylstilbestrol[a]	Theophylline	
Dimethyl sulfoxide	Trypan blue	
Diphenylhydantoin[a]	Urethane	
Diazooxo-L-norleucine	Vinblastine	
	Zinc chloride	

[a] Also a "standard" compound (see Text)

Table 2. Most often, different investigators agreed on the teratogen/non-teratogen classification of these compounds. Where there was discrepancy, the classification made by the majority of investigators was used in the analyses. One compound, sucrose, is listed as a teratogen by this criterion, a classification many teratologists would not agree with. One other compound, amaranth, would have been classified as a teratogen by this criterion but it is considered to be a non-teratogen by Smith et al. (1983, see below) and this latter classification was used in the analyses. The validation performance for each test, using these "common" compounds only, was calculated. The second attempt was to analyse the data available on testing of any of the 47 compounds or conditions selected by a panel of experts as "standard" test agents for teratogenicity tests (Smith et al. 1983).

Given the limitations of all current data, as discussed below, it seems inappropriate to present statistical analyses here on differences between tests for validation performance, although there are highly significant variations. Full lists of all compounds tested for each model system are available from the author.

Results and Discussion

Test Compound Selection

The data analysed represent about 1000 individual compound-tests, the number of agents tested in a single test varying from more than 100 to less than 20, with an average of about 40. Widely disparate groups of test compounds were used, 387 different chemicals or treatments being screened in total. Many of these, perhaps half, are chemicals for which the mammalian data base is not adequate and they are therefore not useful for validation studies. Examination of lists of chemicals tested shows that chemical selection tended to be biased. Many of the commonly tested "non-teratogens" are endogenous or xenobiotic chemicals of an essentially non-toxic nature, e.g. glutamate, lysine, cysteine, ascorbic acid, cyclamate, saccharin (Table 2). By contrast, many of the commonly tested "teratogens" are highly biologically active antimetabolites, alkylating agents and hormones. It seems likely that virtually any cell-biological system would respond differently to two such groups of chemicals. This must be considered a major limitation, since the vast majority of tests did not distinguish between non-specific and developmental toxicities.

Dichotomous Classification Approach

The 14 different tests produce a wide variety of different parameters describing a test result. All tests, excepting the hydra assay, ultimately classify a test chemical as positive or negative based upon their parameters. Studies of these 13 tests based the estimation of validation performance primarily on the dichotomous classification method, although some also used the potency comparison approach (see below). In this presentation of the analyses, it is this final classification of a test result as positive or negative which is considered. It should be realized that some models produce much more information, e.g. highest no-effect concentrations, lowest toxic concentrations, median effective concentrations. In some cases this might allow the calculation of a developmental hazard ratio (see below), but in no case was this reported in the publications cited.

In this most common approach to validation the selection and classification of test chemicals is critically important. A proper interpretation of validation performance requires that "teratogen" and "non-teratogen" are rigidly defined, since to compare performance across tests correctly, the same definitions have to be adopted in all cases. A panel of teratologists has carried out a selection of test compounds, generating a list of 47 chemicals and conditions (Smith et al. 1983). They define a "teratogen" as a compound which, in the absence of maternal toxicity, induces embryolethality, growth retardation, structural abnormality, or perinatal or postnatal functional deficit. They require correctly performed and analysed studies in two mammalian species. This is actually a definition of a developmentally toxic substance and, therefore, validation performance will reflect ability to detect developmental toxins, not specifically teratogens. Also, the stipulation that adverse effects must be induced in the absence of maternal toxicity means that all the selected substances are developmental hazards, although the magnitude of hazard may vary.

Virtually all of the studies analysed did not define the teratogen/non-teratogen classification procedure. It is therefore not clear what the performance data actually reflect. The definition adopted by Smith et al. (1983) is acceptable, although it does not address the problems of how to cope with agents which are highly teratogenic but only in one species, those which are teratogenic in rodents but clearly not in humans, those which require multiple administrations, and so on. In many studies there are also deficiencies in the classification of test results as positive or negative. Often chemicals have been classed as positive when they induced a response, but only with simultaneous toxic action. Chemicals have also been classed as negative when they induced no response of any kind, with testing to an arbitrary top concentration or to maximum solubility. The former type of responses should actually be classed as negative, while the latter should be termed untested, or untestable. The authors' classification of response was used in all analyses reported here.

The procedure of compound selection by Smith et al. (1983) was reasonably logical, the primary requirement being an adequate mammalian data base. The published validation studies analysed here often did not use similarly well-selected lists of compounds. There was frequent use of chemicals with inadequate data concerning mammalian teratogenicity, and disagreements between investigators on the designation of a chemical as a teratogen or non-teratogen were common. In many cases, the chemicals selected do not represent an unbiased sample (see above).

Table 3 summarizes the validation performance of the 13 test systems, calculated for three groups of compounds. The "author" column gives performance data exactly as reported in the original publication. The "common" column gives

Table 3. Validation performance of teratogenicity tests

Test	"Teratogens" Correct/total (% sensitivity)			"Non-teratogens" Correct/total (% specificity)		
	Author	Common	Standards	Author	Common	Standards
WEC	20/20 (100)	14/16 (88)	8/8 (100)	19/20 (95)	6/6 (100)	1/1 (100)
CHEST	–	26/29 (90)	8/8 (100)	–	1/1 (100)	0/2 (0)
FETAX	31/34 (91)	–	–	?/6	–	–
MM CH L	16/17 (94)	10/11 (91)	5/6 (83)	3/4 (75)	2/3 (67)	1/1 (100)
MM R C/L	25/27 (93)	17/19 (89)	6/8 (75)	17/19 (89)	5/6 (83)	3/3 (100)
MM RV C/L	17/18 (94)	12/13 (92)	3/4 (75)	12/13 (92)	3/3 (100)	3/4 (75)
MM M L	19/22 (86)	18/21 (86)	7/9 (78)	5/5 (80)	4/5 (80)	2/2 (100)
CH NCC	10/12 (83)	8/10 (80)	4/6 (67)	4/4 (100)	3/3 (100)	1/1 (100)
DEC	14/17 (82)	21/36 (58)	10/14 (71)	3/3 (100)	4/6 (67)	2/3 (67)
MOT	64/78 (82)	27/41 (66)	11/13 (85)	21/29 (72)	13/20 (65)	2/6 (33)
HEPM	23/35 (66)	19/28 (68)	9/14 (64)	12/20 (60)	10/15 (67)	4/6 (67)
NBLA	34/38 (87)	24/30 (80)	12/14 (86)	14/18 (78)	11/15 (73)	2/3 (67)
Pox virus	57/62 (92)	31/35 (89)	11/11 (100)	9/10 (90)	9/11 (82)	2/2 (100)

The data presented in the "author" columns are exactly as reported in the references listed in Table 1 for each test. The data in the "common" and "standards" columns are for tests on chemicals identified as tested in three or more systems and those selected by Smith et al. (1983), respectively. See section on methods for full details.

performance for those chemicals listed in Table 2, using the majority classification of a chemical as a teratogen/non-teratogen, not necessarily the authors' own
classification in each case. Finally, the "standards" column gives performance
only for the chemicals selected by Smith et al. (1983). Overall, the apparent validation performance is poorer when analysis is restricted to common or standard
compounds, probably because of the elimination of some of the bias in compound
selection. Of the three performances calculated, that for the common compounds
is probably the most useful for comparative purposes, as it represents the testing
of a more homogeneous and better characterized group of compounds than the
authors' full data. The summary of relative performance in the next paragraph
is based on this analysis. Too few standard compounds have been screened in
most tests to allow meaningful comparisons of those performances. It is clear
from all of the validation data that too few acceptable non-teratogenic compounds have been tested in all systems (Table 3).

The DEC, MOT and HEPM tests, each of which monitors a single cellular process, perform poorly for both sensitivity and specificity, giving about 35% false
negatives and false positives. This is clearly an unacceptable performance if these
tests are to be used individually. It remains to be shown whether a battery made
up of several of these tests would perform satisfactorily (Pratt and Willis 1985).
The chick neural creast (CH NCC) and neuroblastoma (NBLA) cell tests show
sensitivities of about 80%. All of the remaining tests perform similarly in terms
of sensitivity, giving about 10% false negative responses. The performance values
for the four micromass systems are remarkably consistent, given the differing
compounds tested and assay conditions. Few conclusions can be made regarding
the specificities of the tests because of the few acceptable "non-teratogens" tested.
In general, validation performance correlates well with the biological complexity
of the model system; the more complex the system, the better the performance.
An interesting exception is the Pox Virus test, which appears to perform better
than might be expected. This may reflect the fact that both host cell and viral integrity are monitored in this system.

Potency Correlation Approach

Publications on the MOT, HEPM and Pox Virus tests included correlations of
effective concentrations in vitro with lowest teratogenic doses in vivo (Braun et
al. 1982; Pratt and Willis 1985; Keller and Smith 1982). Good correlation coefficients were reported in each study. However, this does not prove the validity of
the methods, although in vitro potency may provide a general indication of the
order of magnitude of biologically effective concentrations and is useful for that
purpose. Validity is not proven because effective concentrations of the tested
chemicals varied over several orders of magnitude and a reasonable correlation
would be expected for any two biological effects under such circumstances. For
cxample, LD_{50} values and lowest teratogenic doses would correlate quite well for
a group of compounds of widely different potency, but one would not propose
LD_{50} as a test of teratogenicity, although LD_{50} is an indication of the likely teratogenic dose range. Smith et al. (1983) have discussed other problems of this approach.

Developmental Hazard Approach

This is theoretically the best approach to validation, since developmental hazard is primarily what one wishes an alternative test to detect, as has been discussed. A major problem of this approach is the lack of accepted quantitative estimates of mammalian developmental hazard in vivo. A precise 'Relative Teratogenic Index' has been proposed, but appropriate experimental data which permit its calculation are available for only a few compounds (Fabro et al. 1982). A more approximate index, based on the ratio of minimum adult lethal dose to minimum teratogenic dose, has been used by Johnson (1980, 1981; Johnson and Gabel 1982, 1983). The Hydra assay is the only alternative test designed exclusively to estimate developmental hazard (Johnson 1980). Published information is available on the testing of about 50 chemicals and many more tests have been performed for which data are not yet freely available. It has been claimed that Hydra and mammalian hazard estimates are comparable (Johnson and Gabel 1983), but systematic data to support this relationship have not been presented. Some available information is not supportive. For example, the chemicals isoniazid, saccharin, retinoic acid, ethanol and aspirin are "standard" compounds described from mammalian experimentation as: "negative", "negative", "strong positive", "weak positive" and "strong positive" respectively (Smith et al. 1983). The Hydra hazard ratios are 20, 3, 2, 1.5 and 1.3 respectively (Johnson and Gabel 1983). It can be argued that the mammalian hazard ratios for these chemicals have not been defined and that the designations by Smith et al. may be inappropriate, but on the face of it the Hydra and mammalian data do not seem to correlate well.

The FETAX test also produces a hazard ratio, but this ratio is of embryotoxic/teratogenic concentrations and it has not been compared with mammalian data. Several other test systems are capable of producing an index of hazard (see above). Although there is no published information, the concept of developmental hazard is gaining favour; hazard ratios are now being calculated by several groups and data are likely to be available in the near future.

Conclusions

This analysis shows that all current validation studies of alternative teratogenicity tests are inadequate. The major improvements required are better selection of test compounds and standardized definitions of their teratogenic potential. The list of chemicals selected by Smith et al. (1983) provides a reasonable starting point for compound selection, and several studies using these agents are under way. If the concept of developmental hazard is accepted, then it is clearly not appropriate to classify chemicals as "teratogens" or "non-teratogens" without defining these in terms of hazard. A quantitative measure of developmental hazard in vivo should be calculated for the standard chemicals. Further studies need to be performed in which standard test compounds are screened blind in the test systems and hazard estimates are compared. The true relative performance of tests could then be evaluated.

Acknowledgement. This publication is taken from a critical review, *Alternative Tests for Teratogenicity of Petroleum Products,* carried out by the author under the sponsorship of the American Petroleum Institute, Washington, DC, USA.

References

Bournais-Vardiabasis N, Teplitz RL, Chernoff GF, Seecof RL (1982) Detection of teratogens in the drosophila embryonic cell culture test: assay of 100 chemicals. Teratology 28:109–122

Braun AG, Emerson DJ, Nichinson BB (1979) Teratogenic drugs inhibit tumour cell attachment of lectin-coated surfaces. Nature 282:507–509

Braun AG, Buckner CA, Emerson DA, Nichinson BB (1982) Quantitative correspondence between the in vivo and in vitro activity of teratogenic agents. Proc Natl Acad Sci USA 79:2056–2060

Brown NA, Freeman SJ (1984) Alternative tests for teratogenicity. Alternatives to Laboratory Animals 12:7–23

Dumont JN, Epler RG (1984) Validation studies on the FETAX teratogenesis assay (frog embryos). Teratology 29:38A

Fabro S, Shull G, Brown NA (1982) The relative teratogenic index and teratogenic potency: proposed components of developmental toxicity risk assessment. Teratogen Carcinogen Mutagen 2:61–76

Flint OP, Orton TC (1984) An in vitro assay for teratogens with cultures of rat embryo midbrain and limb bud cells. Toxicol Appl Pharmacol 76:383–395

Flint OP, Orton TC, Ferguson RA (1984) Differentiation of rat embryo cells in culture: response following acute maternal exposure to teratogens and non-teratogens. J Appl Toxicol 4:109–116

Greenburg JH (1982) Detection of teratogens by differentiating embryonic neural crest cells in culture: evaluation as a screening system. Teratogen Carcinogen Mutagen 2:319–323

Guntakatta M, Mathews EJ, Rundell JO (1984) Development of a mouse embryo limb bud cell culture system for the estimation of chemical teratogenic potential. Teratogen Carcinogen Mutagen 4:349–364

Hassell JR, Horigan EA (1982) Chondrogenesis: a model developmental system for measuring teratogenic potential of compounds. Teratogen Carcinogen Mutagen 2:325–331

Jelinek R (1977) The chick embryotoxicity screening test. In: Neubert D, Merker HJ, Kwasigroch TE (eds) Methods in prenatal toxicology: evaluation of embryotoxic effects in experimental animals. Thieme, Stuttgart, pp 381–386

Johnson EM (1980) A subvertebrate System for rapid determination of potential teratogenic hazards. J Environ Pathol Toxicol 4:153–156

Johnson EM (1981) Screening for teratogenic hazards: nature of the problems. Annu Rev Pharmacol Toxicol 21:417–429

Johnson EM (1984) A prioritization and biologic decision tree for developmental toxicity safety evaluations. J Am Coll Toxicol 3:141–155

Johnson EM, Gabel BEG (1983) An artificial 'embryo' for detection of abnormal developmental biology. Fund Appl Toxicol 3:243–249

Keller SJ, Smith MK (1982) Animal virus screens for potential teratogens. I. Poxvirus morphogenesis. Teratogen Carcinogen Mutagen 2:361–374

Mummery CL, van den Brink CE, van der Saag PT, de Laat SW (1984) A short-term screening test for teratogens using differentiating neuroblastoma cells in vitro. Teratology 29:271–279

Neubert D, Blankenburg G, Lewandowski C, Klug S (1985) Misinterpretations of results and creation of "artifacts" in studies on developmental toxicity using systems simpler than in vivo systems. In: Lash JW, Saxen L (eds) Developmental mechanisms normal and abnormal Liss, New York, pp 241–266 (Progress in clinical and biological research, vol 171)

Pratt RM, Willis WD (1985) In vitro screening assay for teratogens using growth inhibition of human embryonic cells. Proc Natl Acad Sci USA 82:5791–5794

Sadler TW, Warner CW (1984) Use of whole embryo culture for evaluating toxicity and teratogenicity. Pharmacol Rev 36:1456S–150S

Schmid BP, Trippmacher A, Bianchi A (1983) Validation of the whole-embryo culture method for in vitro teratogenicity testing. In: Hayes AW, Schnell RC, Miya TS (eds) Developments in the science and practice of toxicology. Elsevier, Amsterdam, pp 563–566

Shepard TH, Fantel AG, Mirkes PE, Greenaway JC, Faustman-Watts E, Campbell M, Juchau MR
    (1983) Teratology testing: I. Development and status of short-term prescreens. II. Biotransforma-
    tion of teratogens as studied in whole embryo culture. In: Macleod SM, Okey AB, Spielberg SP
    (eds) Developmental pharmacology. Liss, New York, pp 147–164 (Progress in clinical and biolog-
    ical research, vol 135)
Smith MK, Kimmel GL, Kochhar DM, Shepard TH, Spielberg SP, Wilson JG (1983) A selection of
    candidate compounds for in vitro teratogenesis test validation. Teratogen Carcinogen Mutagen
    3:461–480
Wilk AL, Greenberg JH, Horigan EA, Pratt RM, Martin GR (1980) Detection of teratogenic com-
    pounds using differentiating embryonic cells in culture. In Vitro 16:269–276

Mechanisms and Models in Toxicology
Arch. Toxicol., Suppl. 11, 115–121 (1987)

The Primate as a Model for Hazard Assessment of Teratogens in Humans

R. Korte, F. Vogel, and I. Osterburg

Hazleton Laboratories Deutschland GmbH, Kesselfeld 29, D-4400 Münster, FRG

Looking at the preclinical guidelines of various countries and international organizations in the field of reproductive toxicology, it is very obvious that the species most used are the rat, the mouse and the rabbit. This prompts the question: why is another species needed at all?

There are several good reasons for the use of a third species in reproductive toxicity studies, especially in teratogenicity studies; five possible examples, of which more could be found, are listed below:

1. One of the two species normally used (rat and rabbit) may not tolerate the application of the compound, so the species cannot be used at all. This is, for example, the case with some antibiotic compounds which induce diarrhoea in rabbits.
2. From time to time it happens that one of the two species normally used shows no teratogenic effect, while the other species may exhibit a higher number of resorptions, i.e. an embryotoxic potential. In this case the third species is needed to evaluate the risk.
3. When hormonal compounds are tested to evaluate their embryotoxic potential, it does not seem advisable to use rats and rabbits on the larger scale at all. In those species the pregnancy is maintained by hormones produced by the ovaries during the whole pregnancy, while in human beings and primates the placenta takes over this function. With some hormonal compounds complete embryonic deaths in rats and rabbits can be induced with doses at or below the human dose levels.
4. Even if teratogenicity studies in rats and rabbits do not show any embryotoxic effect it might be useful to perform a study in a third species in order to minimise the risk for pregnant women, especially if the compounds are intended to be used throughout the entire pregnancy.
5. A compound to be tested may, in one of the species normally used, be subject to a very different metabolism from that in human beings, so it would make no sense to use this species for toxicity studies.

   This leads to the following questions: why should a primate be used as a third species, and what primate species should be used? Dogs, pigs and ferrets, for instance, have been used in teratogenicity studies. However, studies in those species were rare, so that there are not sufficient background data available. On the other hand, all three of these species bring specific difficulties to research, like heat season, volume and stress.

   Cycle length, conception rate, litter size, abortion rate, breeding season and other major factors influence the decision to choose a certain primate species for a teratogenicity study. Hazleton Laboratories Deutschland GmbH was involved in the performance of more than 1100 timed pregnancies in primates, and on the basis of this experience, the cynomolgus monkey (*Macaca fascicularis*) is the animal of choice. The classical animal, the rhesus monkey (*Macaca mulatta*), which was formerly in most common use in research, shows a very clear breeding season. This very distinct breeding season was observed even after 4 years in an indoor breeding colony, and it was also observed in females born in captivity. Female rhesus monkeys menstruate during most of the summer months and, correspondingly, alterations in the testes are histologically detectable in the male animals. In December, for example, all stages of sperm production can be observed while in August only a single germ layer is found.

   The advantages of using the cynomolgus monkey can be summarized as follows:

- They show menstrual cycles throughout the year, so that a teratogenicity study in primates can be initiated at any time during the year.
- They have a fairly stable cycle of 28 days.
- The body weights of 3.0–3.5 kg allow easy handling of the animals.
- Because of the low body weight the cages can be relatively small.
- Small quantities of compounds are needed.
- The availability of the animals is excellent, from the wild or bred. Animals caught in the wild are relatively clean (no tuberculosis) and they are quite cheap.

   For these reasons it is suggested that all teratogenicity studies in primates be carried out with this animal model.

   During recent years more than 860 timed pregnancies have been achieved in the cynomolgus monkey at Hazleton Laboratories Deutschland GmbH. The colony of female cynomolgus monkeys is quite large and the menstrual cycle is monitored in all the animals daily. The amount of bleeding (stage 1 – stage 4) is recorded for each animal on a menstrual cycle card, allowing determination of the middle of its menstrual cycle and thereby increasing mating success.

   Blood samples are collected weekly over the complete period of pregnancy. The progesterone level during early pregnancy is used to confirm pregnancy.

   The dosing period lasts from day 18 post coitum to day 50 post coitum in a normal teratogenicity study in the cynomolgus monkey. This covers the development stages according to Carnegie from 7/8 to 19/20.

   During the complete experimental period of a study, the occurrence of abortions must be expected in both control and/or test animals. Due to the fact that these primates quite often abort overnight and that they eat abortion material, a very careful check has to be carried out every morning to detect blood and/or abortion material in the excrement tray below the cages.

A normal teratogenicity study in primates is terminated on day 100 post coitum caesarian section. This surgery is very simple and easily performed and it does not cause major problems. The normal form of the placenta of the cynomolgus monkey is a placenta bidiscuidalis (meaning that it has two separated disks), but it can also be found that only one disk is visible, or that the two disks are attached to each other. Twins are quite rare in this species. In more than 650 caesarian sections in cynomolgus monkeys, one case of twins was observed.

Rectal palpations over the whole period of pregnancy are performed to measure the size of the uterus. It is absolutely advisable to perform a caesarian section also in those cases in which a believed pregnancy has already been terminated by abortion, although no abortion material was found. In one recent case where caesarian section was performed on day 100 post coitum, a small embryo was

Table 1. Timed pregnancies in control rhesus monkeys

Study number	Positive pregnancy test	False positive pregnancy test	Caesarian section
18	21	0	20
31	25	0	18
55	30	0	23
65	31	0	24
67	27	1	15
72	27	1	21
88	30	1	24
93	66	1	19
129	43	0	29
G	5	0	5
D	1	0	1
Total	306	4	199

Table 2. Abortions in control rhesus monkeys

	Pregnancies	Abortions	%	Day 21–30	Day 31–50	Day 51–70	Later
18	6	0	0.0	0	0	0	0
31	10	1	10.0	0	1	0	0
55	10	1	10.0	0	1	0	0
65	10	1	10.0	0	1	0	0
67	7	1	14.3	0	0	0	1
72	6	1	16.6	0	0	1	0
88	10	0	0.0	0	0	0	0
129	10	1	10.0	0	1	0	0
Total	69	6	8.7	0	4	1	1

Table 3. Annual reproductive rates of rhesus monkeys

Year	Number of females	Pregnancies		Live births		Abortions/ stillbirths	
		Total	Rate	Total	Rate	Total	Rate
1978	249	162	65.1%	145	89.5%	17	10.5%
1979	306	206	67.3%	183	88.8%	23	11.2%
1980	343	205	59.8%	182	88.8%	23	11.2%
Total		573		510	89.0%	63	11.0%

Table 4. Timed pregnancies in cynomolgus monkeys

Study number	Positive pregnancy test	False positive pregnancy test	Caesarian section
1	33	0	26
2	30	1	24
3	42	0	30
4	11	0	8
5	14	0	11
6	42	2	19
7	51	3	32
8	42	1	25
9	5	0	2
10	31	1	19
11	42	1	33
12	43	1	31
13	5	0	0
14	51	2	23
15	20	0	6
16	26	1	20
17	33	2	19
18	1	0	1
19	45	0	37
20	7	1	4
21	13	0	12
22	41	2	17
23	8	0	6
24	32	1	23
25	32	0	16
26	47	0	28
27	23	0	7
28	46	0	25
29	4	0	3
30[a]	36	2	–
31[a]	10	1	–
Total	866	22	507

[a] Studies not completed.

Table 5. Abortions in control cynomolgus monkeys

	Pregnancies	Abortions	%	Day 21–30	Day 31–50	Day 51–70	Later
1	12	3	25.0	2	0	0	1
2	9	2	22.2	1	1	0	0
3	12	3	25.0	0	2	1	0
4	9	0	0.0	0	0	0	0
5	8	1	12.5	0	0	1	0
6	10	2	20.0	0	2	0	0
7	10	1	10.0	0	0	1	0
8	10	0	0.0	0	0	0	0
9	10	1	10.0	0	0	1	0
10	12	2	16.7	1	0	1	0
11	10	0	0.0	0	0	0	0
12	10	2	20.0	1	0	1	0
13	10	4	40.0	1	1	0	2
14	9	3	33.3	1	0	2	0
15	10	3	30.0	0	3	0	0
Total	151	27	17.9	7	9	8	3

Table 6. Annual reproductive rates of cynomolgus monkeys

Year	Number of females	Pregnancies		Live births		Abortions/ stillbirths	
		Total	Rate	Total	Rate	Total	Rate
1978	337	297	88.1%	268	90.2%	29	9.8%
1979	310	275	88.7%	252	91.6%	23	8.4%
Total		572		520	90.9%	52	9.1%

found inside a small uterus; its development was comparable to approximately day 38 of pregnancy. Since that day the embryo must have been dead inside the uterus.

The historical control data for the studies performed in rhesus monkeys are summarized in Tables 1 and 2. The average abortion rate was 8.7% which is an extremely low figure, but the number of 69 control animals was quite limited. Nevertheless, this figure is comparable with the abortion and stillbirths rate (11%) of a former breeding colony (Table 3). The comparable data for the cynomolgus monkeys are summarized in Tables 4 and 5. The average abortion rate for the last 15 studies performed is 17.9%, with a range from 0 to 40%. The figure of 40% is strongly affected by two late abortions after day 70 post coitum. The corresponding figure for abortions and stillbirths in the former breeding colony is 9.1% (Table 6).

Malformations are very rare in untreated macaques. The investigation of still-born fetuses and dead neonates from the former breeding colony revealed only

Table 7. Malformations and retardations in rhesus monkeys

Year	Total number of pregnancies	Examined stillbirths	Examined neonatal deaths	Malformed stillbirths/neonates		Stillbirths/neonates with retardations	
				Total	Rate (to pregnancies	Total	Rate (to pregnancies)
1978	162	11	5	0	0.0%	0	0.0%
1979	206	17	2	1[a]	0.5%	0	0.0%
1980	205	26	3	2[b, c]	1.0%	1[c]	0.5%
Total	573	54	10	3	0.5%	1	0.2%

[a] Slight hydrocephalus.
[b] Bilateral hydrocephalus.
[c] Unilateral hydrocephalus, genital system retarded in development.

Table 8. Malformations and retardations in cynomolgus monkeys

Year	Total number of pregnancies	Examined stillbirths	Examined neonatal deaths	Malformed stillbirths/neonates		Stillbirths/neonates with retardations	
				Total	Rate (to pregnancies	Total	Rate (to pregnancies)
1978	297	29	9	0	0.0%	0	0.0%
1979	275	20	11	0	0.0%	1[a]	0.4%
Total	572	49	20	0	0.0%	1	0.2%

[a] Genital system retarded in development.

Table 9. Classification of test substances

Oestrogen	Antibiotic
Progestogen	Cephalosporin
Combination of oestrogen and progestogen	Sulphonamide
	Fungicide
Anti-androgen	Herbicide
Prostaglandin	Anti-malarial drug
Non-steroidal anti-inflammatory agent	ACE-inhibitor
	Calcium antagonist
Analgesic	Dopamine partial antagonist
Neuroleptic	
Acelaic acid	

three malformed fetuses out of 64 specimens examined in rhesus monkeys, which means approximately 0.5% (Table 7). In all cases, hydrocephalus was observed. This figure agrees quite well with 0.48% from the Sukhumi Primate Center (Lapin 1963) and 0.53% from the Southwest Foundation (Baboons) (Hendrickx 1966). Wilson and Gavan (1967) found 13 malformations out of 2950 pregnancies of different primate species, which is equal to 0.44%. In the former cynomolgus breeding colony, no malformations were observed in stillborn fetuses or dead neonates (Table 8).

Table 9 summarizes the groups of compounds tested, either in rhesus or cynomolgus monkeys. The following compounds have been proved to induce malformations after application to the pregnant female: thalidomide (caused phocomelia); cyproterone acetate (induced feminization); a calcium antagonist, a fungicide and methoxyethanol/ethylene glycol monomethyl ether (led to fore- and hindlimb malformations).

Conclusion

The data presented support the assertion that the primate, especially the cynomolgus monkey, is a valid and available model for hazard assessment of teratogens in humans.

References

Hendrickx AG (1966) Teratological findings in a baboon colony. In: Miller CO (ed) Food and drug administration conference on nonhuman primate toxicology. US Govt. Printing Office, Washington

Lapin BA (1963) Defects in development and malformation. The monkey – subject of medical and biological experiments. Akademia Meditsinskich Nauk SSSR, Sukhumi, p 297

Wilson JG, Gavan JA (1967) Congenital malformations in nonhuman primates: spontaneous and experimentally induced. Anat Rec 158:99–110

Mechanisms and Models in Toxicology
Arch. Toxicol., Suppl. 11, 122–127 (1987)

A Clinician's View of Teratogenesis

R. W. Smithells

Department of Paediatrics and Child Health, Clarendon Wing, General Infirmary at Leeds, Leeds, LS2 9NS, UK

About one baby in every forty is born with a significant birth defect which threatens life, requires surgical correction or conveys lifelong handicap. This figure is derived from observations on babies defined as viable; that is, born at or after the 28th week of pregnancy. In babies born before that time, and especially in very early abortuses, the frequency of structural and genetic defects is very much higher. It is apparent that mechanisms exist which lead to the early eviction of conceptuses that have little or no biological future. The heavy load of birth defects encountered in clinical practice therefore represents only the tip of an iceberg.

Published figures of prevalence of birth defects normally refer only to 'viable' fetuses. Prenatal diagnosis, principally by ultrasound scans and analysis of amniotic fluid, usually leads to termination of affected pregnancies, and this alters, in some cases profoundly, the proportion of affected fetuses attaining 28 weeks' gestation and thereby qualifying for inclusion in statistics.

Although many birth defects are attributable to single gene or chromosomal abnormalities (10%–20%, depending upon the definition of birth defect), the majority are believed to be of multifactorial causation. Very few indeed can be confidently attributed to single, non-genetic determinants. Single gene defects are recognised as such, and their mode of inheritance (autosomal or X-linked, dominant or recessive) derived, by the study of pedigrees. Chromosome abnormalities are identified by cytogenetic studies. As the techniques for staining chromosome preparations continue to improve, smaller and smaller structural defects and rearrangements can be identified.

Multifactorial causation is best studied by epidemiological methods which seek first to identify factors associated with particular defects and then to test the hypothesis that a particular factor is causally related to the defect. The first approach is essentially observational, and may identify people (population subgroups), places (from small locations to entire countries) and time periods (from days to decades) in which particular birth defects are more or less common than in others. Confirmatory studies are usually of the cohort (prospective) or case-control (retrospective) design. Time trends may also be informative (see below).

Turning to everyday clinical problems, the possible relationships between environmental chemicals and human birth defects tend to arise in one of three contexts:

1. Here is a baby with a birth defect. What caused it? Specifically, is it attributable to a chemical to which one or other parent was exposed before or during pregnancy?
2. Here is a chemical (most often a drug). Is it 'safe' to administer to a pregnant woman?
3. Here is a statistically significant association between a chemical and a birth defect. Did the chemical cause the defect?

The parents of a defective baby will strive to find an explanation for the abnormality. This is in part because of strong, if irrational, feelings of guilt, and the hope of expiation by laying the blame at someone else's door. Memories will be searched, relatives quizzed and skeletons dragged from family cupboards in the hope of finding 'the reason'. Since thalidomide, it has been customary to blame 'the tablets', but since many pregnant women avoid taking drugs, alternatives may be suggested, including food additives, occupational and recreational exposures, domestic and gardening products, visual display units, illnesses, anaesthetics, intra-uterine devices, falls, emotional shocks, and so on. The clinician will be asked – was this the cause? Or – even more difficult – could it have contributed to the causation?

If the environmental agent proposed is indeed an acknowledged teratogen, and the defect consistent with what is known about it, the suspicion may be confirmed. If the defect is known to have a genetic cause, the suspicion may be rejected [although phenocopies of genetic disorders are known: punctate epiphyseal dysplasia may be of genetic origin but may also be caused by the anticoagulant drug warfarin (Warkany 1975)].

More often, the clinician can only say whether a causal relationship is possible or impossible. Provided that the time of exposure to the agent under suspicion is known with reasonable accuracy in relation to the stage of gestation, it may be possible to say that the exposure was too late to have been causal. For example, closure of the neural tube to form the primitive brain and spinal cord is normally complete by the 28th day from conception (when the mother is '6 weeks pregnant'). An exposure to a suspected agent at 8 weeks could therefore not be causal for neural tube defects. It cannot be said with equal confidence that an exposure was too early to be causal, because a chemical or its metabolites could – in theory, at least – have a delayed action. Hence the time relationships may enable clinicians to decide between the possible and the impossible (though they may not be believed!). A possibility can never become a certainty in an isolated case. A similar relationship (same chemical, same timing, same defect) in two instances would be suspicious, in three instances suggestive, of a causal link, especially if the chemical was rarely used and the defect rarely seen. But such observations can only raise hypotheses which then need to be tested: except that, if the association is strongly suggestive of a causal relationship, ethical considerations may preclude certain forms of investigation that might otherwise be scientifically desirable.

The first suspicion of environmental teratogens has most often been made by astute clinicians [e.g. rubella (Gregg 1941), X-irradiation (Murphy 1929), thalidomide (McBride 1961; Lenz 1962)], although the birth defects monitoring systems set up worldwide over the last 25 years occasionally pick up something of potential importance [e.g. valproate and spina bifida (Robert and Guibaud 1982)]. The further interpretation of these associations is discussed later.

The investigation of multifactorial defects is perhaps the most difficult of all because there is no one cause. The defect may be the consequence of a dozen or more factors acting synergistically, in which case even the most complex statistical treatments may not demonstrate any significant effect from each of these factors analysed separately. Furthermore, the factors which are relevant in one instance may not be exactly the same as those that are significant in another. Reference has already been made to phenocopies of 'genetic' defects. By the same token, just because six babies are born with cleft palates that are anatomically identical, it should not be assumed that their causations are identical. The most helpful clues are likely to come from epidemiological studies.

What about the safety of drugs and other chemicals? The Medicines Commission and the Committee on Safety of Medicines (CSM) were amongst the many consequences of thalidomide. Their functions include the system of voluntary reporting of suspected adverse reactions (the yellow card scheme), and the scrutiny of all drugs prior to marketing. Drugs already marketed when the CSM was established are being scrutinised in the same way by the Committee on Review of Medicines (CRM). The CSM and the CRM perform some useful functions, but their impact on the risk of drug teratogenicity is almost impossible to assess.

The yellow card scheme, like most voluntary notification schemes, can claim only limited success. Notified associations between drugs taken during pregnancy and birth defects can only give an indication that a particular association needs to be thoroughly investigated. To date, the yellow card scheme has not led to the identification of any teratogenic agent, although some other and important side effects have been brought to light.

So far as the testing of drugs in animals is concerned, this has been described as 'more in the nature of a public relations exercise than a serious contribution to drug safety' (Smithells 1986). That is perhaps a trifle overstated, but the present arrangements in the United Kingdom do seem to put the emphasis in the wrong place.

First, a drug that has teratogenic properties in any animal species will not reach the market and it can therefore never be judged how good a predictor of the human situation the animal tests are. It is known that non-human primates do not always resemble humans more closely than other mammalian species in their responses to drugs.

Secondly, it was not until Somers (1962) gave thalidomide to a New Zealand white rabbit that the human response was reproduced, and it was only because it was known what thalidomide did to humans that these rabbits were shown to be a more appropriate model than rats.

Third, drugs like aspirin and corticosteroids that are clearly teratogenic in some animals (Larsson et al. 1963; Fraser and Fainstat 1951) continue to be used in humans.

Fourth, if a new drug passes its animal reproductive and other studies with fly-ing colours and reaches the market, the data sheet will either counsel against giv-ing the drug in pregnancy because of a theoretical risk of teratogenesis (e.g. a folic acid antagonist) or will advise that it be used with caution in pregnancy. How does one use a drug with caution? Swallow the medicine in small sips, or inject it very slowly? Or should the doctor caution the patient that it is not quite certain what the consequences will be?

But the fifth and greatest paradox lies in what, by and large, is *not* done. Great trouble and expense is involved in animal tests, the significance of which remains largely guesswork. Comes the great day when it is given to humans and what hap-pens? Almost nothing. Of course it would be morally indefensible to give a new drug to several hundred pregnant women in order to find out whether it was ter-atogenic. Nevertheless, it will be given to pregnant women, even if some of them did not realise they were pregnant at the time. The paradox of new drugs has been discussed elsewhere (Smithells 1975). If a clinician wishes to compare a new drug with an old one, or with a placebo, that is research and the approval of the hos-pital's research ethics committee must be sought. However, if the same clinician just finds the salesman so persuasive that he or she throws over previous treat-ment in favour of the new drug, it is not research and nobody need be asked. Per-mission is needed to give it to half the patients attended, but not to give it to them all.

The logical answer is post-marketing surveillance – a system whereby there is close monitoring of every new drug marketed for humans for as many years as it takes to provide the necessary information. It is well known that there is no such thing as absolute safety, because there is no method for excluding very small risks in humans. Furthermore, if the majority of mothers who take a particular drug at the relevant stage of pregnancy give birth to healthy babies,how can it be said that the drug is teratogenic? If there is still a residual association, either the defect is multifactorial and the drug may be one factor in some cases; or a few individual embryos react idiosyncratically to the drug. If 1% of people who take Toxomycin come out in a rash, they are allergic to it. If 1% of women who take it in preg-nancy have babies with spina bifida, the drug is a 'minor teratogen'.

Clinicians are usually in the business of risk/benefit ratios, with the risks and benefits often poorly understood. A woman with pregnancy nausea or vomiting that is not severe is probably wise to avoid drugs, although some of the drugs used for this purpose have, thanks largely to lawsuits, been more thoroughly investi-gated than most. An epileptic woman embarking on a pregnancy is usually wise to remain on treatment, although her drugs and dosage might usefully be re-viewed, and some would advocate a folic acid supplement.

How can the problem of teratogenicity be studied in humans? First, consider drugs that are already in regular clinical use. The three dimensions of epidemiol-ogy are time, place and people. In the time dimension, an association can be sought between the prevalence of defects and the prevalence of the drug. For ex-ample, the limb defects associated with thalidomide were almost unknown in the UK before 1959, increased in birth prevalence through 1960 and 1961, continued to increase until the second half of 1962 (the drug had been withdrawn in November 1961), and then dropped dramatically, with occasional cases only in the first half of 1963 and almost none since (Smithells and Leck 1963). Conversely, the steady increase in the use of Debendox (Bendectin) in Northern Ireland from 1966 to 1978 was not associated with any increase in any birth defect (Harron et al. 1980): nor, does it appear that there has been any decrease since this drug was withdrawn from the market.

Thalidomide also illustrates the place dimension. In the Federal Republic of Germany it was available over the counter, and the related birth defects were widespread. In the UK it was available only on prescription and the problems were less extensive. In the United States of America it did not get beyond the clinical trials stage and cases were very rare.

But at the end of the day it is individual humans that must be studied, and it is unlikely that such a strong – almost obligate – teratogen as thalidomide will be encountered again. The humans studied may be women who take the drug under consideration – a prospective or cohort study – or babies with birth defects – a retrospective or case-control study. In both cases there are two big difficulties: the accuracy of the data and the adequacy of the controls. Clinicians tend to be good at diagnostic accuracy and cavalier about methodology. Epidemiologists and statisticians tend to be obsessional about methodology and have a touching faith in the reliability of other people's data.

Cohort studies begin with a group of women who have taken the study drug early in pregnancy and a second group who have not, and compare the outcome of their pregnancies. The chief advantage is that the drug intake is recorded at the time, and before the outcome of the pregnancy is known. The disadvantages are (a) that large numbers are needed; (b) a quick study is impossible; (c) controls are imperfect, however much 'matching' is done. Confounding variables make interpretation, especially of small differences, difficult. In practice, the timing of administration is often only given as 'first trimester', which is not good enough, and the sophistication of the statistical treatment often exceeds the accuracy of the data.

Case-control studies begin with a group of deformed babies and a second group who have some other defect, or no defect, and compare their mothers' drug histories. The advantages are that relatively small numbers are needed, and a quick study may be possible. The disadvantages are (a) that pregnancy outcome is known and drug histories obtained from mothers may be biased (though contemporary records will not), and (b) again the controls are imperfect.

The tendency of humans to produce offspring one at a time, thereby depriving most people of litter-mates, leads to the conclusion that only randomised studies have adequate controls. This leads to the next paradox. In the UK, the Medical Research Council is currently engaged in a randomised trial of vitamin supplementation in very early pregnancy (Anon. 1985). This is being done to see whether they can confirm observation of a greatly reduced rate of recurrence of neural tube defects in vitamin-supplemented mothers. This and other related studies are ethically acceptable because they start from the premise that they may do good. But if an identical study was proposed as a method of testing vitamins for teratogenicity, it would never be allowed.

The National Health Service in the UK, and particularly the handling of prescriptions by general practitioners, provides a magnificent opportunity to link drugs to birth defects or any other consequence. Prescription pricing bureaux can identify and preserve all prescriptions for a given drug from a given area over a specified time, and the majority can be linked to the patients to whom they were issued. This method was used to investigate meclozine in the early 1960s (Smithells and Chinn 1964), and more recently to study the drug combination Debendox (Smithells and Sheppard 1978), since withdrawn from the market. This approach has been greatly refined and developed by Dr. Inman's unit in Southampton (Inman and Weber 1986).

There will always be a multitude of approaches to the problems of teratogenesis. Clinicians are constantly diverted by the immediacies of patient care. They are on the whole unscientific, unsystematic, disorganised, empirical, mathematically and pharmacologically illiterate. But they do develop antennae, which sometimes twitch.

References

Anon (1985) Prevention of recurrent neural tube defects: Medical Research Council vitamin study. Lancet II:1023

Fraser FC, Fainstat TD (1951) Production of congenital defects in offspring of pregnant mice treated with cortisone. Pediatrics 8:527–533

Gregg N (1941) Congenital cataracts following German measles in the mother. Trans Ophthalmol Soc Austr 3:35–46

Harron DWG, Griffiths K, Shanks RG (1980) Debendox and congenital malformations in Northern Ireland. Br Med J 281:1379–1381

Inman WHW, Weber JCP (1986) Post-marketing surveillance in the general population in the United Kingdom. In: Inman WHW (ed) Monitoring for drug safety, 2nd edn. MTP Press, Lancester, pp 13–47

Larsson KS, Boström H, Ericson B (1963) Salicylate-induced malformations in mouse embryos. Acta Paediatr Scand 52:36–40

Lenz W (1962) Thalidomide and congenital abnormalities. Lancet I:45

McBride WG (1961) Thalidomide and congenital abnormalities. Lancet II:1358

Murphy DP (1929) The outcome of 625 pregnancies in women subjected to pelvic radium or roentgen irradiation. Am J Obstet Gynecol 18:179–187

Robert E, Guibaud P (1982) Maternal valproic acid and congenital neural tube defects. Lancet II:937

Smithells RW (1975) Iatrogenic hazards and their effects. In: Barltrop D (ed) Paediatrics and the environment. Fellowship of Postgraduate Medicine, London, pp 39–43

Smithells RW (1986) Drug teratogenicity. In: Inman WHW (ed) Monitoring for drug safety, 2nd edn. MTP Press, Lancaster, pp 383–390

Smithells RW, Chinn ER (1964) Meclozine and foetal malformations: a prospective study. Br Med J 1:217–218

Smithells RW, Leck I (1963) The incidence of limb and car defects since the withdrawal of thalidomide. Lancet I:1095–1097

Smithells RW, Sheppard S (1978) Teratogenicity testing in humans: a method demonstrating safety of Bendectin. Teratology 17:31–35

Somers GF (1962) Thalidomide and congenital abnormalities. Lancet I:912–913

Warkany J (1975) A warfarin embryopathy? Am J Dis Child 129:287–288

Mechanisms and Models in Toxicology
Arch. Toxicol., Suppl. 11, 128–139 (1987)

Teratogenicity of Valproic Acid and Related Substances in the Mouse: Drug Accumulation and pH$_i$ in the Embryo During Organogenesis and Structure-Activity Considerations*

H. Nau[1] and W. J. Scott[2]

[1] Institut für Toxikologie und Embryopharmakologie, Freie Universität Berlin,
  Garystraße 5, D-1000 Berlin (West) 33, Germany
[2] University of Cincinnati, Children's Hospital Research Foundation, Cincinnati, Ohio 45229, USA

Introduction

The antiepileptic drug valproic acid is a putative human teratogen as suggested by retrospective studies (Robert and Rosa 1983; Lindhout and Meinardi 1984), a number of case reports (reviewed in Tein and McGregor 1985) and prospective investigations (Koch et al. 1983; Jäger-Roman et al. 1986; Nau et al. 1981a). The use of thus drug for seizure control during pregnancy was shown to result in an increased incidence of neural tube defects, in particular spina bifida aperta in addition to numerous other malformations, particularly of the face and the skeletal structures. Clinical doses range between 10–40 mg/kg/day administered as a single daily dose (Rowan et al. 1981) or in divided doses (Gjerloff et al. 1984). The therapeutic range is said to be between 50–100 µg/ml, although peak drug levels may be much higher: Rowan et al. (1981) reported peak levels of 180 µg/ml in a patient treated with a once-a-day dosing regimen. We have recently measured peak levels of 120 and 184 µg/ml in two epileptic patients during the first trimester of pregnancy (Jäger-Roman et al. 1986).

Valproic acid is also teratogenic in mouse (Nau et al. 1981b; Kao et al. 1981; Eluma et al. 1984; Nau 1985; 1986), hamster (Moffa et al. 1984), rat (Ong et al. 1983), rabbit (Petrere et al. 1986) and monkey (Mast et al. 1985; 1986). Skeletal objects were observed in all animal species, but neural tube defects only in the mouse and the hamster. The doses needed to ellicit a teratogenic response in the animals were about 5–10 times higher than the therapeutic doses in man. Peak drug levels in the mouse (Nau 1985; 1986) and the monkey (Mast et al. 1986), resulting in significant teratogenicity, were about 300 µg of total valproic acid per ml maternal plasma if the drug was administered once a day throughout organogenesis. Because of lowered plasma protein binding at these high teratogenic drug levels (only about 40–60% of the drug was protein-bound at these high concentrations), the teratogenic peak concentrations of free drug were between 120–200 µg/ml. Thus, also the free drug concentration peaks – which

---

Dedicated to Prof. Dr. H. Herken on the occasion of his 75th birthday.

are of particular importance in regard to teratogenicity as discussed below – are considerably higher in experimental animals than those expected during therapy (the subject of species differences in pharmacokinetics and teratogenicity was recently by Nau 1986b).

In this paper it is shown that valproic acid, as well as some other acids drugs, accumulates in the early mouse embryo during organogenesis because of the alkaline embryonic milieu. Studies with substances related to valproic acid demonstrate a strict structural requirement of teratogenic activity.

Material and Methods

Teratological Studies

Female NMRI mice were mated with males for a period of 2 h (from 8–10 a.m.). The following day was designated day 0 if vaginal plugs were found. Altromin 1324 diet and tap water were given ad libitum. All acidic drugs were administered as the sodium salts, ethosuximide and valpromide (valproic acid amide) as such. The vehicle was water except for valpromide, where 50% ethanol was used as solvent. The doses used and the administration regimens are explained in the legends to the Figure and Tables.

Teratological examinations were performed on day 18 of gestation. Implantation sites were counted and each fetus was weighed individually and inspected for the presence of neural tube defects. Internal malformations were evaluated with Wilson's slicing technique (Wilson 1965).

Placental Transfer Studies

At various times after injection of the drugs on day 9 of gestation (morning) a maternal blood sample was taken from the abdominal aorta and the embryos were removed from the uterus. Maternal plasma was prepared by centrifugation, the embryos were accurately weighed, and all samples were then stored at $-30\,°C$ until analysis.

Measurement of Intracellular pH

$[^{14}C]$Dimethadione (100 μCi/mouse; specific activity 50 mCi/mmol) was injected i.p. One hours after injection, when the drug had reached transplacental equilibrium, radioactivity was determined in maternal plasma and embryo by liquid scintillation spectrometry, and the pH of the maternal blood was measured with a blood gas analyzer. The extracellular embryonic space (55–58%) was determined via measurements of the chloride concentrations in maternal plasma and embryo. Embryonic pH was calculated by the formula of Waddell and Butler (1959).

Test Compounds

Valproic acid (sodium salt), 2-en-valproic acid, valpromide and ethosuximide
were obtained from Desitin Werk Carl Klinke, Hamburg (Dr. H. Schäfer).

CH$_3$–CH$_2$–CH$_2$
                    ⟩CH–COOH
CH$_3$–CH$_2$–CH$_2$

valproic acid

CH$_3$–CH$_2$–CH$_2$
                    ⟩CH–CONH$_2$
CH$_3$–CH$_2$–CH$_2$

valpromide

CH$_3$–CH$_2$–CH
                  ⟩C–COOH
CH$_3$–CH$_2$–CH$_2$

2-en-valproic acid

            O
            ‖
CH$_3$–CH$_2$–C
                  ⟩CH–COOH
CH$_3$–CH$_2$–CH$_2$

3-keto-valproic acid

              CH$_3$
               |
CH$_2$–C–CH$_2$–CH$_3$
        | ⟩C=O
    O⟍C–NH
     O

ethosuximide

Analytical Measurements

All drugs and their metabolites were extracted and analyzed by a gas chromatography-mass spectrometry-computer method (Nau et al. 1981b) with appropriate
selection of ions to be monitored ($M^+ - 15$ ions). Protein binding was measured
by ultrafiltration using YMT membranes (Amicon, Danvers, Mass) as described
by Wittfoht et al. (1984).

Results and Discussion

Placental Transfer in the Mouse on Day 9 of Gestation

Valproic acid concentrations in the embryo exceeded corresponding free maternal plasma levels after injection of the drug both i.p. (Fig. 1) and s.c. (Fig. 2), by
a factor of about 2. Plasma protein binding was about 40%–50%, so that the maternal plasma concentrations of the total drug (not shown) were in the same range
as the embryo levels (Nau and Scott 1986). Metabolite levels were very low, both
in plasma and embryo (see 2-en-valproic acid in maternal plasma in Fig. 2 as an
example).

    Following administration of the main plasma metabolite 2-en-valproic acid, this
substance was also found to accumulate in the embryo (Fig. 3). The embryo concentrations of 2-en-valproic acid at 1 and 2 h were slightly lower than of the parent
drug. Since the free maternal plasma concentrations of both compounds were
similar, the accumulation of the metabolite in the embryo was lower than of the
parent drug. After 1 h the drug concentrations of the metabolite decreased much
more rapidly than those of the parent drug. Interestingly, small amounts of valproic acid were also produced via metabolism of 2-en-valproic acid (Fig. 3); anal-

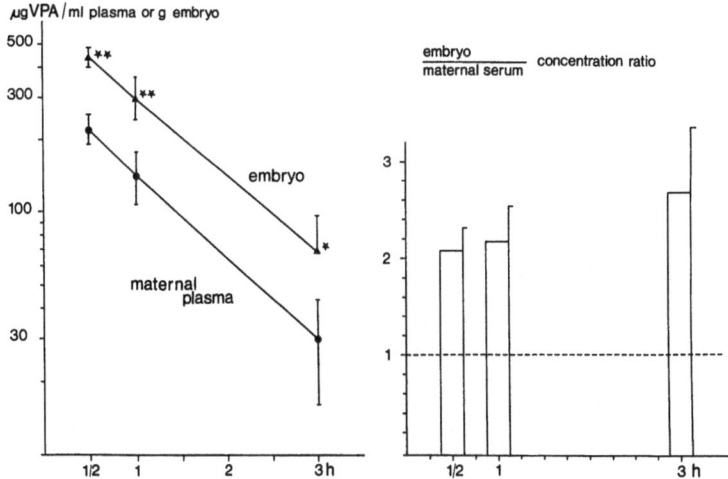

Fig. 1. Valproic acid concentrations in embryo proper and maternal plasma following a single dose i.p. of 300 mg sodium valproate/kg body wt. on day 9 of gestation

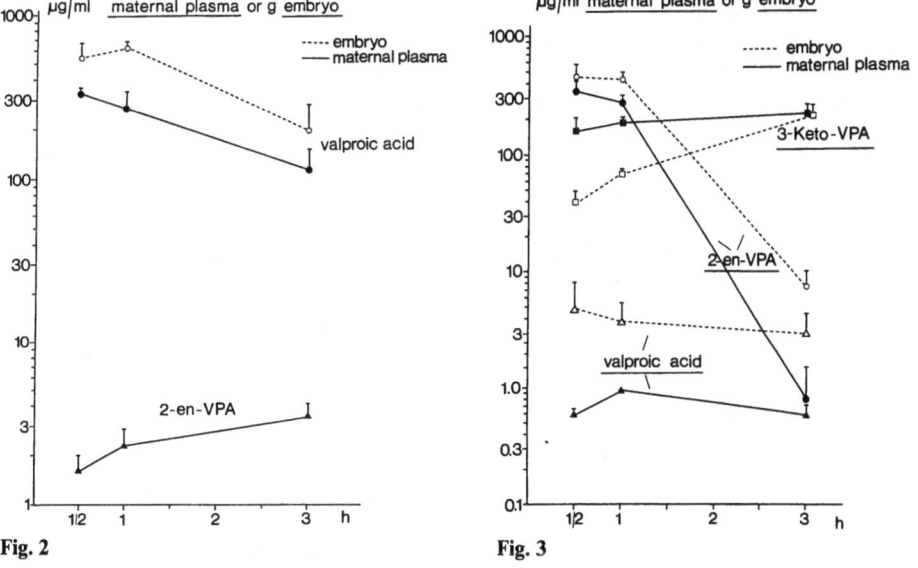

Fig. 2. Valproic acid concentrations in embryo proper and maternal plasma following a single dose s.c. of 400 mg sodium valproate/kg body wt. on day 9 of gestation. At ½ h, 1 h, and 3 h the weights of the embryos were 1.4 ± 0.54 mg, 1.5 ± 0.92 mg, and 1.9 ± 0.95 mg; the somite counts were 18 ± 2.6, 18 ± 2.6, and 18 ± 3.6; the maternal blood pH was 7.19 ± 0.06, 7.20 ± 0.01, and 7.18 ± 0.09, respectively (mean$\pm$S.D.; $n=5$)

Fig. 3. 2-en-valproic acid concentrations in embryo proper and maternal plasma following a single dose s.c. of 400 mg sodium 2-en-valproate/kg body wt. on day 9 of gestation. At ½ h, 1 h, and 3 h the weights of the embryos were 1.4 ± 0.9 mg, 1.6 ± 0.9 mg, and 1.7 ± 0.4 mg; the somite counts were 14 ± 2.9, 17.5 ± 3.9, and 17 ± 1.7; the maternal blood pH was 7.29 ± 0.03, 7.27 ± 0.02, 7.46 ± 0.02, respectively (mean$\pm$S.D.; $n=4$)

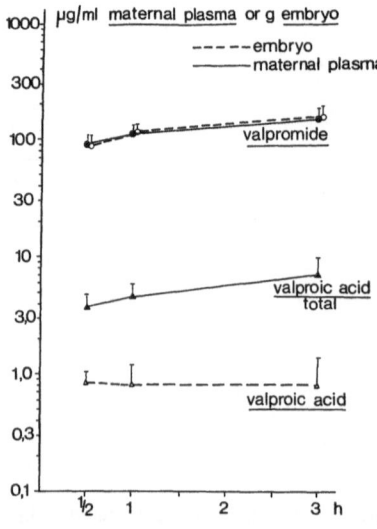

Fig. 4. Valpromide (valproic acid amide) concentrations in embryo proper and maternal plasma following a single dose s.c. of 400 mg/kg body wt. on day 9 of gestation. At ½ h, 1 h, and 3 h the weights of the embryos were 1.0 ± 0.4 mg, 1.4 ± 0.5 mg, and 1.6 ± 1.0 mg; the somite counts were 14 ± 1.7, 17 ± 1.7, and 18 ± 3.5; the maternal blood pH was 7.18 ± 0.07; 7.13 ± 0.05; and 7.08 ± 0.04, respectively (means$\pm$S.D.; $n=4$)

ysis of the 2-en-valproic acid administered did not show any trace of valproic acid. The main metabolite of 2-en-valproic acid is the 3-Keto-valproic acid which is present in large and increasing amounts both in maternal plasma and embryo. Apparently, this more polar metabolite is more slowly transferred to the embryo; the embryo concentrations increased during the time studied to approach the maternal plasma levels at 3 h (Fig. 3).

In contrast to the two acidic compounds discussed above, the essentially neutral valpromide reached very similar concentrations in plasma and embryo (Fig. 4). Only small amounts of valproic acid were produced via hydrolysis of the amide bond. Also, the essentially neutral drug ethosuximide reached similar concentrations in maternal plasma and embryo (Nau and Scott 1986).

Structure and Teratogenicity

Valproic acid was highly teratogenic in the mouse, and neural tube defects (exencephaly) were produced in a dose- and concentration-dependent manner. Probit analysis of maternal plasma concentration–response curves showed that a 10% incidence of exencephaly in live fetuses was produced by peak drug concentrations of 445 µg/ml (single injection s.c. on day 8 of gestation, the time of maximum sensitivity for this malformation), of 322 µg/ml (injection once daily), of 273 µg/ml (injection twice daily) or of 225 µg/ml (injection four times daily); steady levels of 248 µg/ml were needed (via osmotic minipump administration) to produce the same incidence of exencephaly (Nau 1985).

A number of malformations in addition to exencephaly were produced by a single administration of valproic acid between day 7½ and day 9 (Table 1). Particularly noteworthy are the malformations of the uterine horn, the kidney, and the limbs. Other malformations such as cleft palate are produced in a much higher incidence at later treatment periods. Skeletal defects are also very prominent (Kao et al. 1981).

Table 1. Malformations produced by valproic acid in the mouse as determined by Wilson's slicing technique (Wilson 1965)

	Saline injection		Administration of a single dose of 600 mg sodium valproate/kg body wt.							
	Day 8		Day 7.5		Day 8		Day 8.5		Day 9	
Hypoplastic uterine horn	0/ 51	0	0/49	0	6/ 51	12%	6/42	16%	2/36	6%
Agenesis uterine horn	0/ 51	0	0/49	0	3/ 51	6%	5/42	12%	0/36	0
Misplaced ovaries	0/ 51	0	0/49	0	1/ 51	2%	0/42	0	0/36	0
Hypoplastic ovaries	0/ 51	0	0/49	0	0/ 51	0	1/42	2%	0/36	0
Cryptorchid	0/ 53	0	0/47	0	2/ 56	4%	0/46	0	0/43	0
Stage 3 hydronephrosis	0/104	0	0/96	0	4/107	4%	5/88	6%	8/79	10%
Hydronephrosis	0/104	0	0/96	0	7/107	7%	3/88	3%	1/79	1%
Agenesis kidney	0/104	0	0/96	0	1/107	0.9%	1/88	1%	0/79	0
Agenesis ureter	0/104	0	0/96	0	1/107	0.9%	2/88	2%	0/79	0
Abnormal limbs	1/104	1%	0/96	0	1/107	0.9%	10/88	11%	15/79	19%
Folded retina	3/104	3%	1/96	1%	6/107	6%	0/88	0	0/79	0
Microphthalmia	0/104	0	0/96	0	5/107	5%	0/88	0	0/79	0
Cleft palate	0/104	0	0/96	0	0/107	0	0/88	0	1/79	1%
Facial cleft	0/104	0	0/96	0	4/107	4%	2/88	2%	0/79	0
Hypoplastic ureter	0/104	0	0/96	0	0/107	0	1/88	1%	0/79	0
Heart defect	0/104	0	0/96	0	0/107	0	0/88	0	1/79	1%
Agenesis of tail	0/104	0	1/96	1%	0/107	0	0/88	0	0/79	0
Short tail	0/104	0	0/96	0	0/107	0	0/88	0	2/79	3%
Curly tail	0/104	0	0/96	0	0/107	0	1/88	1%	0/79	0

The data are presented as follows: number of fetuses affected/number of fetuses examined and % of incidence.

A recent study involving 18 substances demonstrated that the teratogenicity of valproic acid in the mouse in vivo gives evidence of very strict structural requirements (Nau and Löscher 1986). Homologous compounds with shorter or longer alkyl chains were less teratogenic. Substitution of the α-H atoms (e.g., 2-methyl-2-ethylhexanoic acid) abolished the teratogenic response. Introduction of a double bond in the ω-position (4-en-valproic acid) did not change the malformation rate, a ω-2 double bond (2-en-valproic acid) abolished teratogenicity. Straight-chain acids (octanoic acid) and the antiepileptic drugs valpromide and ethosuximide, also in clinical use in humans, did not induce neural tube defects.

The reasons for the high specificity of the teratogenic response of this class of compounds are not known. Pharmacokinetics differences are probably only part of the answer. It may be that some of these drugs with low teratogenic potency do not reach the embryo in concentrations sufficient to result in a teratogenic response. Straight-chain acids such as octanoic acid are very efficiently cleared in the organism and it is feasible that this rapid elimination prevents the buildup of adequate embryonic concentrations.

Such considerations do not hold true in the case of 2-en-valproic acid. This compound was shown to be efficiently transferred to the embryo both in vivo in the mouse (Nau 1986c; Nau and Scott 1986; see also Fig. 3) and in rat embryos in vitro (Lewandowski et al. 1986). This compound may therefore become an excellent tool for studying the mechanism of valproic acid-induced teratogenicity. Furthermore, since 2-en-valproic acid exhibits anticonvulsant activity similar to valproic acid in several animal models, albeit at somwhat higher sedation (Nau et al. 1984; Löscher et al. 1984), this metabolite may lead the way to the development of compounds with the desired anticonvulsant properties, but lower teratogenic potency.

It may be hypothesized that maternal plasma protein binding may be an important parameter of teratogenicity, since only the free concentrations (not bound to proteins) can equilibrate with the embryo and thus elicit a direct teratogenic response. Indeed, at low concentrations great differences exist in regard to the protein binding of the acidic drugs discussed here. For one example, 2-en-valproic acid is much more highly bound (98.5%) than valproic acid (67%) at plasma concentrations of 10 µg/ml in the mouse (Nau and Löscher 1986). At higher concentrations, which are significant in regard to teratogenicity in vivo (>200 µg/ml), the plasma protein binding of acidic drugs in this class becomes more and more similar because of a strong concentration dependence. Acidic drugs usually have two high-affinity binding sites on albumin. Therefore, above 200–250 µg/ml both binding sites will be occupied. Thus, at 300 µg/ml maternal plasma, the protein binding of valproic acid was 42%, of 2-en-valproic acid 47%, of octanoic acid 68%, and of 2-butylhexanoic acid 72% (Nau and Löscher 1986). Thus, the extent of protein binding may explain some quantitative difference in teratogenic potency of the various acidic drugs, but cannot explain the drastic differences observed.

Therefore, structural considerations must play an important role. It is hypothesized that 2-en-valproic acid may be nonteratogenic because of the absence of a α-H atom. Some other acids lacking an α-H atom were therefore tested and indeed also found to be nonteratogenic: 2-methyl-2-ethyl-hexanoic acid; 2,2-dimethyl-pentanoic acid; 1-methyl-1-cyclohexanoic acid. Detailed placental transfer studies with one of these compounds will therefore be performed in the future to see if indeed – as is the case with 2-en-valproic acid – the intrinsic teratogenic activity of these substances is low, or if the compound does not reach the embryo in adequate concentrations.

Intracellular pH of Mouse Embryo During Organogenesis

It was recently demonstrated that the intracellular pH (pH$_i$) of the rodent embryo during early organogenesis is surprisingly high (Scott et al. 1987; Scott and Nau 1985; Nau and Scott 1986). The pH$_i$ of the mouse embryo on days 8 and 9 of gestation was found to be almost 0.4 units above maternal blood pH (Table 2). The pH$_i$ subsequently drops to reach a value similar to maternal blood pH on day 11 and was below maternal blood pH at later gestational stages (Table 2).

These significant differences between embryonic pH$_i$ and maternal blood pH have important consequences in regard to transplacental distribution and possibly teratogenicity of weakly acidic drugs. If it can be assumed that only the nonionized form of the drug is able to traverse membranes, then the degree of ionization on both sides of the placental membranes will determine the transplacental concentration gradient. An acidic drug such as valproic acid will be ionized to a

Table 2. Intracellular pH of mouse embryo as compared to maternal plasma pH between day 8 and day 12 of gestation[a]

Day of gestation	Somites (range)	n	Maternal blood pH	Embryonic pH$_i$
8	3– 6	4	7.34±0.03	7.70±0.10
9	10–23	4	7.27±0.10	7.65±0.02
10	31–33	5	7.33±0.06	7.46±0.06
11	40–46	4	7.24±0.06	7.22±0.06
12	49–53	5	7.30–0.10	7.12±0.10

[a] For a detailed discussion of stage-specific changes of embryonic pH$_i$, see Scott et al. (1987).

higher degree in the relatively basic milieu of the early embryo than in maternal plasma. Based on the pK_a of valproic acid (4.7), the pH partition hypothesis would predict a concentration of the drug in the embryo twice as high as in maternal plasma (Fig. 5; Nau and Scott 1986). This was indeed found to be true experimentally, as demonstrated in Figs. 1 and 2. Accumulation in the embryo was also found for valproic acid and methoxyacetic acid, a metabolite of methoxyethanol, in the early rat embryo.

Also, 2-en-valproic acid concentrations were higher in the mouse embryo than in maternal plasma (see Fig. 3), and dimethadione accumulation in rat and mouse embryo was used to calculate embryonic pH$_i$ (Scott et al. 1987; Nau and Scott 1986).

A thalidomide metabolite (a glutamic acid derivative; Keberle et al. 1965) as well as a halothane metabolite (probably trifluoroacetic acid; Danielsson et al. 1984) were also found to accumulate in the rabbit blastocyst and mouse embryo, respectively (Table 3). It has been hypothesized that such polar metabolites may be trapped in the embryo after they have been produced via metabolism of the parent drugs; but the pH partition hypothesis is just as likely to provide an explanation for the embryonic accumulation of these acidic metabolites. The distribu-

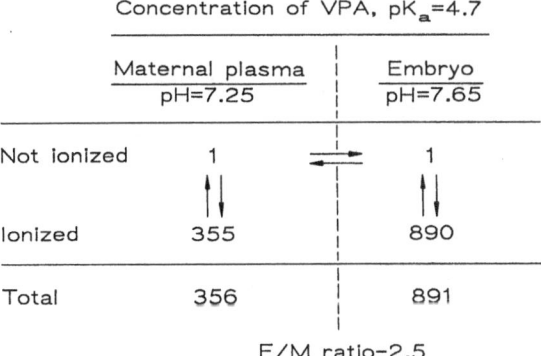

Fig. 5. Distribution of valproic acid across membranes at postdistribution equilibrium via nonionic diffusion. Calculations by the Henderson–Hasselbach equation was based on the pK_a of valproic acid and the maternal plasma pH and embryonic pH$_i$

Table 3. Summary of available data on the teratogenicity and embryo/maternal (E/M) plasma concentration ratios of acidic substances and related compounds with low ionizing potential

Drug	Species	Placental transfer		Terato-genic	Reference
		Period of gestation	E/M ratio		
Valproic acid	Mouse	Day 9	1.6–2.3 (Fig. 1,2)	Yes	Nau and Scott (1986); Kao et al. (1981); Nau et al. (1981c); Scott and Nau (1985)
Valproic acid	Rat	Day 11	1.5–1.7	Yes	Mast et al. (1985); Nau and Scott (1986); Ong et al. (1983)
Salicylic acid	Rat	Day 10	1.3–1.7	Yes	Tagashira et al. (1981)
Thalidomide (acid metabolite)	Rabbit	Day 8 (blastocyst)	1.2	Yes	Keberle et al. (1965)
Dimethadione	Mouse	Day 9	1.4–1.7	Yes	Scott et al. (1986); Fabro et al. (1984)
	Rat	Day 11		Yes	
Halothane (trichloroacetic acid)	Mouse	Day 11	Accumulation of radioactivity	Yes	Danielsson et al. (1984)
Methoxyethanol (methoxyacetic acid)	Rat	Day 12	2	Yes	Brown et al. (1984); Ritter et al. (1985)
Hydrochloric acid (acidified sea water)	Sea urchin embryo, in vitro	5 h (32 cells)	–	Yes	Pagano et al. (1985)
2-n-Valproic acid	Mouse	Day 9	1.2–1.5 (Fig. 3)	No (minimally)[a]	Nau and Scott (1986); Nau et al. (1984)
Valpromide	Mouse	Day 9	1 (Fig. 4)	No	Nau and Scott (1986); Nau and Löscher (1986)
Ethosuximide	Mouse	Day 9	1	No	Nau and Scott (1986); Nau and Löscher (1986)

[a] The highest dose used (600 mg/kg i.p.), which already approached the LD_{50} (Löscher and Nau 1985) resulted in a 10% resorption rate and 3.5% incidence of exencephaly (background level of exencephaly 0–1.5%).

tion of essentially neutral drugs such as the anticonvulsants valpromide (see Fig. 4) and ethosuximide (see Table 3) should not be affected by transplacental pH gradient; indeed concentrations of these two drugs in the embryo were essentially the same as corresponding concentrations in maternal plasma.

It should be pointed out in this context that a number of human teratogens or their metabolites are weakly acidic substances: valproic acid, trimethadione (metabolite dimethadione), phenytoin, thalidomide (glutamic acid derivatives as metabolites), warfarin, isotretinoin, etretinate (metabolite etretin), among others. Basic drugs are not represented in lists of human teratogens.

It may be that the predominance of acidic drugs in the list of human teratogens and possibly experimental teratogens as well (Freese et al. 1979) stems from the fact that these substances, as demonstrated here, accumulate in the early embryo, resulting in unexpectedly high "exposure" of the embryo as compared to the maternal organism. It may – alternatively or additionally – be that some weak acids are teratogenic because they can alter the pH_i of the embryonic cell, which is attractive as a general mechanism of teratogenesis because hydrogen ion activity controls or is associated with a number of cellular functions including proliferation and intercellular communication (cf. Aerts et al. 1985). Such pH_i changes have not yet been detected in embryos cultured *in vitro* (Brown 1987). However, preliminary experiments by Collins et al. (1986) showed that the pH_i of rat embryos actually was increased by maternal administration of teratogenic doses of valproic acid, acetazolamide, ethylhexanoic acid, and dimethadione. This rise, although quite contrary to expectation, was consistent and of considerable magnitude (0.15–0.30 pH units). Further studies with substances such as 2-en-valproic acid and possibly 2-methyl-2-ethyl-hexanoic acid – substances which are able to reach the embryo, but with low teratogenic potency – should demonstrate whether this alteration of embryonic pH_i has any significance in regard to teratogenicity.

Certainly, the fact that some related substances without an acid function do not accumulate in the embryo and exhibit very low teratogenic potency supports the hypothesis of a special significance of the acid function in regard to teratogenicity. Already Willhite and Shealy (1984) have shown that the amides of all-*trans* and 13-*cis*-retinoic acid were much less teratogenic in the hamster than the corresponding acids. The present authors have also demonstrated that valpromide and ethosuximide, both neutral substances, are essentially not teratogenic.

Acknowledgements. This work was supported by the Deutsche Forschungsgemeinschaft by a grant to the Sonderforschungsbereich 174. The preparation of the manuscript by Mrs. R. Ebbinghaus and N. Nau is gratefully acknowledged.

References

Aerts RJ, Durston AJ, Moolenaar WH (1985) Cytoplasmic pH and the regulation of the dictyostelium cell cycle. Cell 43:653–657

Brown NA (1987) Teratogenicity of carboxylic acids, distribution studies in whole embryo culture. In: Nau H, Scott WJ (eds) Pharmacokinetics in teratogenesis. CRC Press, Boca Raton, Florida (in press)

Brown NA, Holt D, Webb M (1984) The teratogenicity of methoxyacetic acid in the rat. Toxicol Lett 22:93–100

Collins MW, Scott W, Pitter E, Nau H, Wittfoht W (1986) Correlation of teratogenic potency with alteration of intracellular pH by C-8 carboxylic acids. Teratology 33:45C

Danielsson BRG, Ghantous H, Dencker L (1984) Accumulation in murine amniotic fluid of halothane and its metabolites. Acta Pharmacol Toxicol (Copenh) 55:410–417

Eluma FO, Sucheston ME, Hayes TG, Paulson RB (1984) Teratogenic effects of dosage levels and time of administration of carbamazepine, sodium valproate, and diphenylhydantoin on craniofacial development in the CD-1 mouse fetus. J Craniofac Genet Dev Biol 4:191–210

Fabro S, Shull G, Brown NA (1984) The teratogenicity of trimethadione and dimethadione. Teratogenesis Carcinog Mutagen 2:61–76

Freese E, Levin BC, Pearce R, Sreevalsan T, Kaufman JJ, Koski WS, Semo NM (1979) Correlation between the growth inhibitory effects, partition coefficients and teratogenic effects of lipophilic acids. Teratology 20:413–440

Gjerloff I, Arentsen J, Alving J, Secher BG (1984) Monodose versus 3 daily doses of sodium valproate: a controlled trial. Acta Neurol Scand 69:120–124

Jäger-Roman E, Deichl A, Jakob S, Hartmann AM, Koch S, Rating D, Steldinger R, Nau H, Helge H (1986) Fetal growth, major malformations and minor anomalies in infants born to women receiving valproic acid. J Pediatr 108:997–1004

Kao J, Brown NA, Schmid B, Goulding EH, Fabro S (1981) Teratogenicity of valproic acid: in vivo and in vitro investigations. Teratogenesis Carcinog Mutagen 1:367–382

Keberle H, Loustalot P, Maller RK, Faigle JW, Schmid K (1965) Biochemical effects of drugs in the mammalian conceptus. Ann NY Acad Sci 123:252–265

Koch S, Jäger-Roman E, Rating D. Helge H (1983) Possible teratogenic effect of valproate during pregnancy. J Pediatr 103:1007

Lewandowski C, Klug S, Nau H, Neubert D (1986) Pharmacokinetic aspects of drug effects in vitro: effects of serum protein binding on concentration and teratogenicity of valproic acid and 2-en-valproic acid in whole embryos in culture. Arch Toxicol 58:239–242

Lindhout D, Meinardi H (1984) Spina bifida and in utero exposure to valproate. Lancet II:396

Löscher W, Nau H (1985) Pharmacological evaluation of various metabolites and analogues of valproic acid. Neuropharmacology 24:427–435

Löscher W, Nau H, Marescaux C, Vergnes M (1984) Comparative evaluation of anticonvulsant and toxic potencies of valproic acid and 2-en-valproic acid in different animal models of epilepsy. Eur J Pharmacol 99:211–218

Mast TJ, Hendrickx AG, Nau H (1985) Teratology and pharmacokinetics of valproic acid in the rhesus monkey. Teratology 31:25A

Mast TJ, Cukierski MA, Nau H, Hendrickx AG (1986) Predicting the human teratogenic potential of the anticonvulsant, valproic acid, from a non-human primate model. Toxicology 39:111–119

Moffa AM, White JA, Mackay EG, Frias JL (1984) Valproic acid, zinc and open neural tubes in 9 day-old hamster embryos. Teratology 29:47A

Nau H (1985) Teratogenic valproic acid concentrations: infusion by implanted minipumps vs. conventional injection regimen in the mouse. Toxicol Appl Pharmacol 80:243–250

Nau H (1986a) Valproic acid teratogenicity in mice after various administration and phenobarbital-pretreatment regimens: the parent drug and not one of the metabolites assayed is implicated as teratogen. Fundam Appl Toxicol 6:662–668

Nau H (1986b) Species differences in pharmacokinetics and drug teratogenesis. Environ Health Persp in press

Nau H (1986c) Transfer of valproic acid and its main active unsaturated metabolite to the gestational tissue: correlation with neural tube defect formation in the mouse. Teratology 33:21–27

Nau H, Löscher W (1986) Pharmacologic evaluation of various metabolites and analogs of valproic acid: teratogenic potencies in mice. Fundam Appl Toxicol 6:669–676

Nau H, Scott WJ (1986) Weak acids as teratogens: drug accumulation in the basic milieu of the early mammalian embryo. Nature 323:276–278

Nau H, Rating D, Koch S, Häuser I, Helge H (1981a) Valproic acid and its metabolites: placental transfer, neonatal pharmacokinetics, transfer via mother's milk and clinical status in neonates of epileptic mothers. J Pharmacol Exp Ther 219:768–777

Nau H, Wittfoht W, Schäfter H, Jakobs C, Rating D, Helge H (1981b) Valproic acid in several metabolites: quantitative determination in serum urine, breast milk and tissues by gas chromatography-mass spectrometry using selected ion monitoring. J Chromatogr 226:69–78

Nau H, Zierer R, Spielmann H, Neubert D, Gansau C (1981 c) A new model for embryotoxicity testing: teratogenicity and pharmacokinetics of valproic acid following constant-rate administration in the mouse using human therapeutic drug and metabolite concentrations. Life Sci 29:2803–2814

Nau H, Löscher W, Schäfer H (1984) Anticonvulsant activity and embryotoxicity of valproic acid. Neurology 34:400–401

Neubert D, Chahoud I (1985) Significance of species and strain differences in pre- and perinatal toxicology. Acta Histochem [Suppl] (Jena) 31:23–35

Ong LL, Schardein JL, Petrere JA, Sakowski R, Jordan H, Humphrey RR, Fitzgerald JE, de la Iglesia F (1983) Teratogenesis of calcium valproate in rats. Fundam Appl Toxicol 3:121–126

Pagano G, Cipollaro M, Corsale G, Esposito A, Ragucci E, Giordano GG (1985) pH-Induced changes in mitotic and developmental patterns in sea urchin embryogenesis. I. Exposure of embryos. Teratogenesis Carcinog Mutagen 5:101–112

Petrere JA, Anderson JA, Sakowski R, Fitzgerald JE, de la Iglesia FA (1986) Teratogenesis of calcium valproate in rabbits. Teratology 34:263–269

Ritter EJ, Scott WJ, Randall JL, Ritter JM (1985) Teratogenicity of dimethoxyethyl phthalate and its metabolites methoxyethanol and methoxyacetic acid in the rat. Teratology 32:25–31

Robert R, Rosa F (1983) Valproate birth defects. Lancet II:1142

Rowan AJ, Overweg J, Meijer JWA (1981) Monodose therapy with valproic acid: 24 h telemetric EEG and serum level studies. In: Dam M, Gram L, Penry JK (eds) Advances in epileptology. Raven, New York, pp 533–539

Scott WJ, Nau H (1985) Weak acids as human teratogens: accumulation in the young mammalian embryo. Teratology 31:25A

Scott WJ, Duggan CA, Schreiner CM, Collins MD, Nau H (1986) Intracellular pH of rodent embryos and its association with teratogenic response. In: Welsch F (ed) Approaches to evaluate mechanisms in teratogenesis. Hemisphere, Washington

Tagashira E, Nakao K, Urano T, Ishikawa U, Hiramori T, Yanaura S (1981) Correlation of teratogenicity of aspirin to the stagespecific distribution of salicylic acid in rats. Jpn J Pharmacol 31:563–571

Tein I, MacGregor DL (1985) Possible valproate teratogenicity. Arch Neurol 42:291–293

Waddell WJ, Butler TC (1959) Calculation of intracellular pH from the distribution of 5,5-dimethyl-2,4-oxazolidinedione (DMO). Application to skeletal muscle of the dog. J Clin Invest 38:720–729

Willhite CC, Shealy YF (1984) Amelioration of embryotoxicity by structural modification of the terminal group of cancer chemopreventive retinoids. JNCI 72:689–695

Wilson JG (1965) Embryological considerations in teratology. In: Wilson JG, Warkany J (eds) Teratology: principles and techniques. University of Chicago Press, Chicago

Wittfoht W, Duwe K, Kuhnz W, Nau H (1984) Microscale ultrafiltration technique for determining free drug in 50-μl serum samples. Clin Chem 30:878

Mechanisms and Models in Toxicology
Arch. Toxicol., Suppl. 11, 140–142 (1987)

Embryotoxic Action of β-Aminopropionitrile During Early Organogenesis in Rats

M. N. Simpson, S. J. Freeman, and C. E. Steele

Department of Toxicology, Smith Kline and French Research Limited, The Frythe, Welwyn, Herts., AL6 9AR, UK

Introduction

The lathyrogen β-aminopropionitrile (β-APN) has been shown to be teratogenic in rats after administration to the dam at the late organogenesis stage of gestation, commonly inducing cleft palate and a variety of skeletal malformations in fetuses (Wilk et al. 1972; Barrow and Steffek 1974). Unusually among teratogens, however, β-APN has been reported not to affect embryos during the early organogenesis stage of development, when sensitivity to teratogenic insult is often maximal (Barrow and Steffek 1974). This observation is in contrast to that made in the hamster, in which administration of β-APN to the dam during early organogenesis resulted in the induction of neural tube defects (Wiley and Joneja 1976). Furthermore, it has been demonstrated (Steele and Marlow 1985; Simpson et al. 1986) that the cultured early organogenesis stage rat embryo is susceptible to dysmorphogenesis when β-APN is present in the culture medium.

This report re-evaluates the effect of β-APN on the early organogenesis rat embryo in vivo and presents data that demonstrate a dysmorphogenic action of β-APN on development at this early stage.

Methods

Pregnant Olac Wistar rats were dosed orally (2000 mg/kg body wt.) with solutions of either β-APN fumarate (Sigma Chemical Company Ltd.) or with distilled water, at both 9.5 and 10.5 days of gestation (mating timed from the midnight preceding the morning on which a vaginal plug was found). These doses were chosen to match exactly those used by Wilk et al. (1972). On pregnancy day 11.5, embryos were explanted and their development and growth assessed by the following criteria: normal axial rotation, closure of neural tube, number of somites, presence of limb buds, optic and otic vesicles, and the number of pharyngeal arches. Crown–rump and head lengths, somite number and embryo protein content (Lowry et al. 1951) were determined and were statistically analysed by Student's t test. All other parameters were analysed by χ^2 test with Yates' correction.

Results and Discussion

Embryos from β-APN-treated dams showed significant alterations in several developmental parameters (Table 1): decreased frequency of normal rotation and closure of posterior neuropore (both $p < 0.05$); a difference in the numbers of embryos possessing 2 or 3 pharyngeal areches ($p < 0.05$ and < 0.001, respectively); a reduction in the number of somites per embryo ($p < 0.001$).

Furthermore, embryos from β-APN-treated dams showed significant growth retardation (Table 2), as indicated by decreased protein content and crown–rump and head lengths (all $p < 0.001$). Other deviations from normal development noted were expansion of the pericardium (30% incidence) and enlargement of the amniotic cavity (13% incidence).

There was at least one abnormal embryo from each of the seven litters treated, whereas there were no abnormal embryos in the three control litters.

In contrast to a previous report (Barrow and Steffek 1974), the present data indicate that during early organogenesis, as at later stages (Wilk et al. 1972), the rat embryo is susceptible to the toxic effects of β-APN. These observations are also in accord with the in vitro findings of Steele and Marlow (1985).

The discrepancy between these findings and those of Barrow and Steffek (1974) could be attributed to the different time at which the pregnancies were terminated

Table 1. Effect of maternal administration of β-APN on embryos: morphogenetic parameters

Parameters	Distilled water control ($n = 39$) (3 litters)	β-APN ($n = 92$) (7 litters)
Normal axial rotation	39 (100%)	86 (93%)[a]
Presence of:		
Optic vesicles	39 (100%)	91 (99%)
Otic vesicles	39 (100%)	92 (100%)
Limb buds	39 (100%)	89 (97%)
No. of pharyngeal arches: 0	0	0
1	0	5 (5%)
2	0	14 (15%)[a]
3	39 (100%)	73 (79%)[b]
Allantois fused with chorion	39 (100%)	89 (97%)
Anterior neuropore closed	39 (100%)	91 (99%)
Posterior neuropore closed	37 (100%)[c]	83 (90%)[a]
No. of somites ($x \pm$ S.E.)	25 ± 0.3	23 ± 0.3 ($n = 91$)[b]

[a] Significantly different from control, $p < 0.05$.
[b] Significantly different from control $p < 0.001$. There was at least 1 abnormal embryo from each treated litter.
[c] Group of 37.

Table 2. Effect of maternal administration of β-APN on embryos: growth parameters

Parameters	Distilled water control	β-APN
Crown-rump length (mm) (mean ± S.E.)	3.7 ± 0.07 (n = 25)	3.3 ± 0.09[a] (n = 33)[b]
Head length (mm) (mean ± S.E.)	2.1 ± 0.03 (n = 26)	1.7 ± 0.07[a] (n = 34)
Protein content (µg) (mean ± S.E.)	288 ± 7 (n = 39)	161 ± 4[a] (n = 92)

[a] Significantly different from control; $p < 0.001$.
[b] Severe abnormality: not possible to measure in 1 embryo.

Crown-rump and head length measurements were made during the later experiments only.

(day 21 in the Barrow and Steffek study). The developmental defects reported here may have been transient phenomena and subject to subsequent repair. An alternative explanation could be a difference in sensitivity to β-APN during early organogenesis in the two strains of rats.

It has to be established whether the abnormal action of β-APN in the present experiments is due to its lathyrogenic properties.

References

Barrow MV, Steffek AJ (1974) Teratologic and other embryotoxic effects of β-aminopropiotrile in rats. Teratology 10:165–172

Simpson MN, Marlow R, Steele CE (1986) Use of cultured rat embryos to evaluate the teratogenic activity of sera: β-aminopropionitrile and cyanoacetic acid. Fd Chem Toxic 24:634

Steele CE, Marlow R (1985) An in vitro study of the teratogenicity of β-aminopropionitrile. Hum Toxicology 4:104

Wiley MJ, Joneja MG (1976) The teratogenic effects of β-aminopropionitrile in hamsters. Teratology 14:43–52

Wilk AL, King CTG, Horigan EA, Steffek AJ (1972) Metabolism of β-aminopropionitrile and its teratogenic activity in rats. Teratology 5:41–48

Mechanisms and Models in Toxicology
Arch. Toxicol., Suppl. 11, 143–147 (1987)

Valproic Acid Teratogenesis and Embryonic Lipid Metabolism

D. O. Clarke and N. A. Brown

Experimental Embryology and Teratology Unit, MRC Laboratories, Woodmansterne Road, Carshalton, Surrey, SM5 4EF, UK

Introduction

The anticonvulsant drug valproic acid (2-propylpentanoic acid) is teratogenic in laboratory species (Kao et al. 1981) and probably in humans (Anon. 1982). Whole embryo culture studies have shown that valproic acid and some other short-chain carboxylic acids (SCCA) directly affect embryogenesis (Brown and Coakley 1984; Rawlings et al. 1985) but their mechanism(s) of action is or are unknown. An experimental protocol has been designed to examine initial embryonic responses during teratogenic exposure to short-chain carboxylic acids (Fig. 1). Using this protocol, the present study reports significant effects of valproic acid on embryonic lipid synthesis. In addition to valproic acid, the actions of butyric acid and mevinolinic acid on embryonic lipid synthesis are reported. Butyrate is the most potent of all SCCA examined for teratogenic potential in whole embryo culture (Brown and Coakley 1984). Mevinolinic acid is a specific inhibitor of the rate-limiting hydroxymethylglutaryl-coenzyme A (HMG-CoA) reductase reaction in cholesterol biosynthesis (Alberts et al. 1980) and was used as a positive control in the present study.

Materials and Methods

Valproic acid and butyric acid (each >98% pure; Aldrich, UK) were neutralised with sodium hydroxide and diluted in minimum essential medium Eagle (MEM) with Earle's salts (Imperial Laboratories, UK). Sodium mevinolate was prepared from mevinolin (donated by Dr. A. W. Alberts, Merck Institute for Therapeutic Research, New Jersey, USA) by alkaline hydrolysis in ethanolic solution, and diluted in MEM.

Abbreviations: SCCA, short-chain carboxylic acids; MEM, minimum essential medium Eagle; TLC, thin-layer chromatography.

[³H]Acetic acid (sodium salt in ethanol; NEN Du Pont, UK) was evaporated to dryness and redissolved in MEM before use. Conceptuses from F344 rats were explanted at 9.5 days' embryonic age and cultured in a medium of 75% immediately-centrifuged, heat-inactivated rat serum and 25% MEM (3 conceptuses per culture bottle). At 16 h of culture [³H]acetate (125 µCi/ml, 100–130 µCi/µmol) was added, with or without teratogenic agent, bringing the total culture medium volume to 4 ml per bottle. After an 8-h exposure, conceptuses were removed from culture, washed, and dissected into embryos proper and visceral yolk sacs. Tissues were homogenised and aliquots taken for determination of protein content (Lowry et al. 1951). Rat liver homogenate was added as carrier, and total lipid preparations of embryos proper and visceral yolk sacs were obtained by the solvent extraction and washing procedures of Folch et al. (1957). Separation into neutral lipid classes was achieved by thin-layer chromatography (TLC) on silica gel G plates (Merck, BDH Chemicals, UK), using petroleum ether: diethyl ether: glacial acetic acid (80:20:1 by vol.; Wood et al. 1964). Plates were developed in iodine and lipid classes identified using reference standards (Sigma, UK). (Resolution of cholesterol and 1,3-diglyceride, and of lanosterol and fatty acid alcohols, were not obtained, whilst resolution of cholesterol esters and squalene was only partial). Incorporated radioactivity was quantitated by elution of TLC fractions and scintillation counting.

Results and Discussion

Rat conceptuses explanted at 9.5 days and exposed to 1–1.5 mM valproic acid for 8 h, from the 16th h of culture, develop somite abnormalities observable at 48 h (Brown and Colhoun 1984). These defects appear to be identical to those induced by valproic acid treatments in vivo, which lead to rib and vertebral malformations at term. Since valproic acid is not incorporated by the developing conceptus in vitro and freely diffuses out of the embryonic compartment upon the removal of treatment (Brown 1987), these structural defects must be a result of insult(s) initiated during the exposure period. Thus, the initial biochemical changes in the pathway to malformation should be detectable by the end of this treatment period. The protocol outlined in Fig. 1 has been used in previous studies, which have

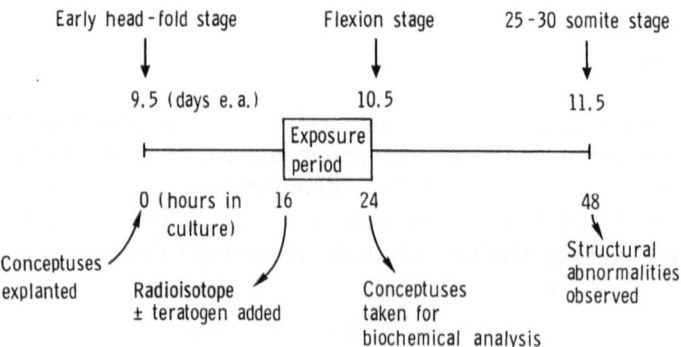

Fig. 1. Experimental protocol used to examine initial embryonic biochemical responses during a teratogenic exposure to short-chain carboxylic acids

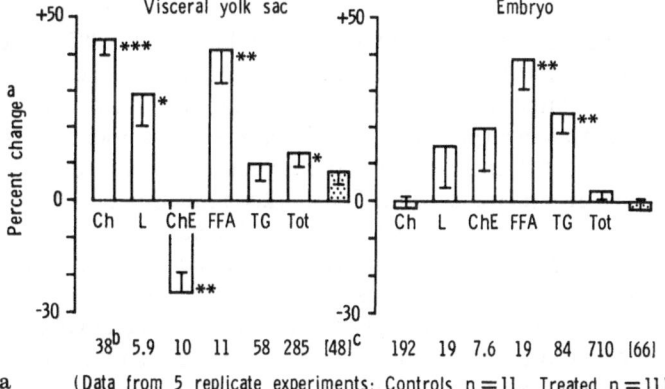

a   (Data from 5 replicate experiments; Controls n = 11, Treated n = 11)

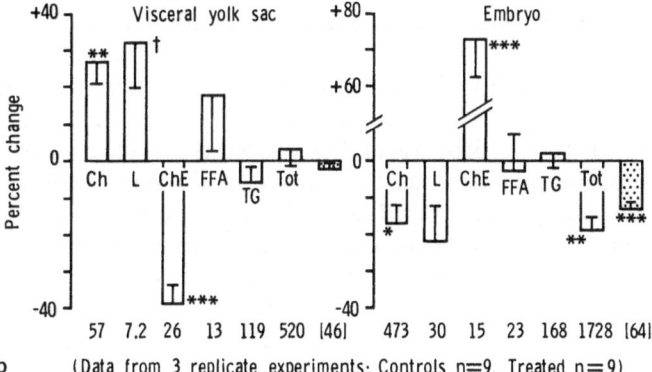

b   (Data from 3 replicate experiments; Controls n = 9, Treated n = 9)

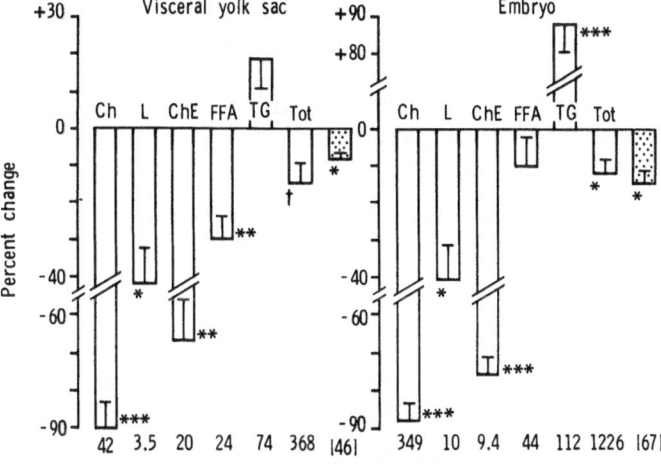

c   (Data from 2 replicate experiments; Controls n = 6, Treated n = 6)

Fig. 2. Effects of **a** valproate (1.25 mM), **b** butyrate (0.75 mM), and **c** mevinolate (6.0 μM) on the incorporation of [³H]acetate into visceral yolk sac and embryo lipids of 10.5-day rat conceptuses cultured in vitro. TLC fractions: *Ch*, cholesterol; *L*, lanosterol; *ChE*, cholesterol esters; *FFA*, free fatty acids; *TG*, triacylglycerols; *Tot*, total lipids; ▦, μg protein. [a]dpm per μg protein expressed as the 'percentage change' from mean control values; [b]mean control values; [c]mean μg protein. †$p<0.1$, *$p<0.05$, **$p<0.01$, ***$p<0.001$, analysis of variance

established that valproic acid does not affect glycolysis, DNA and protein synthesis, acetyl coenzyme A levels or yolk sac pinocytosis (Coakley et al. 1987). The significant effects found on [³H]acetate incorporation (Fig. 2a) suggest that changes in embryonic lipid synthesis may be an early event in the teratogenic effect. Although [³H]acetate was incorporated into all major neutral lipid classes, only certain classes were affected, indicative of specific actions of valproic acid and butyrate, rather than a general toxic insult. The marked reduction of [³H]acetate incorporation into embryonic cholesterol (-90%) and related lipids induced by mevinolate is the expected response to an HMG-CoA reductase inhibitor and demonstrates the sensitivity of the techniques used.

The common effects induced by valproic acid and butyrate on visceral yolk sac sterol synthesis may be of importance. Incorporation of [³H]acetate into cholesterol and lanosterol fractions was increased, whilst incorporation into the cholesterol ester fraction was concomitantly decreased. These observations might be explained by alterations in sterol acylation/esterase reaction equilibrium, and/or altered rate of cholesterogenesis. In addition, valproic acid, but not butyrate, increased [³H]acetate incorporation into free fatty acids, and into embryo proper triacylglycerols. Although it is plausible that valproic acid inhibits embryonic fatty acid oxidation, previous work (Brown et al. 1985) suggests that the biochemical mechanism responsible would differ from that causing inhibition of fatty acid oxidation in adult hepatocytes (Coudé et al. 1983). Moreover, butyrate, but not valproic acid, induced changes in embryo sterols. Unlike valproic acid, butyrate is incorporated by rat conceptuses in vitro (Brown 1987); thus, the different changes induced on embryo lipids by these two SCCA might be explained by competition between acetate and butyrate for metabolism by the developing embryo.

These effects of valproic acid on [³H]acetate incorporation into lipids might reflect a consequence of other initial effects of valproic acid, rather than a direct effect on embryonic lipid biosynthesis: for example, actions on membrane transport processes or the redirection of acetate into or away from other pathways. Nevertheless, the specific responses induced, coupled with the previous negative findings using this experimental design, suggest a promising lead in the search for the initial teratogenic insult of valproic acid.

Acknowledgement. The authors gratefully acknowledge the support of D.O.C. by a Saunders Foundation Research Studentship.

References

Alberts AW, Chen J, Kuron G et al. (1980) Mevinolin: a highly potent competitive inhibitor of hydroxymethylglutaryl-coenzyme A reductase and a cholesterol-lowering agent. Proc Natl Acad Sci USA 77:3957–3961

Anon (1982) Valproate and malformations. Lancet II:1313–1314 (editorial)

Brown NA (1987) Teratogenicity of carboxylic acids: distribution studies in whole embryo culture. In: Nau H (ed) Pharmacokinetics in teratogenesis. CRC Press (in press)

Brown NA, Coakley ME (1984) Valproic acid teratogenesis. II. Actions of related acids and potential antagonists and the role of coenzyme A. Teratology 29:20A

Brown NA, Colhoun CW (1984) Valproic acid teratogenesis. I. In vivo/in vitro comparisons and effects on somite morphogenesis. Teratology 29:20A–21A

Brown NA, Farmer PB, Coakley M (1985) Valproic acid teratogenicity: demonstration that the bio-chemical mechanism differs from that of valproate hepatotoxicity. Biochem Soc Trans 13:75–77

Coakley ME, Rawlings SJ, Brown NA (1987) Short chain carboxylic acids, a new class of teratogens: studies of potential biochemical mechanisms. Environ Health Perspect (in press)

Coudé FX, Grimber G, Pelet A, Benoit Y (1983) Action of the antiepileptic drug, valproic acid, on fatty acid oxidation in isolated rat hepatocytes. Biochem Biophys Res Commun 115:730–736

Folch J, Lees M, Sloane Stanley GH (1957) A simple method for the isolation and purification of total lipides from animal tissues. J Biol Chem 226:497–509

Kao J, Brown NA, Schmid B, Goulding EH, Fabro S (1981) Teratogenicity of valproic acid: in vivo and in vitro investigations. Teratogenesis Carcinog Mutagen 1:367–382

Lowry OH, Rosebrough NJ, Farr AL, Randall RJ (1951) Protein measurement with the Folin phenol reagent. J Biol Chem 193:265–275

Rawlings SJ, Shuker DEG, Webb M, Brown NA (1985) The teratogenic potential of alkoxy acids in postimplantation rat embryo culture: structure-activity relationships. Toxicol Lett 28:49–58

Wood P, Imaichi K, Knowles J, Michaels G, Kinsell LW (1964) The lipid composition of human plasma chylomicrons. J Lipid Res 5:225–231

Mechanisms and Models in Toxicology
Arch. Toxicol., Suppl. 11, 148–151 (1987)

Prenatal Exposure to Methylazoxymethanol (MAM) Acetate: Effects on Ultrasonic Vocalization and Locomotor Activity in Rat Offspring

R. Cagiano [1], M. De Salvia [1], G. Renna [1], G. Racagni [2], and V. Cuomo [1]

[1] Institute of Pharmacology, University of Bari, Piazza G. Cesare, 70124 Bari, Italy
[2] Institute of Pharmacology and Pharmacognosy, University of Milan, Via A. del Sarto 21, 20129 Milan, Italy

Introduction

Methylazoxymethanol (MAM), a potent alkylating agent, produces marked microencephaly as well as long-term learning impairments in the progeny of rats injected at the beginning of the 3rd week of pregnancy (Spatz and Laqueur 1968; Vorhees et al. 1984). Interestingly, neurochemical studies have shown that prenatal exposure to MAM can lead to notable alterations of the central dopaminergic system in offspring of exposed dams (Balduini et al. 1984). The experiments reported here were performed in order to investigate, in infant rats, the effects of prenatal administration of MAM on behavioural models which are partly linked to dopaminergic mechanisms. In particular, the effects of prenatal MAM exposure on ultrasonic vocalization elicited by the removal of rat pups from their nest were evaluated. In this regard, we recently demonstrated that ultrasonic calling in rat pups may be considered as an early sensitive indicator of subtle changes produced by the developmental administration of drugs influencing the dopaminergic system (Cagiano et al. 1986).

The locomotor activity of young rats prenatally exposed to MAM was also measured.

Materials and Methods

Pairs of primiparous female Wistar rats were housed with single male rats in the late afternoon and vaginal smears were taken on the following morning at 9.00 a.m. The day on which sperm was present was designated day 1 of gestation. Females were then randomly assigned to treatment groups and individually housed in standard cages. A single dose of either MAM acetate (20 mg/kg body wt. i.p.; Aldrich, USA) dissolved in saline or else an equivalent volume of saline was injected on day 13 of gestation.

All litters were reduced to a standard size of eight pups per litter (four males and four females, where possible) within 24 h of birth and weaned 3 weeks later.

Ultrasonic calling (rate, frequency, intensity, duration) of rat pups was measured according to the method recently described by Cagiano et al. (1986). Locomotor activity was measured with an apparatus (toggle-floor boxes) previously used for the study of locomotion in rats (Racagni et al. 1982).

Results

The results show that prenatal exposure to MAM altered the ultrasonic vocalization elicited by the removal of rat pups from their nest. In particular, a significant decrease in the duration of ultrasonic calls was found in both male and female MAM-treated pups (Figs. 1, 2). Other parameters of ultrasonic emission (rate of calling, frequency, sound pressure level) were not influenced by prenatal administration of this alkylating agent (data not shown). As far as locomotor activity is concerned, the results of the present study (Table 1) show that prenatal exposure to MAM induced significant hyperactivity in 21-day-old female rats; con-

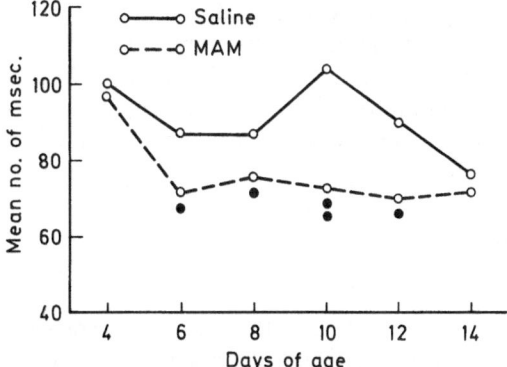

Fig. 1. Duration of ultrasonic calls in male rat pups after prenatal exposure to MAM. Each group consisted of 12 pups. MAM vs saline: $\bullet p < 0.02$; $\bullet\bullet p < 0.001$ (Mann–Whitney U test)

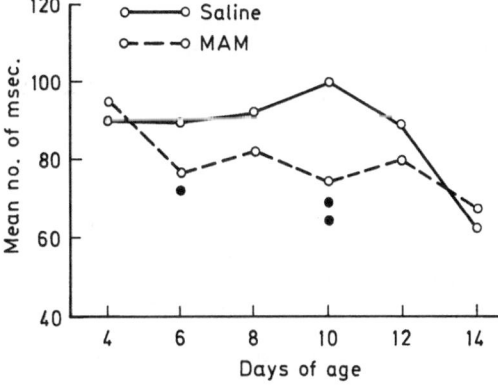

Fig. 2. Duration of ultrasonic calls in female rat pups after prenatal exposure to MAM. Each group consisted of 12 pups. MAM vs saline: $\bullet p < 0.02$; $\bullet\bullet p < 0.01$ (Mann–Whitney U test)

Table 1. Effects of prenatal exposure to MAM on locomotor activity
(mean no. of crossings $\pm$ S.E.) in 21-day-old rats (15 min session)

Sex	Saline	MAM
Males	14.2$\pm$1.36 ($n=8$)	18.8$\pm$2.71 ($n=8$)
Females	17.4$\pm$2.36 ($n=7$)	24.0$\pm$1.34[a] ($n=8$)

[a] $p<0.05$ vs saline (Student's t test).

versely, locomotor activity levels of males were not affected by prenatal treatment
with MAM.

Finally, offspring exposed to MAM showed no increase in mortality but
weighed less than controls up to the 21st day of life (data not shown).

Discussion

The present study shows that prenatal exposure to MAM produced subtle but significant alterations of the ultrasonic vocalization in rat pups removed from their
nest. These data further confirm that ultrasonic emission in infant rats may represent an useful test in studies of developmental toxicity. In this regard, in fact, recent findings have showed that ultrasonic calling during early postnatal life is a
sensitive indicator of subtle adverse effects produced by perinatal exposure to
drugs and environmental chemicals (Adams 1982; Adams et al. 1983; Cagiano et
al. 1986). Moreover, ultrasonic vocalizations represent one of the few response
patterns emitted by rat pups which may be quantitatively evaluated and which
may be produced by quantifiable stimuli.

Finally, the results of the present experiments indicate that only female rats exposed to MAM during gestation exhibited a significant increase in spontaneous
locomotor activity. In this regard, these data are in agreement with those of other
authors showing sex differences in some behavioural changes produced by prenatal MAM administration (Rabe and Haddad 1972; Vorhees et al. 1984).

In summary the present findings contribute to further characterizes MAM-
induced behavioural alterations that are considered by Vorhees et al. (1984) to be
a potentially useful animal model of congenital microencephaly and associated
mental retardation, as well as a valuable tool as a positive control treatment in
the area of behavioural teratology.

References

Adams J (1982) Ultrasonic vocalizations as diagnostic tools in studies of developmental toxicity: an
    investigation of the effects of hypervitaminosis A. Neurobehav Toxicol Teratol 4:299–304
Adams J, Miller DR, Nelson CJ (1983) Ultrasonic vocalizations as diagnostic tools in studies of devel-
    opmental toxicity: an investigation of the effects of prenatal treatment with methylmercuric chlo-
    ride. Neurobehav Toxicol Teratol 5:29–34
Balduini W, Abbracchio MP, Lombardelli G, Cattabeni F (1984) Loss of intrinsic strial neurons after
    methylazoxymethanol acetate treatment in pregnant rats. Dev Brain Res 15:133–136

Cagiano R, Sales GD, Renna G, Racagni G, Cuomo V (1986) Ultrasonic vocalization in rat pups: effects of early postnatal exposure to haloperidol. Life Sci 38:1417–1423

Rabe A, Haddad RK (1972) Methylazoxymethanol-induced microencephaly in rats: behavioral studies. Fed Proc 31:1536–1539

Racagni G, Mocchetti I, Renna G, Cuomo V (1982) In vivo studies on central noradrenergic synaptic mechanisms after acute and chronic antidepressant drug treatment: biochemical and behavioural comparisons. J Pharmacol Exp Ther 223:227–234

Spatz M, Laqueur GL (1968) Transplacental chemical induction of microencephaly in two strains of rats. Proc Soc Exp Biol 129:705–710

Vorhees CV, Fernandez K, Dumas RM, Haddad RK (1984) Pervasive hyperactivity and long-term learning impairments in rats with induced microencephaly from prenatal exposure to methylazoxymethanol. Dev Brain Res 15:1–10

Mechanisms and Models in Toxicology
Arch. Toxicol., Suppl. 11, 152–154 (1987)

The Comparative Effects of Cytotoxic Agents on the Numbers of Oocytes in Mice

N. Abu-Khalaf[1], J. A. Double[2], and T. G. Baker[1]

[1] School of Biomedical Sciences, University of Bradford, Bradford, BD7 1DP, UK
[2] School of Clinical Oncology, University of Bradford, Bradford, BD7 1DP, UK

Introduction

The treatment of cancer with cytotoxic agents is gradually becoming more effective and the eventual curing of some less common cancers is now a real possibility. It is therefore pertinent that more attention now be paid to the chronic as well as the acute toxicity problems arising from the administration of cytotoxic agents. Where practical, studies to determine potential chronic as well as acute toxicities of new agents are now being introduced in the preclinical evaluation of prospective anticancer agents. The majority of standard and investigational agents are poorly selective and have the potential to kill all dividing cells. The process of oogenesis involves considerable cell division before birth, but in adults the germ cells are all blocked at the diplotene stage of meiotic prophase. Nevertheless, these follicular oocytes are known to be sensitive to irradiation and cytotoxic drugs, and the granulosa cells are actively dividing. Before instituting a model for use in determining potentially damaging effects of new agents, it is first necessary to evaluate it by observing the effects of standard established agents whose clinical toxicities are well documented and to show that there is a good correlation between the clinical and experimental situation. This study investigates the effects on follicular oocytes in the mouse by standard and investigational cytotoxic agents.

Materials and Methods

Seven-week-old female pure strain NMRI (Naval Medical Research Institution) mice from the Clinical Oncology Unit's own breeding colony were used throughout this study. They were allowed food (CRM Labsure, UK) and water ad libitum.

Cyclophosphamide, isophosphamide, and 5-fluorouracil were dissolved in isotonic saline. MeCCNU [methyl N-(2-chloroethyl-N'-cyclohexyl-N-nitroso-urea] was dissolved in 10% ethanol/arachis oil and mitozolomide suspended in arachis oil. The concentrations were such that the required dose could be administered in 0.1 ml/10 g body wt. All injections were intraperitoneal. Ovaries were dissected, fixed in Bouin's fluid, and 5 μm serial sections were stained with haematoxylin and eosin. After completion of counts from every 10th section, the total numbers of follicles per ovary were determined.

Results

Figure 1 shows the effects of single maximum tolerated dose of cyclophosphamide and isophosphamide on the numbers of oocytes compared with age-matched controls for a period of 140 days after treatment. It can be clearly seen that both agents reduce the numbers of oocytes, and that at equitoxic doses cyclophosphamide was the more potent agent.

Figure 2 illustrates the effects of a single maximum tolerated dose of 5-fluorouracil. Oocyte numbers are reduced by the action of the drug but this was the least toxic of the agents tested.

Figure 3 compares the effects of MeCCNU with mitozolomide. In clinical use MeCCNU has a very steep dose-response curve and frequently produces some

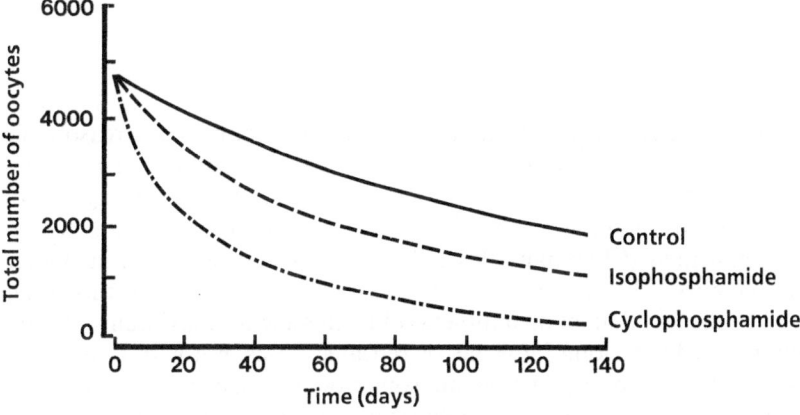

Fig. 1. The effect of cyclophosphamide and isophosphamide on the total numbers of oocytes

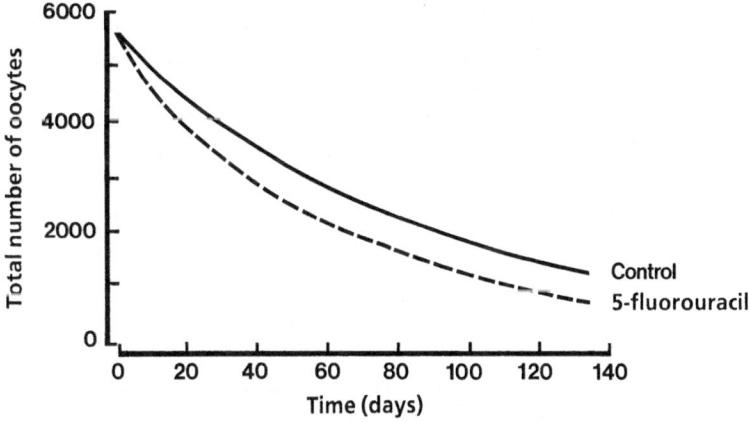

Fig. 2. The effect of 5-fluorouracil on total numbers of oocytes

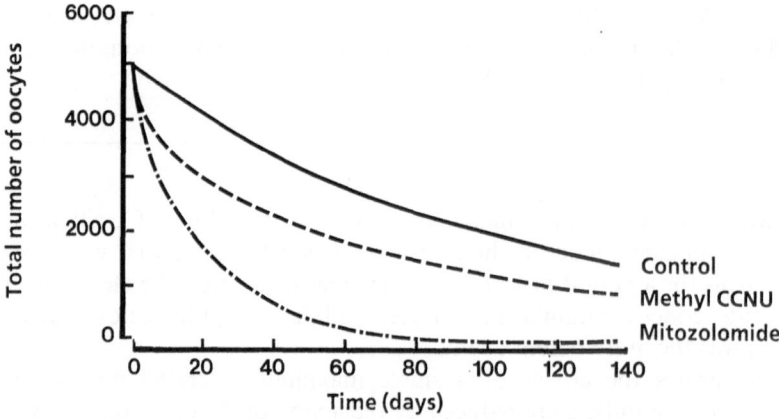

Fig. 3. The effect of Me CCNU and mitozolomide on the total numbers of oocytes

haemopoietic toxicity, but in this experiment mitozolomide has a far more toxic action on the ovaries.

Discussion

The results of this study have shown that female NMRI mice may be a reasonable model in which to study potential ovarian toxicity. Cyclophosphamide, an alkylating agent, and 5-fluorouracil, an antimetabolite, are established agents in cancer chemotherapy, and their toxic effects on female reproduction are reasonably well documented (Chapman 1984). Both agents induced a fall in oocyte numbers in the mice. The fall with 5-fluorouracil was only slight, but this could be explained by the fact that, as an antimetabolite, this agent's maximum cytotoxicity is only reached with long infusions or repeated doses, not with a single injection, as used here. Isophosphamide, an isomer of cyclophosphamide in which there is considerable clinical interest (Hellmann and Carter 1983), was less toxic to the ovaries, and this may prove of clinical significance.

The result with mitozolomide is perhaps the most significant of all, especially when compared with MeCCNU, to which it may have a similar mechanism of action. Mitozolomide has shown a wide range of anti-tumour activity in experimental tumour systems, similar to that previously shown by the nitrosoureas. The agent is currently in phase II clinical trials but its ultimate clinical role will depend very much on the level of toxicity it produces. The results presented here indicate that potential ovarian toxicity may limit its clinical usefulness, but further experimental studies with clinically equivalent dose regimes should be conducted in order to give a more definitive prediction of toxicity and clinical limitations.

References

Chapman RM (1984) Effects of cytotoxic therapy on sexuality and gonadal function. In: Perry MC, Yarbro JW (eds) Toxicity of chemotherapy. Grune and Stratton, Orlando, pp 343–363
Hellmann K, Carter SK (1983) Ifosfamide and mesna. Cancer Treat Rev 10 [Suppl A]

Mechanisms and Models in Toxicology
Arch. Toxicol., Suppl. 11, 155–158 (1987)
© by Springer-Verlag 1987

Development of a Method for Assessing the Acute Toxicity of Chemicals on Early Post-Implantation Embryos

F. Beck, E. Mensah-Brown, and M. K. Pratten

Department of Anatomy, Leicester University Medical School, University Road, Leicester, LE1 7RH, UK

Introduction

The whole-embryo culture technique developed by New (1978) is being increasingly used in investigating the mode of action of embryopathic agents. Appropriately devised experiments make it possible to decide whether a substance can act directly on the conceptus (McGarrity et al. 1981) or whether its embryotoxic effect requires maternal mediation (Fantel et al. 1979). In some cases it has even proved possible to assess the relative effects of a drug and its principal human metabolites (Beck et al. 1984). However, growing rat embryos within their yolk sacs and adding putative embryopathic agents to the culture serum does not enable the investigator to distinguish a direct effect on embryonic tissue from one on the extra-embryonic membranes. Furthermore, when a substance crosses the extra-embryonic membranes in only small quantities there is difficulty either in investigating the capacity of the embryonic tissues to detoxify and metabolise it or in developing a comprehensive picture of its pharmacokinetics and of possible target sites in the embryo. In an attempt to overcome these problems, and, in addition to assess acute direct embryotoxicity, a method was devised of injecting materials directly into the vitelline vessels of embryos in culture and observing their effect over a culture period of up to 6 h.

Materials and Methods

Embryos within their yolk sacs were dissected from the decidua of rats at 11.3 days of a timed gestation. The parietal layer of the yolk sac was carefully stripped away to expose the vascularised visceral yolk sac. Using a mechanically drawn micropipette and a graduated delivery system, various volumes of fluid between 1 μl and 5 μl were then injected into a tributary of the main vitelline vein. The injections were carried out at 37 °C under a dissecting microscope using fibre-optic illumination, with the embryo placed in a fluid-filled well made in an agar block separated from a copper-plated stage by a film of Hanks solution. After injection, but before removal of the pipette tip, the segment of vitelline vessel injected was closed proximally and distally by a diathermy system. After injection embryos were cultured for 6 h in immediately centrifuged, homologous, heat-inactivated serum, gassed with 40% O_2/5% CO_2/55% N_2, using a standard roller culture system (New 1978). Observations, following the injection of Hanks' solution as well as various markers in appropriately buffered and ionically balanced isosmotic carriers, are presented here.

Experimental Observations

Figure 1 a demonstrates complete perfusion of the vitelline vessels obtained after incubation for 30 min following injection of colloidal carbon, and Fig. 1 b illustrates equally satisfactory penetration of the embryonic circulation. Light microscopy revealed an exclusively intravascular location of the injected material, but serial sections of embryos 6 h after injection showed some uptake by cells of the vascular endothelium. Similar results were obtained when fluorescent latex beads (diameter 0.5 μm) were injected.

Table 1 shows the effects on embryonic growth 6 h after injection of increasing quantities of Hanks' solution. As can be seen, 1 μl is well tolerated, but 2 μl lead to a slower heart rate and a sluggish circulation. At higher doses the peripheral vessels appear empty and the heart beat is slow though still present even after 5 μl.

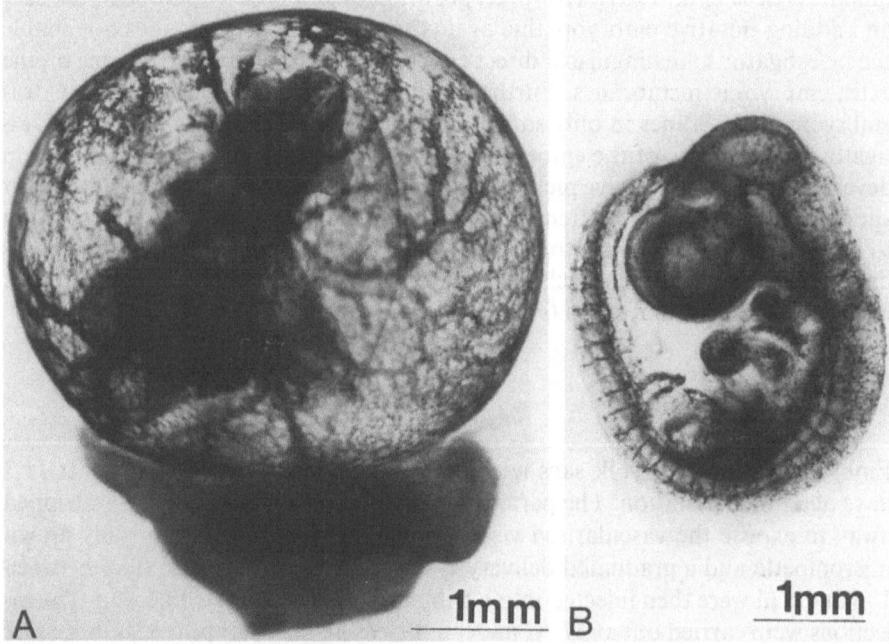

Fig. 1. Cultured rat embryo 30 min after injection of colloidal carbon into vitelline vein. **A** Complete perfusion of the vitelline circulation; **B** complete perfusion of the embryonic tissues

Table 1. Effect of vascular injection of Hanks solution on embryonic growth

Volume injected	(n)	Crown–rump length	Somite no.	Protein (µg)	Circulation
Embryo grown in vivo	(5)	4.25 ± 0.07	27.63 ± 0.27	426.84 ± 9.31	+ + +
Grown in vitro for 6 h without injection	(5)	4.30 ± 0.07	27.27 ± 0.027	428.32 ± 22.46	+ + +
Sham injection, then grown in vitro for 6 h	(5)	4.27 ± 0.06	27.00 ± 0.21	410.80 ± 12.95	+ + +
1.0 µl injected	(5)	4.28 ± 0.10	27.66 ± 0.33	403.44 ± 11.95	+ + +
2.0 µl injected	(5)	4.08 ± 0.15	26.00 ± 0.57[a]	400.80 + 7.02[a]	+ +
3.0 µl injected	(5)	3.74 ± 0.07[a]	24.50 ± 0.67[a]	382.00 ± 18.70[a]	+
5.0 µl injected	(5)	3.61 ± 0.10[a]	24.16 ± 0.30[a]	356.58 + 3.57[a]	+
Control at time of explantation	(5)	3.28 ± 0.08[a]	23.36 ± 0.41[a]	256.24 + 5.07[a]	+ + +

[a] $p < 0.05$ compared to sham injected series.

Injection of a soluble macromolecule (^{125}I-labelled polyvinylpyrrolidone) suggests that rapid equilibration with the extra-embryonic coelomic fluid takes place (within a few minutes), followed by uptake from the circulatory compartment into the embryonic tissues. The study of this activity is continuing.

Injection of rat IgG labelled with colloidal gold indicated rapid accumulation (within 2 h) of the marker in vacuoles of the endothelial cells (Fig. 2). The uptake may well be ligand-mediated, because addition of unlabelled IgG to a concentration 10 000 times that of labelled IgG was found to reduce dramatically the number

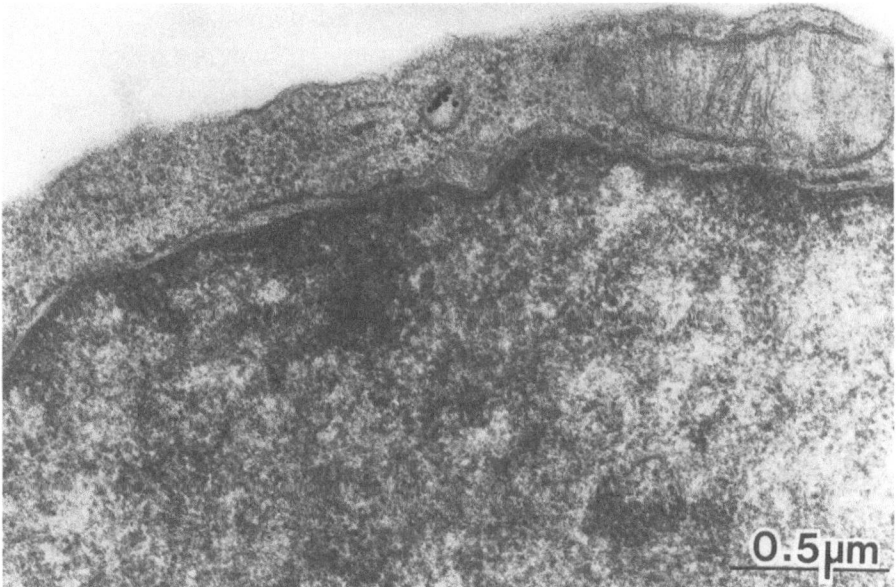

Fig. 2. Colloidal gold-labelled IgG present in a vacuole in the endothelial cell 2 h after injection into the vitelline vein. Bar = 0.5 µm

of gold-containing vacuoles visible in endothelial cells. A quantitative study is in progress. Further evidence in favour of specific IgG-binding is suggested by the observation that a similar concentration of gold-labelled albumin produces a much smaller number of labelled vesicles than does labelled IgG (about one-third in a preliminary semi-quantitative study), while colloidal gold alone is not absorbed to any significant extent at all.

Acknowledgement. The authors are grateful to the Wellcome Trust for a grant in aid of research.

References

Beck F, Huxham IM, Gulamhusein AP (1984) In: Porter et al. (eds) Mechanisms of alcohol damage in utero. Pitman, London, pp 218–233 (Ciba Foundation symposium 105)

Fantel AG, Greenway JC, Juchau MR, Shephard TM (1979) Teratogenic bioactivation of cyclophosphamide in vitro. Life Sci 25:67–72

McGarrity C, Samani N, Beck F, Gulamhusein A (1981) The effect of sodium salicylate on the rat embryo in culture: an *in vitro* model for the morphological assessment of teratogenicity. J Anat 133:(2)257–269

New DAT (1978) Whole embryo culture and the study of mammalian embryos during organogenesis. Biol Rev 53:81–122

Mechanisms and Models in Toxicology
Arch. Toxicol., Suppl. 11, 159–162 (1987)

The "Giant" Yolk Sac: A Model for Studying Transport Across Extra-Embryonic Membranes

M. K. Pratten, A. Dunton, and F. Beck

Department of Anatomy, Leicester University Medical School, University Road, Leicester, LE1 7RH, UK

For over a decade it has been possible to maintain in culture post-implantation rat embryos removed between day 9.5 and day 11.5 of gestation, such that growth and differentiation are identical to those observed in vitro (New 1978). In order to prolong the culture period it is necessary to culture embryos in hyperbaric oxygen concentrations and under somewhat unphysiological conditions (New 1978). During these stages of gestation, before the formation of the chorioallantoic placenta, the major nutritional requirements of the embryo are supplied by the uptake, digestion and transport functions of the visceral yolk sac (Freeman et al. 1981). A technique has recently been developed for the culture of the visceral yolk sac as a closed vesicle from the 9.5th day of gestation until term: the "giant" yolk sac. Morphological studies indicate the presence of tight junctions and functional similarities to the in vivo yolk sac (Dunton et al. 1986). This system has been used to study vectorial transport of materials from the external milieu to the embryonic environment.

Methods

The culture method for giant yolk sacs was as described by Dunton et al. (1986). Briefly, embryos were explanted from female Wistar rats at 9.5 days gestation and cultured in homologous, heat-inactivated, immediately-centrifuged serum at 37 °C in roller culture. At the start of culture the incubation bottles were gassed with 5% O_2, 5% CO_2, 90% N_2 and thereafter daily with 20% O_2, 5% CO_2, 75% N_2. Fresh serum was introduced every 48 h and the volume of serum per yolk sac was increased appropriately as the tissue expanded. Under these conditions the embryo died and was partially autolysed, whilst the yolk sac continued to mature. (An alternative technique permits removal of the embryonic pole of the conceptus prior to culture, under which circumstances the yolk sac develops as a closed vesicle without the complication of the dead embryo.)

Uptake and transport of macromolecules was investigated by incubation of giant yolk sacs in either homologous serum or medium 199 in the presence of ^{125}I-labelled polyvinylpyrrolidone (2 μg/ml), formaldehyde-denatured ^{125}I-labelled bovine serum albumin (10 μg/ml) or ^{125}I-labelled IgG (1 μg/ml). Incubations were carried out at 37 °C in an atmosphere of either 20% O_2, 5% CO_2, 75% N_2 or 95% O_2, 5% CO_2 for periods up to 5 h. At the end of incubations the yolk sacs were washed three times in 1% NaCl. Samples of culture medium, giant yolk sac fluid and yolk sacs were counted for total radioactivity. In addition, for protein substrates, the quantity of trichloroacetic acid (TCA) soluble radioactivity was estimated as a measure of the amount of material that had been digested. Protein estimations were carried out on yolk sacs using a modification of the method of Lowry et al. (1951). The uptake of ^{125}I-labelled substrates by yolk sacs obtained direct from the mother at 17.5 days gestation ("in vivo") was also measured for comparison using the method of Williams et al. (1975). Uptake was expressed as an "Endocytic index", defined as the volume of culture medium (μl) whose contained radioactivity has been captured per mg yolk sac protein per h.

Results and Discussion

Uptake of ^{125}I-labelled polyvinylpyrrolidone was linear with time for both in vivo yolk sacs and giant yolk sacs. There was no evidence of transfer of the polymer into the fluid contained within the giant yolk sac. Table 1 shows the Endocytic indices obtained under different incubation conditions. When ^{125}I-labelled bovine serum albumin was used as a substrate, the tissue-associated radioactivity tended to reach a plateau after 1 h, especially in in vivo yolk sacs, whilst there was a steady release of TCA-soluble digestion products (Fig. 1). There was some evidence of a preferential release of digestion products to the inside of the giant yolk sac, compared with the amount released to the culture medium. No intact albumin was detected in giant yolk sac fluid. ^{125}I-labelled IgG was captured very avidly by both systems. When yolk sacs were preloaded with ^{125}I-labelled IgG and then reincubated in fresh medium, approximately equal amounts of intact protein and digestion products were released to the culture medium. In addition, the giant yolk sac fluid was generally found to contain slightly more intact protein than digestion products at each time point (Fig. 2).

Table 1. Uptake of ^{125}I-labelled polyvinylpyrrolidone by rat visceral yolk sac cultured in vitro

Culture conditions		Endocytic index(μl/mg protein/h)	
Medium	Gas mixture	In-vivo yolk sac	Giant yolk sac
Rat serum	20% O_2/25% CO_2/75% N_2	0.43 ± 0.04	0.46 ± 0.06
Rat serum	95% O_2/5% CO_2	1.05 ± 0.09	0.94 ± 0.014
Medium 199	20% O_2/5% CO_2/75% N_2	0.76 ± 0.03	0.51 ± 0.02
Medium 199	95% O_2/5% CO_2	2.65 ± 0.11	0.96 ± 0.04

Results are expressed as an "Endocytic index", defined as the volume of culture medium whose contained substrate has been captured per mg yolk sac protein per h. Each result is the mean of at least 25 yolk sacs ±SEM.

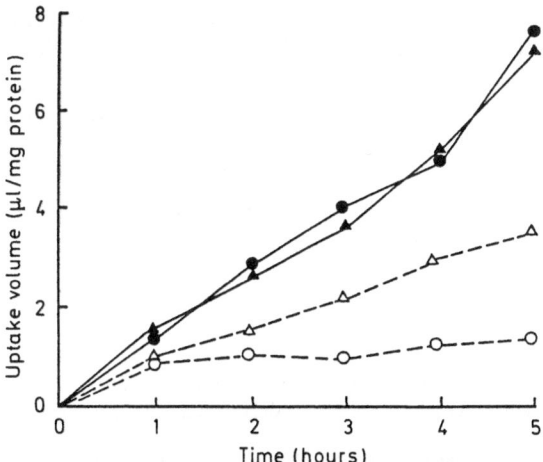

Fig. 1. Uptake of ^{125}I-labelled bovine serum albumin by rat visceral yolk sacs cultured in vitro. Each point represents the mean from at least three yolk sacs. Total uptake by yolk sacs obtained direct from the mother at 17.5 days gestation (●—●) and cultured in vitro from 9.5 days gestation (▲—▲) is shown. In addition, the tissue-associated radioactivity for "in vivo" (○---○) and "giant" (△---△) yolk sacs is shown

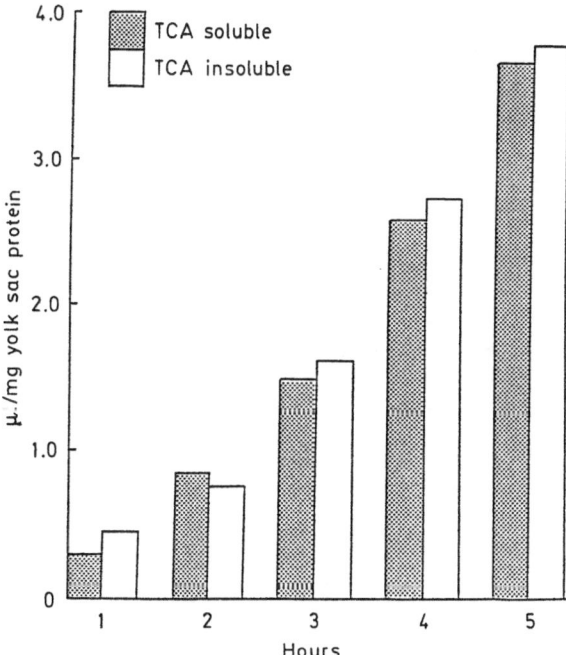

Fig. 2. Release of material to the inside of giant yolk sacs cultured in vitro at 17.5 days gestation after incubation with ^{125}I-labelled IgG. The histogram shows transport of intact (TCA-insoluble) and digested (TCA-soluble) substrate

A large volume of data has been published which indicates that the rat visceral yolk sac is highly active in pinocytosis (as reviewed by Duncan and Pratten 1985). The data presented here indicate that the giant yolk sac system shares this property. The nature of the transport of protein substrates, either intact or as digestion products, is clearly demonstrated by the giant yolk sac system.

Acknowledgements. Thanks are due to the Wellcome Trust and Unilever for their generous support of this work.

References

Duncan R, Pratten MK (1985) Pinocytosis: mechanism and regulation. In: Dean RT, Jessup W (eds) Mononuclear phagocytes: physiology and pathology. Elsevier-North Holland, Amsterdam, pp 27–51

Dunton A, Al-Alousi L, Pratten MK, Beck F (1986) The giant yolk sac: a model for studying early placental transport. J Anat 145:189–206

Freeman SJ, Beck F, Lloyd JB (1987) The role of the visceral yolk sac in mediating protein utilisation by rat embryos cultured *in vitro*. J Embryol Exp Morphol 6:223–234

Lowry DH, Rosebrough NJ, Farr AL, Randall RJ (1951) Protein measurement with Folin phenol reagent. J Biol Chem 193:265–275

New DAT (1978) Whole embryo culture and the study of mammalian embryos during organogenesis. Biol Rev 53:81–122

Williams KE, Kidston ME, Beck F, Lloyd JB (1975) Quantitative studies of pinocytosis. I. Kinetics of uptake of ^{125}I-polyvinylpyrrolidone in rat yolks sacs cultured *in vitro*. J Cell Biol 64:113–122

Mechanisms and Models in Toxicology
Arch. Toxicol., Suppl. 11, 163–167 (1987)

The Effect of Ethanol on the Growth of Rat Embryos: The Role of Stage Dependency and Hyperosmolality

A. M. Clode, M. K. Pratten, and F. Beck

Department of Anatomy, Leicester University Medical School, University Road, Leicester, LE1 7RH, UK

Introduction

Clinical studies and experimental research have established the teratological relationship between constant ethanol consumption throughout pregnancy, and the occurrence of alcohol embryopathy (AE) in the offspring of alcoholics (as reviewed by Abel, 1982). The implication of social or "binge" drinking is of specific interest because confusion exists concerning advice given to pregnant women about their drinking habits.

In order to investigate the role of such drinking patterns, it is useful to establish an animal model which has relevance to the human condition in respect of dose and duration of ethanol exposure. This has been achieved with in-vivo models using mice (Kronick 1976; Webster et al. 1980; Sulik et al. 1981), and to a lesser extent with rats (Tze and Lee 1975; Henderson et al. 1979; Abel and Dintcheff 1978). The use of in-vitro models, such as in the roller culture technique of New (1978), allows controlled conditions of ethanol exposure for a great part of the the period of organogenesis, which is normally particularly sensitive to teratological insult. Many workers using rat embryos in culture have shown embryo-sensitivity only above ethanol concentrations of 400 mg%, and with long exposure periods of up to 48 h (Brown et al. 1979; Popov et al. 1982; Priscott 1982, Wynter et al. 1983); this would be equivalent to an almost lethal dose and several weeks' gestation in humans. However, Beck et al. (1984) exposed 9.5-day-old rat embryos for 4 h to serum from human donors who had consumed whisky. The serum contained approximately 120 mg% ethanol, and significant retardation of growth together with abnormal development was found.

Based on this result; the potential of the in-vitro culture technique as a model for AE was investigated, using embryos cultured in rat serum supplemented with ethanol. Two factors were concentrated on: the stage dependency of the response, and the role of increased serum osmolality associated with the presence of ethanol.

Materials and Methods

Rat embryos were obtained on the 9th day of gestation and assessed for development, in order to be differentiated into three categories: the head-process stage (pre-neural groove; Fig. 1 a), the early head-fold stage (Fig. 1 b), and the late head-fold stage (Fig. 1 c). The embryos were cultured for 48 h by the method of New (1978) in hyperosmotic rat serum containing either ethanol, glycerol, NaCl, or concentrated Hanks' salts; or iso-osmotic sera containing the same solutes plus 27% distilled water (as described below).

Embryos at each of the three stages were cultured for 4 h in 300 mg% (65.5 mM) ethanol, and then for 44 h in normal rat serum, in order to establish the stage dependency of the response. Since addition of ethanol to serum raises serum osmolality, the importance of osmolality can be investigated by mimicking hyperosmotic serum by the addition of other solutes to serum. Therefore, rat serum was supplemented with 65.5 mM glycerol, 32.8 mM NaCl or 7% concentrated ($\times$4) Hanks' salts. A second series of embryos at the head-process and

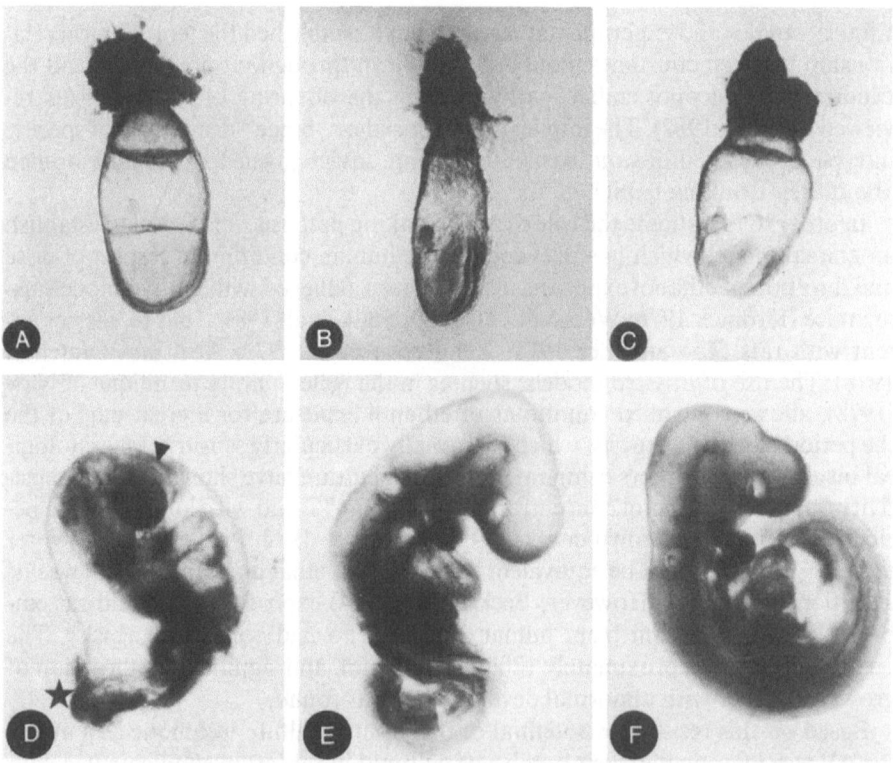

Fig. 1. A Egg-cylinder at the head-process (pre-neural groove) stage of development. **B** Egg-cylinder at the early head-fold stage of development. **C** Egg-cylinder at the late head-fold stage of development. **D** A grossly retarded and abnormal embryo, exposed to ethanol at the head-process stage of development, showing the characteristic open neural tube (▼) and dorsally convex tail (★). **E** A slightly retarded embryo exposed to ethanol at the early head-fold stage of development, with the characteristic "spiral" tail. **E** A normal embryo exposed to ethanol at the late head-fold stage

early head-fold stages were cultured for 4 h in each of these sera and then transferred to normal rat serum for the remaining 44 h. Correction of osmolality and dilution of the solute concentration occur when distilled water is added to hyperosmotic serum in proportion to the increase in osmolality. In order to keep the final solute concentration constant, excess ethanol (82.5 mM), glycerol (82.5 mM) and NaCl (41.3 mM) were added initially, and the osmolality was corrected by adding 27% distilled water. A further series of embryos at the head-process and the early head-fold stages were cultured for 4 h in these media and then transferred to normal rat serum for the rest of the culture period. In addition the dose response to a 4-h exposure to ethanol at the head-process stage was investigated. Again embryos were exposed for 4 h to ethanol in doses of 50–300 mg%, and then were placed for the remainder of the culture period in normal rat serum.

Embryos were assessed for growth and development by their crown–rump length, protein content, morphological score, etc.; specific abnormalities such as open neural tubes were also noted.

Results and Conclusions

Nine-day-old rat embryos showed a stage-dependent response to a 4-h exposure to 300 mg% ethanol (Table 1). The embryos showed significant retardation of growth and development at the most sensitive head-process stage, but this effect was virtually absent by the late head-fold stage some 5 h later (Fig. 1 d–f). This offers an explanation for the apparent resistance of rat embryos to teratogenic insult by ethanol as previously reported by Brown et al. (1979), Popov et al. (1982), Priscott (1982), and Wynter et al. (1983).

Exposure to either hyperosmotic serum, or corrected hyperosmotic serum resulted in greater abnormalities at the head-process stage, than at the early head-fold stage (Fig. 2), again showing stage-dependency. Hyperosmotic serum con-

Table 1. The effect of 300 mg% ethanol on the embryonic growth of 9.5-day-old rat embryos grown in culture at different stages of gestation (mean ± SEM)

Gestational stage	Abn. + Ret./ n	Morphological score	Crown–rump length	Protein (μg)	% Open neural tube
Head-process					
control	0/20 (0%)	42.90 ± 0.26	3.29 ± 0.04	203.06 ± 8.72	0
ethanol	9/15 (60%)	36.90 ± 1.80[a]	2.99 ± 0.10[a]	166.90 ± 13.39[a]	40
Early head-fold					
control	0/19 (0%)	43.11 ± 0.16	3.28 ± 0.05	185.80 ± 5.18	0
ethanol	7/20 (35%)	42.10 ± 0.26[a]	3.02 ± 0.06[a]	161.50 ± 6.51[a]	0
Late head-fold					
control	0/31 (0%)	43.17 ± 0.13	3.20 ± 0.05	222.58 ± 5.55	0
ethanol	2/28 (7%)	43.30 ± 0.14	3.29 ± 0.06	204.25 ± 5.73[b]	0

[a] Significantly different at $p \leq 0.01$.
[b] Significantly different at $p \leq 0.05$.
Abn. = abnormal embryo; Ret. = retarded embryo.

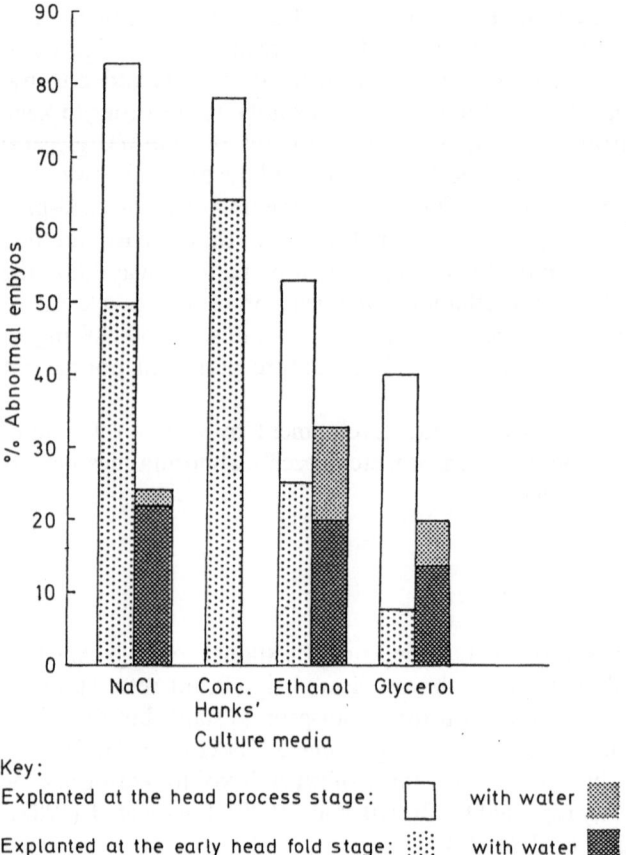

Key:

Explanted at the head process stage: ☐ with water ▦

Explanted at the early head fold stage: ⬚ with water ◼

Fig. 2. The effect of developmental stage and osmolality on the percentage of abnormal embryos

taining glycerol mimicked to some extent the effects of ethanol, but the embryos were not so adversely affected. Embryos cultured in serum containing NaCl or concentrated Hanks' salts were more severely affected than those exposed to ethanol, many optic abnormalities being observed. Addition of distilled water partially reversed the embryopathic effect of each of the hyperosmotic sera, although a residual effect remained. Thus, the effect of ethanol can be partially attributed to increased osmolality. However, there are some effects that cannot be abrogated by normalising the osmotic effect.

Preliminary investigations into the dose response to a 4-h exposure of ethanol at the head-process stage have shown that an embryopathic effect only occurs at doses at or above 150 mg%.

Acknowledgement. Thanks are due to Wellcome Trust for their generous support of this work.

References

Abel EL (1982) Consumption of alcohol during pregnancy: a review of effects on growth and development of offspring. Hum Biol 54:421–453

Abel EL, Dintcheff B (1978) Effects of pre-natal alcohol exposure on growth and development in rats. J Pharmacol Exp Ther 207:916–921

Beck F, Huxham IM, Gulamhusein AP (1984) Growth of rat embryos in the serum of alcohol drinkers. In: Porter et al. (eds) Mechanisms of alcohol damage in utero. Pitman, London, pp 218–233 (CIBA Foundation Symposium 105)

Brown NA, Goulding EH, Fabro S (1979) Ethanol embryotoxicity: direct effects on mammaliam embryos *in vitro*. Science 206:573–575

Henderson GL, Hoyumpa A, McClain C, Schenker S (1979) The effects of chronic and acute alcohol administration on the fetal development in the rat. Alcoholism Clin Expt Res 3:99–106

Kronick JB (1976) Teratogenic effects of ethyl alcohol administered to pregnant mice. Am J Obstet Gynecol 124:678–680

New DAT (1978) Whole embryo culture and the study of mammalian embryos during organogenesis. Biol Rev 53:81–122

Popov VB, Vaisman BL, Puchkov VF, Ignat'eva TV (1982) Toxic action of ethanol and its biotransformation products on post-implantation rat embryos in culture. Bull Eksp Biol Med 72:1707–1710

Priscott PK (1982) The effects of ethanol on rat embryos developing in vitro. Biochem Pharmacol 31:3641–3643

Sulik KK, Johnston MC, Webb MA (1981) Fetal alcohol syndrome: embryogenesis in a mouse model. Science 214:936–938

Tze WJ, Lee M (1975) Adverse effects of maternal alcohol consumption on pregnancy and foetal growth in rats. Nature 257:479–480

Webster WS, Walsh DA, Lipson AH, McEwen SE (1980) Teratogenesis after acute alcohol exposure in inbred and outbred mice. Neurobehav Toxicol 2:227–234

Wynter JM, Walsh DA, Webster WS, McEwen SE, Lipson AH (1983) Teratogenesis after acute exposure in cultured rat embryos. Teratogenesis Carcinog Mutagen 3:421–428

Mechanisms and Models in Toxicology
Arch. Toxicol., Suppl. 11, 168–171 (1987)

Modification of Teratogenic Action In Vitro Due to Reduced Culture Medium Serum Content

D. W. Young and S. J. Freeman

Department of Toxicology, Smith Kline and French Research Limited, The Frythe, Welwyn, Herts., AL6 9AR UK

Introduction

The ability to control the environment in which embryos are growing and developing by using whole post-implantation embryo culture techniques has led to significant advances in the basic understanding of how teratogens exert their effects on morphogenesis (Sadler and Warner 1984). In the present paper, the effect of altering the serum content of the culture medium on the actions of two teratogens, anti-visceral yolk sac antiserum (anti-VYS) and suramin, is reported. The results indicate that embryos cultured in medium containing as little as 40% rat serum grow and develop as well as embryos cultured in standard medium containing 75% rat serum, and that decreasing the serum content of the culture medium results in an increased potency of the two agents.

Methods

In all experiments, early to mid head-fold stage rat embryos of the Olac Wistar Strain (Olac 1976 Ltd., UK) were explanted at 9.5 days' gestation (pregnancy timed from the midnight preceding the morning on which a vaginal plug was found) and cultured for 48 h by the method of New (1978). Culture medium comprised homologous rat serum (75%, 50% or 40% by volume) and Eagle's minimal essential medium (MEM). Anti-VYS, prepared as described previously (Freeman and Brown 1986) but omitting the Con-A–Sepharose purification step, or suramin (a gift from Professor J. B. Lloyd, University of Keele, UK) was added to cultures in MEM and was present throughout the 48 h.

At harvesting, embryonic development was assessed by the criteria of Brown and Fabro (1981) and embryonic protein content determined (Lowry et al. 1951).

Results and Discussion

Table 1 compares the morphological scores and protein contents of embryos cultured in medium containing different proportions of rat serum. The data demonstrate that in culture medium containing as little as 40% serum, embryos apparently grew and developed as well as in standard culture medium containing 75% serum. However, the susceptibility of embryos to teratogenic insult increased in low-serum-containing medium. The incidence of embryonic dysmorphogenesis and extent of growth retardation (protein content) after culture in the presence of anti-VYS (Fig. 1) was greater in medium containing 50% and 40% serum than in medium containing 75% serum. Similarly, 1000 µg/ml suramin caused considerably more growth retardation and dysmorphogenesis in medium containing 40% or 50% serum than in medium containing 75% serum, although 500 µg/ml suramin produced little effect when the medium serum content was decreased (Fig. 2). The extent and severity of malformations observed in low-serum medium was also greater (data not shown).

Both of these teratogens are thought to exert their effects through an action on yolk sac-mediated embryotrophic nutrition (Freeman et al. 1982; Freeman and Lloyd 1985). Suramin is known to be extensively protein-bound in serum (Hawking 1978). A decrease in serum protein concentration might result in an increase in the free suramin concentration in the medium and hence a more severe toxic effect on the embryo.

Anti-VYS immunoglobulins have been postulated (Freeman and Brown 1986) to act on yolk sac by cross-reaction with a specific plasma membrane antigen. A decrease in the serum protein concentration of the culture medium might reduce non-specific competition for binding to this antigen and increase the potency of anti-VYS.

Alternatively, the reduction in medium serum may have induced microscopic changes in embryonic tissues, rendering them more susceptible to toxic insult.

Table 1. Comparative growth and development of rat embryos cultured in medium containing different proportions of serum[a]

Percentage serum by volume	Morphological score[b] ($\pm$ SD)	Protein (mg) ($\pm$ SD)
75% (control)	41.3 $\pm$ 1.2 ($n=18$)	235.7 $\pm$ 34.4 ($n=16$)
50%	41.5 $\pm$ 1.3 ($n=23$)	247.2 $\pm$ 47.1 ($n=13$)
40%	41.2 $\pm$ 1.0 ($n=30$)	220.1 $\pm$ 34.6 ($n=24$)

[a] No significant differences were detected between values determined in culture medium containing 50% and 40% serum and control (75% serum) as judged by Student's t test.
[b] Morphological score was derived by the method of Brown and Fabro (1981).

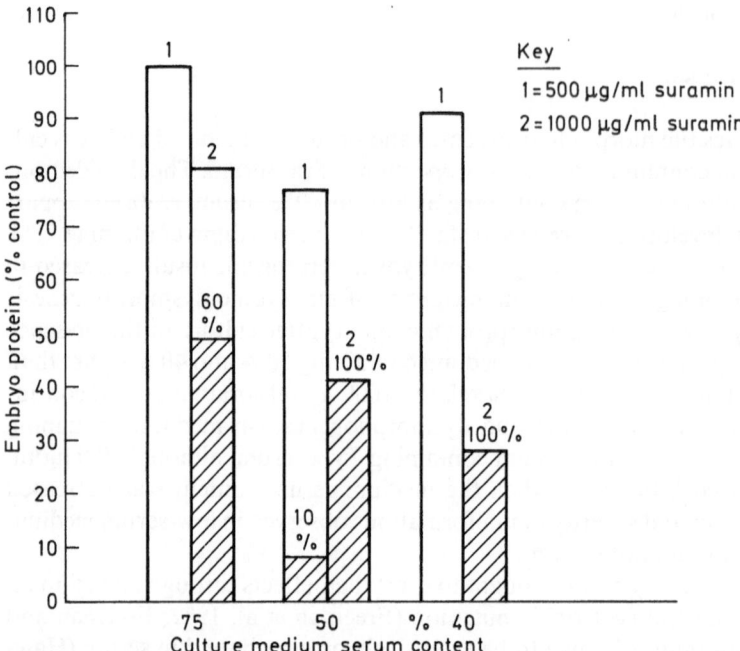

Fig. 2. Effect of suramin on embryonic development in vitro in medium containing different proportions of serum. Hatched areas of columns indicate the percentage (enumerated at the top of the hatched areas) of embryos in the group that were abnormal

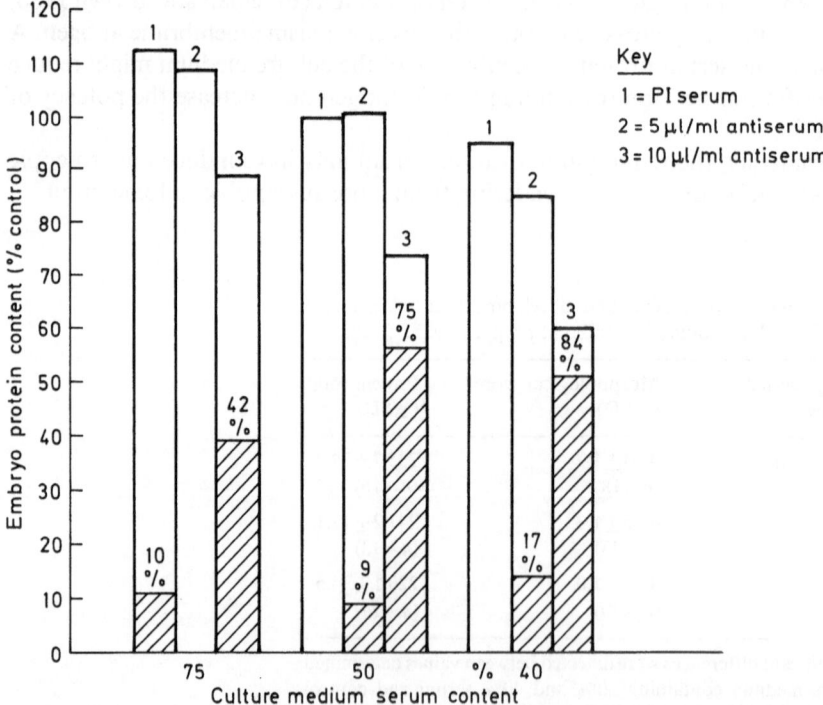

Fig. 1. Effect of anti-VYS and rabbit pre-immunization serum (PI; 25 μl/ml) on embryonic development in vitro in medium containing different proportions of serum. Hatched areas of columns indicate the percentage (enumerated at the top of the hatched areas) of embryos in the group that were abnormal

References

Brown NA, Fabro S (1981) Quantitation of rat embryonic development in vitro: a morphological scoring system. Teratology 24:65–78

Freeman SJ, Brent RL, Lloyd JB (1982) The effect of teratogenic antiserum on yolk sac function in rat embryos cultured in vitro. J Embryol Exp Morphol 71:63–74

Freeman SJ, Brown NA (1986) An in vitro study of teratogenicity in the rat due to antibody-induced yolk sac dysfunction. Identification of the yolk sac antigen involved. Roux's Archiv Dev Biol 195:236–242

Freeman SJ, Lloyd JB (1985) Interference with embryonic nutrition as the teratogenic mechanism of action of suramin and aurothiomalate in rats. Biochem Soc Trans 13:196–197

Hawking F (1978) Suramin: with special reference to onchocerciasis. Adv Pharmacol Chemother 15:289–322

Lowry OH, Rosebrough NJ, Farr AL, Randall RJ (1951) Protein measurement with the Folin phenol reagent. J Biol Chem 193:265–275

New DAT (1978) Whole embryo culture and the study of mammalian embryos during organogenesis. Biol Rev 53:81–122

Sadler TW, Warner CW (1984) Use of whole embryo culture for evaluating toxicity and teratogenicity. Pharmacol Rev 36:1455–1505

Mechanisms and Models in Toxicology
Arch. Toxicol., Suppl. 11, 172–174 (1987)

In Vitro Teratogenicity of Parbendazole

C. L. Wildgoose and C. E. Steele

Department of Toxicology, Smith Kline and French Research Limited, The Frythe, Welwyn, Herts., AL6 9AR, UK

Introduction

In order to determine the value of whole embryo culture (WEC) as a screen for teratogens, an attempt was made to reproduce in this system the teratogenic effects seen in routine in vivo reproductive toxicity studies. Parbendazole (SKF 29044) was found to be teratogenic in vivo in the dose range 10–50 mg/kg body wt. Litters of pregnant Wistar rats dosed during mid-gestation exhibited malformations which indicated effects in both early (exencephaly, anophthalmia, etc.) and late (retina folding, fused ribs, etc.) organogenesis. The former malformations are such that they could be demonstrated in WEC.

Parbendazole (2-carbomethoxyamino-5-*n*-butylbenzimidazole; formerly marketed as "Helmatac", a veterinary antihelmintic agent) is only available in the form of a suspension. Rats were therefore dosed with the suspension and bled at the time of peak plasma concentration. Serum prepared from the blood samples was used to provide the embryo culture medium.

The results show that the use of WEC as a screen for teratogens would have predicted the adverse effects of parbendazole observed in vivo.

Methods

Olac Wistar rat embryos (head-fold stage) were explanted into Hanks' saline on day 9.5 of gestation (day 0.5 being midday on the day a positive vaginal smear or a vaginal plug was found). The embryos were transferred into culture medium consisting of serum (1 ml per embryo) containing antibiotics. The embryos were cultured in a roller apparatus (New 1978) in an incubator maintained at a temperature of 37 °C. They were assessed 48 h after the start of culture (see Table 1).

Serum was prepared from the blood of non-pregnant SKF Wistar rats. All blood samples were immediately centrifuged at ca. 1550 g for 10 min and the serum heat-inactivated at 56 °C for 30 min (Steele and New 1974). Control serum

Table 1. Effect on embryonic development of culture in serum prepared from the blood of rats dosed with parbendazole

Dose	No. of embryos	At end of culture		Turning[a]			Optic vesicles	Oto-cysts	Pharyngeal pouches			Neuro-pore closed (anterior)	Fusion of allantois with chorion	Limb buds	No. of somites $(x \pm SE)$	Protein $(x \pm SE)$ (µg)
		Heart beat	Yolk sac circulation	U	U–C	C			1	2	3					
B Control vehicle	9	9	9	0	1	8	9	9	0	0	9	6	9	9	25±0	123±6
C 25 mg/kg[b]	9	–	–	–	–	–	–	–	–	–	–	–	–	–	–	29±4[c]
A Control serum	4	4	4	0	0	4	4	4	0	0	4	4	4	4	24±0	192±9
B Control vehicle	7	7	7	0	2	5	7	7	0	0	7	6	7	7	24±0	142±25
C 12.5 mg/kg[b]	10	–	–	–	–	–	–	–	–	–	–	–	–	–	–	126±20[c]
A Control serum	10	10	10	1	1	8	9	10	0	1	9	9	10	10	24±1	182±7
B Control vehicle	13	13	13	1	1	11	13	13	0	1	12	13	13	12	25±1	179±12
C 11 mg/kg[d]	16	6	0	16	0	0	3	5	5	2	0	1	5	6	12±1	47±5
A Control serum	18	18	18	0	3	15	18	18	0	0	18	17	17	18	24±0	146±10
B Control vehicle	28	28	26	2	4[g]	22[g]	28	28	0	3	25	27	28	28	24±1	150±12
C 10 mg/kg	32	29[e]	29[f]	3	4[h]	25[h]	32	32	0	3	29	30	30[i]	32	24±0	149±13
B Control vehicle	4	4	4	0	3	1	4	4	0	0	4	4	4	3	23±2	179±36
C 10 mg/kg	4	3	1	1	0	3	3	3	1	0	3	3	3	1	23±1	131±13
C 7 mg/kg	4	2	1	0	2	2	4	4	0	1	3	4	4	3	22±3	174±37
C 4 mg/kg	3	3	3	0	3	3	3	3	0	0	3	3	3	3	26±1	237±33
C 1 mg/kg	3	3	3	0	0	3	3	3	0	0	3	3	3	3	26±1	233±29

[a] "Turning" is the process by which the embryo adopts the characteristic fetal position. U, unturned; C, turned; U–C, partially turned.

[b] Embryos too poorly formed to assess.

[c] Compared with A or B, all parameters are significantly different ($p < 0.001$).

[d] Embryos not dissected from membranes.

[e] Significantly different from A and B, $p < 0.05$.

[f] Significantly different from A, $p < 0.05$.

[g] Significantly different from A, $p < 0.01$ (U–C and C combined).

[h] Significantly different from A, $p < 0.05$ (U–C and C combined).

[i] Significantly different from B, $p < 0.05$.

(A) was obtained from untreated rats. Treated serum was obtained from rats dosed orally by gavage, 2–3 h prior to bleeding, with either the excipient of the parbendazole suspension (B, vehicle control) or with 10 ml/kg parbendazole suspension (C). Final doses were in the range 1–25 mg/kg.

The data were analysed statistically by Student's t test (somites, protein) or χ^2 (all other parameters).

Results

There were very few abnormalities in control embryos (group A). Vehicle control embryos (group B) were significantly different ($p < 0.01$) from control embryos in only one parameter measured, degree of turning (see Table 1).

In contrast, group C embryos cultured in serum from rats dosed with 25 or 12.5 mg/kg parbendazole were dead and disintegrating by the end of the culture period. Those cultured in serum from rats receiving 11 mg/kg exhibited retardation of differentiation (somite number), growth (protein content) and all parameters assessed (see Table 1). At 10 mg/kg or less, development in group C embryos exhibited little or no difference from that of groups A and B.

Discussion

An adverse effect was obtained in vitro at the lower end (11 mg/kg) of the in vivo teratogenic range (10–50 mg/kg). This is presumably due to the long-term (48-h) exposure to the peak concentration in vitro, compared with the short-term (1–6-h) peaks in vivo. The close approximation in the present experiments of the highest no-effect level (10 mg/kg) and the lowest embryotoxic concentration (11 mg/kg) is noteworthy. The large difference in the effects seen at these doses suggests that these two values could be further defined. In this instance embryo culture is clearly a sensitive test for embryotoxicity at the stage of early organogenesis. It is not possible to compare the abnormalities seen in vitro in group C embryos with those seen in vivo because of the general retardation in all parameters assessed. This could possibly be rectified by using a dose of 10.5 mg/kg parbendazole, in which case the embryos might be less dramatically affected and a comparison be made. An alternative would be to reduce the time of exposure of the embryos to culture medium containing parbendazole

References

New DAT (1978) Whole-embryo culture and the study of mammalian embryos during organogenesis. Biol Rev 53:81–122

Steele CE, New DAT (1974) Serum variants causing the formation of double hearts and other abnormalities in explanted rat embryos. J Embryol Exp Morphol 31:707–719

Safety Evaluation of Biotechnology Products

Mechanisms and Models in Toxicology
Arch. Toxicol., Suppl. 11, 177–181 (1987)

Predictive Tests for Occupational Allergies

W. E. Parish

Environmental Safety Laboratory, Unilever Research and Engineering,
Colworth House, Sharnbrook, Bedford, MK 44 1LQ, UK

The workplace may present special allergic hazards not normally occurring in the general environment. Staff may be exposed for long periods to chemicals not encountered by the general public – or not in the same amounts – or there may be prolonged exposure to normal substances by an abnormal route, as, for instance, the inhalation of dusts of cereals, yeasts and additives by bakers, sometimes resulting in asthma.

Most natural substances and chemicals of high molecular weight are antigenic, inducing replication of specifically primed lymphocytes and usually formation of antibody. Some low-molecular-weight substances, usually below 400 daltons, are not antigenic but become so on binding strongly to the body proteins, particularly, but not exclusively, by covalent links. These haptens are a major source of allergens inducing lymphocyte-mediated hypersensitivity, usually manifested as contact dermatitis, though they may also stimulate formation of antibody.

People respond immunologically to most antigens to which they are exposed, but despite formation of sensitized lymphocytes and antibody they show no abnormal response on further exposure. Furthermore, even persons who become sensitized and respond to a skin prick test by a weal-and-flare anaphylactic response frequently show no adverse effect on normal or occupational exposure.

Every type of allergic response can result from occupational exposure, but the two of most frequent concern are anaphylactic sensitivity, usually manifested as asthma, and less frequently, contact urticaria and the lymphocyte-mediated, delayed hypersensitivity presenting as contact dermatitis. The following is a brief account of laboratory predictive tests for anaphylactic allergic potential and for contact dermatitis sensitization.

Prediction of Allergenic Potency

Past History

The most valuable indication of the potential of a substance to induce allergy is the information on exposure to it or to similar substances available in publications and computer data banks.

Structure/Activity Relationships

Studies to predict allergic potential have as yet little application. In atopic (spontaneous anaphylactic) sensitivity, there is much variation in allergic potency of substances; for example, in cow's milk containing 32 or more antigens, only four are normally considered to be allergens, and one in particular, β-lactoglobulin, is the major allergen. There are data to implicate lysine–sugar sequences in a highly reactive (or reducing) form as the critical epitopes in a wide range of natural allergens (Berrens 1971).

In studies of hapten allergens inducing delayed hypersensitivity, within a group of similar chemicals the relative allergic potency may be predicted by determining their alkylating properties (Roberts and Williams 1982; Goodwin and Roberts 1986). By determining in vitro properties of the chemical – the alkylation rate constant measured against a standard nucleophile, molar dose, and the partition coefficient measured between a standard polar/non-polar solvent – it was found possible to predict the sensitization potential within a series of sultones (Goodwin et al. 1983) and within a series of p-nitrobenzyl compounds (Roberts et al. 1983). Thus some limited prediction of sensitization potential may be obtained from in vitro data.

In Vitro Predictive Tests

There are no in vitro procedures applicable to prediction of antigenic or allergenic potential, though in vitro tests on lymphocytes or antibodies may be used to extend observations from animal tests (Parish 1986) in the manner as used to study human allergies.

Predictive Tests for Anaphylactic Allergenic Potential

The antibody mediating most human anaphylactic responses (asthma, allergic rhinitis, and much acute urticaria) is IgE. Any individual may, on appropriate exposure, form IgE antibody, but about 15% of the population have a particular susceptibility to forming IgE antibodies to environmental antigens (e.g. grass pollen and fungal spores) well tolerated by the majority. There is no equivalent of this atopic susceptibility in small laboratory animals.

There is no adequate animal model to predict anaphylactic potential of substances for man except in inhalation tests. On antigenic stimulation most laboratory animals form IgG antibodies, some subclasses of which contain the main anaphylactic antibodies. Formation of IgE antibodies can be induced by concomitant stimulation with adjuvants, e.g. *Bordetella pertussis* antigen in rats and mice. There is no good evidence that this treatment enables clear differentiation between allergens with and without a particular ability to induce anaphylactic sensitization in man. Differences in responses of guinea-pigs and rats to induced anaphylactic sensitivity compared to the sensitivity occurring in man by environmental exposure is presented in Table 1.

The regimen of induction and examination of sensitization in vitro or in vivo compared with that of a standard allergen is described elsewhere (Parish 1981). Though induction by injection does not provide good evidence of anaphylactic

Table 1. Anaphylactic sensitivity induced in guinea-pigs and rats: differences from that occurring in man. (From Parish 1981)

Guinea-pigs and rats	Man
The usual response to experimental antigenic stimulation is formation of anaphylactic IgG antibodies.	Most anaphylactic antibody is IgE; a small proportion of people form IgG anaphylactic antibodies (IgG S-TS).
To induce formation of IgE antibodies are needed adjuvants and special treatment regimen.	IgE is formed spontaneously, especially in atopic subjects.
Some strains of actively sensitized animals show increased "releasability" of histamine from tissue and blood, but few other susceptibilities to mediators of anaphylaxis.	Atopic subjects, and some non-atopic sensitized subjects, show increased "releasability" of histamine and other mediators, and increased susceptibility to the effects of mediators.
Inhalation tests are probably comparable to human exposure (though effects are not usually mediated by IgE). Sensitization by injection and feeding has not been shown to be comparable to human anaphylactic disease.	

potential, such tests do enable the immunogenic (general antigenic) potential to be assessed in comparison to selected standard substances.

Tests by inhalation exposure according to a similar protocol provide a more relevant prediction of human anaphylactic sensitization potential by the same route of exposure. There are, however, several examples of occupational asthma in which the allergic aetiology is unknown and controversial, and for which animal experiments have provided little support, e.g. in the case of toluene diisocyanate (TDI) (Bernstein 1982; Davies 1984), or have been derived from tests on man and have not predicted the activity, i.e. in the case of platinum (Pepys 1984).

Delayed Hypersensitivity Contact Dermatitis

Allergic contact dermatitis is a frequently occurring occupational disorder. In this manifestation of delayed hypersensitivity, chemical haptens or antigens penetrating the skin react with specifically sensitized lymphocytes, stimulating them to generate and release their products (lymphokines), which mediate the tissue changes. There are several predictive tests of varying discriminating potential (see Marzulli and Maibach 1977; Ritz and Buehler 1980; Parish 1981).

The most discriminating is the maximization test of Magnusson and Kligman (1970), in which guinea-pigs are first treated with the test substance in Freund's complete adjuvant to induce any sensitization, and later challenged by a non-irritant concentration of the substance in a patch test, as in routine diagnostic tests on man. Since the first requirement is to determine *any* potential for sensitization, it is appropriate to use the most critical procedure available. Thus the maximization test was the method of choice in 10 out of 14 laboratories participating in an ECETOC study group (ECETOC 1980), and is the preferred method of the United Kingdom Health and Safety Commission Code of Practice (Health and Safety Commission 1982).

Table 2. Relevance of animal models to prediction of allergenic potential of substances for man

Type of allergy	Route of induction/challenge	Prediction of allergenicity for man
Anaphylactic	Injection	Poor
Anaphylactic	Injection plus adjuvants for IgE formation	Poor
Anaphylactic	Inhalation	Quite good
Immune-complex mediated	Injection or inhalation	Very poor
Delayed hypersensitivity (contact dermatitis)	Injection and/or application	Very good

The results of the test provide evidence of hazard. For evaluations of risk much experience is necessary to assess the influence of several properties and conditions of use, including the allergic potency of the substance, concentration in use, frequency of use, persistence on or penetration through skin, cross-reactivity with other substances in use, and the number of people exposed. The number of people exposed should not be a determining feature; if even one person is sensitized, the product is at fault in that respect. However, evidence of sensitization in a population may only become apparent after many are exposed for long periods.

The relevance of animal models to the prediction of allergenic potential of substances for man is summarized in Table 2.

References

Bernstein IL (1982) Isocyanate-induced pulmonary diseases: a current perspective. J Allergy Clin Immunol 70:24–31

Berrens L (1971) The chemistry of atopic allergens. Basel, Karger

Davies RJ (1984) Respiratory hypersensitivity to diisocyanates. In: Pepys J (ed) Occupational respiratory allergy. Saunders, London, pp 103–123

ECETOC (1980) Skin sensitization. European Chemical Industry Ecology and Toxicology Centre. Brussels (task force report)

Goodwin BFJ, Roberts DW (1986) Structure–activity relationships in allergic contact dermatitis. Fd Chem Toxic (in press)

Goodwin BFJ, Roberts DW, Williams DL, Johnson AW (1983) Skin sensitization potential of saturated and unsaturated sultones. In: Gibson GG, Hubbard R, Parke DV (eds) Immunotoxicology, Academic, London, pp 443–448

Health and Safety Commission (1982) Methods for the determination of toxicity. Her Majesty's Stationery Office, London (Health and Safety Commission Approved Code of Practice)

Magnusson B, Kligman AM (1970) Allergic contact dermatitis in the guinea-pig. Identification of contact allergens. Thomas, Springfield

Marzulli FN, Maibach HJ (eds) (1977) Dermatotoxicology and pharmacology. Wiley, New York

Parish WE (1981) Immunological tests to predict toxicological hazards to man. In: Gorrod JW (ed) Testing for toxicity. Taylor and Francis, London, pp 297–315

Parish WE (1986) Evaluation of in vitro predictive tests for irritation and allergic sensitization. Fd Chem Toxic 24:481–494

Pepys J (1984) Occupational allergy due to platinum complex salts. In: Pepys J (ed) Occupational respiratory allergy. Saunders, London, pp 131–157

Ritz HL, Buehler EV (1980) Planning, conduct and interpretation of guinea-pig sensitization patch tests. In: Drill VA, Lazar P (eds) Current concepts in cutaneous toxicity, 2nd edn. Academic, New York, pp 25–40

Roberts DW, Williams DL (1982) The derivation of quantitative correlations between skin sensitisation and physio-chemical parameters for alkylating agents, and their application to experimental data for sultones. J Theor Biol 99:807–825

Roberts DW, Goodwin BFJ, Williams DL, Jones K, Johnson AW, Alderson JCE (1983) Correlations between skin sensitization potential and chemical reactivity for p-nitrobenzyl compounds. Fd Chem Toxic 21:811–813

Mechanisms and Models in Toxicology
Arch. Toxicol., Suppl. 11, 182–190 (1987)
© by Springer-Verlag 1987

Toxicological Evaluation of Biotechnology Products: A Regulatory Viewpoint *

R. Bass and E. Scheibner

Institut für Arzneimittel, Bundesgesundheitsamt (Federal Health Office), Seestr. 10, D-1000 Berlin (West) 65, Germany

Introduction

Many large pharmaceutical companies have already decided to move into the area of biotechnology; others will certainly follow. This first important decision has already been taken and products have begun to show up at the other end of the research and development pipeline. Regulatory decisions allowing the marketing of these products have been seemingly easy up until now. The development of future products, which may, it is hoped, allow treatment of causes of illness, requires information on how regulatory agencies will fulfil their legal obligation to protect the consumer while not hindering the development and use of important products. Last but not least, to take into account the need to protect animals, which might be in conflict with the growing desire for non-human primate data must be taken into account. The present situation of safety testing resembles the malicious, confused and confusing conception of double-blind trials. The doctor does not know who he is aiming at and the patient does not know what he is receiving. Since either role can be played successfully by the company or the regulatory agency, they should act together.

From the viewpoint of a regulatory agency this must be achieved by acting according to the following script:
- Pre-existing rules for drug safety testing
- Reasons for toxicological studies with biotechnological products
- Criteria stemming from
  type of production employed
  type of product obtained
  type of effect (dose) aimed at
- Toxicological approaches leading to registration
- Experience

---

* This paper presents the opinion of the authors. Views presented were derived in part from discussions of the Safety Working Party (chairman: first author) of the European community's Committee for Proprietary Medicinal Products (CPMP). No official statement describing toxicological testing of biotechnology products is available.

Pre-Existing Rules for Drug Safety Testing

In a member state of the European Community, the EC rules and regulations for marketing new proprietary medicinal products (Council Directives and Council Recommendations 1983, 1984) are cited in place of other national or international regulations. In principle, the ground they cover includes safety testing of biotechnologically produced compounds, unless superseded by special rules. As regards biotechnology, the major aims of EC safety regulation are to guarantee sufficient proof of safety, to avoid duplicate experiments, to harmonize requirements and decisions, to speed up development and registration of products, and to widen the definition of "drug" to additionally accommodate vaccines, blood products and in vitro diagnostics, in order to fully cover biological medicines (Proposal for a Council Directive 1984). This paper restricts itself to the requirement for the guarantee of safety, which is handled by the Safety Working Party of the Committee for Proprietary Medicinal Products.

Until specific guidance for biotechnological products becomes available, there are two options. The first is to perform all the toxicological studies in the book (Notes for Guidance in Council Directive 1983 and Proposal for a Council Recommendation 1984) prior to marketing, excepting only those studies which are obvious inappropriate. Even many regulatory agencies seem unhappy with this strategy. The second is to perform studies on a case by case basis. But what studies? Before the EC has produced 'Points to Consider' or 'Notes for Guidance', member states are trying to protect their agencies or help industry by writing or drafting national requirements (France, United Kingdom). Of course, other countries, like USA, Japan and Sweden did so some time ago. As far as the authors are aware, these countries either adhere to one of the two options above or are noncommital.

Guidance on quality aspects of biotechnological products has developed gradually and remains manageable by both industry and regulatory authorities; guidance on pharmacological experimentation clearly states what needs to be proved; and proper design, performance and monitoring of careful clinical trials become obvious. However, the toxicological experimentation and guidance which are needed both for safety of the patient and registerability of the drug are relatively underdeveloped. It must be said that regulation at the toxicological level can be only as good and precise as the scientific state of the art will allow; the developmental state of the art, however, relies on research-and-development companies. Many biotechnological products are antineoplastic agents. For these drugs one would be well advised to adjust toxicological testing to the indication claimed, and then decide about additional needs in order to avoid competition between the treatment-oriented approach employed for cytostatics and the broad safety approach to be employed for biotechnological products. Unfortunately, rules for preclinical and clinical requirements for antineoplastics have not been drafted, published or internationally harmonized to a satisfying extent.

Biotechnological products are classified in the EC as 'New Drugs', even if they are not considered to be a new chemical entity. This is done, in part, in order to protect the pharmaceutical company concerned and its know-how.

Today's Reasons for Toxicological Studies with Biotechnological Products

Testing according to strategies deduced from existing (toxicity, pharmacokinetics) or upcoming Notes for Guidance of the EC (safety pharmacology, antineoplastic agents) may prove suitable to cover a considerable part of today's
safety requirements for biotechnological products. One difficulty in predicting
the type of experiments and results needed for registration is caused by the apparent misuse of toxicological experimentation for quality control measures. Some-
how there has been a return to the old days of pharmaceutical manufacture, when
synthesis, weighing and analysis of pure chemical compounds was unheard of.
Toxicological determination of the lethality of digitalis preparations by frog-
doses was the established means for the determination of quality, stability, purity
and content of this active component in the batch of the plant extract. Therefore,
use of such methods for biotechnological compounds was nothing new; it derived
from experience. In view of progress achieved in the past, however, the use of in
vitro models instead of in vivo techniques should be aimed at for such purposes,
even for compounds produced differently. It will have to be decided at a later
stage and by category of compound whether this type of quality control will be
transient or is impossible to replace.

Safety pharmacology is a kind of pharmacological screening for anticipated
substance-related effects on the large systems and functions of the body which
employs high, unpharmacological (i.e., potentially toxic) doses in experiments of
short duration. Such studies are used as a substitute for clinically testing high
doses in humans. Such studies may be performed by either pharmacologists,
toxicologists, or, best of all, both working together. Small groups of animals, of
several species if necessary, can easily be assessed for central nervous system, cardiovascular, lung, kidney and hormonal function and interactions. The methods
employed are clearly pharmacologically oriented, but are carried out from a
toxicological viewpoint. When such experiments are performed in the right species, they are more likely to also detect immune reaction related syndromes or
parts thereof which are known to occur in humans, like the 'acute phase syndrome' or 'flu syndrome' (see Table 1). It is important to mention that here and
later on that the targets are those which have already been established by experience in animal or man, e.g. with reference substances. Precise questions can
therefore be formulated and addressed by in vitro or in vivo model systems.

Table 1. Some examples for reactions described as occurring after
administration of biotechnological products in humans or animals

Acute reactions	Chronic reactions
Acute phase syndrome	Neutropenia
Flu syndrome	Thrombocytopenia
Fever, leucopenia	Hepatotoxicity
Aching joints, malaise	Glomerulonephritis
Fatigue, headache	Neurotoxicity
Anaphylactic reactions	Gastrointestinal toxicity
Urticaria	

After prolonged administration, other toxic effects or syndromes have to be ascertained and quantified (Table 1). Bone marrow, liver, kidney, gastrointestinal tract and the nervous system, in addition to the organs therapeutically aimed at, are among the possible or expected immune targets. Here again, pharmacological and clinical experience is used as a guide to subchronic and chronic testing. This necessitates repeated-dose administration experiments whose major emphasis is not predominantly on routine analysis, as is on other products. Although pure compounds which have so far reached the new drug application (NDA) stage do not have inherent mutagenic or carcinogenic potential, short-term testing for mutagenicity and carcinogenicity is generally thought necessary in order to cover other aspects such as, for example, cytotoxicity. Reproductive toxicity studies have been performed, some of them using primate species. The outcome may seem clear; however, the impact and the cause of toxicity described are still hard to interpret. Pharmacokinetic studies are, of course, desirable. The methods used will depend on the analytical methods that can be applied under in vivo conditions. For low blood levels of natural human proteins, assessment of activities vs time may be mor helpful. This is again an approach borrowed from (clinical) pharmacology.

Investigation and assessment of immune responses and of immunotoxicity beyond pathomorphological manifestations present a different set of problems which cannot be discussed here. Only when the scientific development in immunology and toxicology has progressed can in vivo or in vitro methods be defined and plugged into a general testing schedule. Until then the questions asked by safety pharmacology and repeated-dose administration must be answered. In addition, each biotechnological product will produce its own immunological problems, which must be solved as development of the individual drug proceeds, and which might possibly require individually developed methods of testing.

Type of Production Employed

The first parameter which determines the type and extent of testing required is the type of production employed. Use of recombinant DNA techniques obviously requires data on the exclusion of bacterial contaminants from the finished product and exclusion of products other than the one therapeutically wanted. For the production process, proof of DNA stability is required, otherwise the characteristics of the product may be altered. Investigations of pyrogenicity and of adjuvant activity are also necessary. Such a list could be lengthened almost indefinitely, but would overlap more and more with the proof of quality needed for registration.

Use of hybridoma techniques in the production of monoclonal antibodies poses different problems. Lymphoma cell constituents (DNA, virus particles) and host constituents (virus) have to be assayed. The possibility that non-DNA peptide sequences can possibly act as oncogenes has to be considered.

Use of aneuploid continuous cell lines, e.g. in the preparation of vaccines, involves the possibility of potentially oncogenic DNA being transmitted. Removal of DNA must, therefore, be shown.

Table 2. Classification of biotechnological products and uses

Type of product obtained	Type of use (dose and effect) aimed at)
Natural human proteins (hormones, enzymes, cytokines, transmitters) and their active sequences	Physiological/unphysiological
Analogues of human proteins [different species derived, modifications, (ex)changes]	Physiological/unphysiological, unknown
Novel oligopeptides	Unphysiological, unknown
Isosteric peptides	Unphysiological, unknown

For all types of production, including that of synthetic peptides, problems show up which are new and not yet adequately considered by toxicological or any other regulation so far. Toxicologists have yet to stake their claims on the basis of the power of their methods.

Type of Product/Type of Use

The next parameters which determine toxicological requirements are those of (non-)identity with natural human proteins and of physiological or unphysiological effects aimed at or obtained involuntarily (Table 2).

Hormones, enzymes, cytokines and other transmitters in their original human characteristics can be employed at low doses for substitution therapy. Higher doses used to induce unphysiological pharmacological effects are also possible. Analogues of human proteins can be derived from various species, and can be modified, purposely or otherwise. Modifications at the terminal and those within the amino acid sequence may have different consequences. Additions, exchanges and deletions are possible. Use of such products may occur at the physiological or unphysiological dose level, or the substance itself can be unphysiological. Novel oligopeptides and isosteric peptides will probably be applied for unphysiological pharmacological therapies and may induce as yet unknown effects.

This classification of products according to the therapeutic aim or dose and the unknown effects to be expected allows a graduated set of test requirements. Substances and effects close to human physiological conditions will require less testing for registration than those farther away.

Classification of Safety Testing

From the classification of products outlined above, three categories for safety testing requirements can be developed, category I requiring the least and category III requiring the most extensive testing for registration (Table 3). Although requirements are stepped up with increasing distance of the product from its natural human analogue, no direct correlation with any of the categories is set.

For category I, it is proposed that those tests needed to aid in establishing the identity of the product with its natural human counterpart, and the purity of the

Table 3. Safety testing requirements for the three categories of biotechnology products

---

Category I
  Identity, purity
  Pharmacology
  Safety pharmacology

Category II
  Category I plus:
  Detailed analysis of pharmacological actions vs. quality problems
    (human, animal)
  Relation between plasma concentrations and antibody titer
    (human, animal, in vitro), tolerance
  Selected toxicological testing

Category HI
  Categories I and II plus:
  Studies guided by indication
  Studied guided by duration of treatment

---

final product be performed. Changes or variations in three-dimensional structure
have been claimed to occur; they are most interesting with respect to the epitope
region determining antigenicity. The determination of pharmacological activity
at physiological doses as well as safety pharmacological studies as outlined above
should be performed.

For category II, a detailed analysis of quality problems via pharmacological
actions is suggested. Futhermore the relation between plasma concentration and
the development of antibodies, and tolerance towards the action of the drug,
should be studied by employing suitable animal and in vitro models. The results
should be compared with human data. Finally, some toxicological testing will be
required.

For category III, additional studies should be performed in relation to the proposed indication, dosage and duration of treatment. Studies should be adjusted
to the needs and requirements of other regulations, e.g. those for antineoplastic
agents.

It is apparent from what has been discussed so far that the clear-cut separation
and time sequence of preclinical and clinical development possible elsewhere cannot be used for biotechnology products. More and earlier interaction between
preclinical and clinical trials is acceptable and will have feedback on nonclinical
testing designed to solve suspected problems in suspected possible targets which
show up in clinical trials. Since neither the 'case by case' nor the 'everything in
the book except ...' approaches may provide the necessary amount of guidance
for the swift development and registration of a product, one should try to employ
paramctcrs relevant to risks which can be deduced from the type of product obtained, the type of production employed, and the type of use intended, together
with the three categories of safety testing, to derive what may be called a structured or pre-selective approach to toxicity testing, with allowances for case by
case deviations.

Structured Approach to Toxicity Testing

Performance of Safety Pharmacology Studies

These studies should be performed with all products at the beginning of toxico-logical investigations. If studies with pharmacologically active doses give no indi-cation of particular sensitivity in one species, several animal species should be screened, ranging from rodents to primate, to determine the most sensitive. Tests for impurities should then be carried out in this species.

Performance of Acute Toxicity and Mutagenicity Studies

These studies are performed routinely on all test compounds. Since lethality from acute exposure to proper biotechnology products does not seem to represent the major hazard for man, the possibility that safety pharmacology studies can wholly or partly replace acute toxicity studies should be investigated.

Mutagenicity studies should perhaps be performed, not only to detect mutage-nicity but also to detect cytotoxicity and stability of the manufacturing process and of the product (Galbraith, in press). The Note for Guidance for testing for mutagenic potential (proposal for a Council Recommendation 1984) can be ap-plied. Short-term tests to assess carcinogenic potential can be performed at this or a later stage.

Detailed Analysis of Safety Pharmacology in Short-term Experiments

For many products, pre-existing knowledge stemming from related products or from first clinical studies will indicate the necessity of assessing general bodily reactions, functions and interactions of organ systems, and reactions at unex-pected target organs. Pre-existing or accumulated knowledge will also indicate problems not accessible to solution by these studies. Further information from clinical studies may change this. Direct toxic reactions should be separated from those secondary to therapeutic effects. Hormonal interactions, action on repro-ductive organs, or unphysiologically high doses used in humans may require the assessment of specific periods of reproduction.

Impurities should be further searched for in the most sensitive species. A com-parison of plasma levels with (neutralizing) antibody formation vs time should be carried out.

Controversial Studies

Further studies should be governed by the proposed use (life-threatening or not), the distance of the product from natural human analogues, and the dosage and duration of treatment proposed. Chronic studies may have to be terminated be-cause of antibody formation. For this reason antibody formation should be moni-tored. Reproductive toxicity studies may become necessary. Where carcinogenic-ity studies become necessary but cannot be performed, short-term tests should be substituted, models like the nude mouse considered, and possible carcinogenic properties of the product reassessed.

Selection of Species

Until more knowledge that can be used for biotechnological product testing accumulates and until knowledge about the specific product allows decisions, a tendency towards using primate species for testing will increase. If this is deemed necessary, small, bred species should be employed for preference, and their selection should be based, on, e.g., the inducibility of pharmacological effects. Since the studies to be performed are mostly of the 'safety pharmacology' type (and of short duration), small-sized groups are feasible, and animals do not always need be killed.

Selection of Dosages

Since usable dosages may seem 'unlimited' because acute lethality is unlikely to occur, dose-selection should be determined according to the expected clinical dose. If clinical demands later require higher dosages, reassessment of the dosages tested in animals may require new studies. These will usually be designed differently because of further clinical experience.

Experience

It is not possible to report in detail on the types of studies performed, on their outcome, and on the arguments used by the pharmaceutical manufacturers; the EC has had very little experience with marketed biotechnological products. Countries with an IND (investigational new drug) procedure grasp the opportunity of influencing the developmental process leading to registration, and gain early knowledge about the studies performed, their results and problems. In the Federal Republic of Germany, federal regulation begins at the NDA stage. Insulins, thymus-stimulating preparations, and LHRH analogues have been granted marketing authorization. Not all of these products are biotechnologically derived, but they have all posed similar questions both to the company concerned and to regulatory authorities. The standings of clinical investigations and the registration process for other products are largely known in the scientific community. The overall situation leading to the risk–benefit decision for the granting of a marketing authorization may be different in various countries concerned.

Conclusions

If true guidelines for the toxicological testing of biotechnological products were to be written today, they would look exactly like those for other products. It would then become almost impossible to reason against some type of study for a specific product. From experience gained in the pharmaceutical industry, their subsidiaries, and in research laboratories, it has been learned that prolonged testing may prove impossible because of antibody formation. Other toxic reactions may show up in the early stages of clinical trials or use, and thus possibly indicate means for their assessment by subsequent animal or in vitro experimentation.

Structuring the demands of regulatory agencies and aligning them with the scientific requirements has become possible to some extent.

References

Council Directive 83/570/EEC (1983) Office J Eur Commun L 332, vol 26. Annex 1: Note for guidance on repeated dose toxicity (pp 12–19). Annex 2: Note for guidance on reproduction studies (pp 20–22). Annex 3: Note for guidance on carcinogenic potential (pp 23–28)

Galbraith WM (1986) New challenges in the safety evaluation of drugs and biologics

Proposal for a council directive 84/293/C (amending council directive 83/570/EEC) (1984) Office J Eur Commun C 293, vol 27. (Biotechnological/high technology products, pp 1–3)

Proposal for a Council Recommendation 84/293/C (1984) Office J Eur Commun C 293, vol 27. Annex 1: Note for guidance on single dose toxicity (pp 9–11). Annex 2: Note for guidance on testing of medicinal products for their mutagenic potential (pp 11–14)

Mechanisms and Models in Toxicology
Arch. Toxicol., Suppl. 11, 191–193 (1987)
© by Springer-Verlag 1987

Myco-Protein: Safety Evaluation of a Novel Food

G. L. Solomons

RHM Research Ltd., Lincoln Road, High Wycombe, Bucks., HP13 3QR, UK

In 1963, RHM Research Ltd. initiated a research programme aimed at developing a novel human food, based upon the production of a filamentous fungus, grown in continuous culture on a carbohydrate substrate.

Filamentous microfungi have a limited use in European foods, especially for developing unique flavours in cheeses (e.g. Stilton, Camembert). In the Far East many mould-fermented foodstuffs, (e.g. miso, tempeh) form part of the staple diets of large populations. However, in no case is the organism consumed in substantial quantities, its presence being due to its use as a flavouring or texture-modifying agent (proteolytic enzyme producer).

If a novel source of a high-protein food is to be introduced into the UK diet, there are three basic requirements:

1. The products would have to be attractive to eat and be in an acceptable price range.
2. They would have to possess good nutritional qualities.
3. They would have to be demonstrably safe to eat.

When the research started there were well-established toxicological protocols for the examination of a wide range of chemicals, pharmaceuticals and food additives, but the concept of testing the safety of a major food ingredient had not been developed. Conventional toxicology rested, and in large measure still rests, on the principle of measuring the response in animals and other test systems, of feeding or applying the test substance at a 'no effect level' of 100 times the level expected per unit of bodyweight. Moreover, in animal feeding trials it is usually assumed that the addition of the test substance, which rarely constitutes more than a very low fraction of the diet even at the most elevated levels tested, will have little or no influence on the nutritional value of the test diet or in any way alter the nutrient balance of the diet. It rapidly becomes evident that with a foodstuff, the clear distinction between nutritional and toxicological responses become obscured.

Since human intakes of up to 40 g dry wt./day in a total diet of approximately 300 g dry wt./day were anticipated, it immediately became obvious that the conventional 100/1 test margin was inappropriate. In addition, there was no prospect of testing a complex food material containing proteins, lipids and carbohydrates, in high concentration, without its greatly affecting the nutritional balance of the diet, if it was merely added to a conventional laboratory animal diet. To resolve these issues a series of semisynthetic diets was constructed, in which Myco-protein supplied either all of the animals' protein requirement or half of the protein requirement, the other half being supplied by casein. These two diets were then compared to a diet in which all the protein was supplied by casein (the semisynthetic control diet) and a diet formulated from conventional animal diet constituents (the conventional control). It must be emphasized that these diets were formulated individually; Myco-protein was never added to an already complete control diet. The individual ingredients within each diet were adjusted so as to maintain the levels of all controllable nutrients.

Thus, all the test programmes were based upon feeding four different diets, but in the light of experience it can now be said that exact balancing of these diets to nutritional equivalence was a difficult task and was to lead to the most significant problems experienced in the testing programme.

To judge the safety of the material, it had to be tested for the following major responses:

1. Acute toxicity
2. Chronic toxicity
3. Carcinogenic potential
4. Effects on reproduction
5. Teratogenicity
6. Immunological effects

In conventional toxicological studies, acute toxicity is preliminarily assessed by obtaining an LD_{50} value. For a food, such a determination is meaningless. In its place however, the Net Protein Utilization (NPU) was used as an indicator of both protein value and acute oral toxicity. It is of interest to note that of the 75 or so organisms which were screened in this manner, only one produced acute toxic effects, causing animal deaths.

Most of these trials were carried out using the rat as the test animal. Studies included 1-, 3- and 6-month subchronic rat trials; a 3-month subchronic study in baboons; a life-span trial in rats, with in utero exposure; a 4-generation reproduction rat study, with the addition of multiple matings of the last generation; teratology studies in the rat and New Zealand rabbits; and studies on neonates using calves.

All of the normal toxicology procedures were followed, including gross pathology, examination of all major organs, histology, examination of blood haematology and biochemistry. Details of food and water consumption and changes in animal body weight were routinely examined. Data was also obtained for skin and eye sensitivity.

The nutritional quality of Myco-protein was evaluated in a number of domestic species, including the broiler chicken, the laying hen, the pig and the calf. The nutritional requirements are well defined and sensitive to dietary change or toxicity. For example, much is known of the nutritional requirements of the hen for egg production, which is very sensitive to adverse dietary factors.

Finally, trials were carried out on human volunteers to study tolerance and immunological response. During the testing phase, some 4500 individuals consumed the material and only one positive response was observed. This person experienced nausea, sickness and stomach pains, but was normal in 24 h. Immunological studies indicated that she was a sensitive atopic whose reaction to the test material was a cross-reaction to other fungal species.

All of these studies were reinforced with extensive chemical and bacteriological data and particular emphasis was placed on mycotoxin analysis. No mycotoxins were found except in one case, when low levels of zearalenone were detected. This was, however, shown to be present in the batch of food-grade maize starch used in the culture medium preparation.

In the entire testing programme, which has occupied 12 years, no response was found which could, on examination, have been toxicological in origin. The main problem experienced was in not achieving exact nutritional balance in some diets, especially early in the programme when the nutritional knowledge of Myco-protein was still developing. The presence of high levels of phosphorus in Myco-protein resulted in a Ca:P:Mg imbalance which led to problems of nephrocalcinosis and associated kidney problems. This effect was also found by others investigating yeast protein and bacterial proteins. When this mineral balance was corrected, no further problems were found.

The result of some 15 years of investigation was submitted to the United Kingdom Ministry of Agriculture, Fisheries and Food. This body of evidence comprised some 28 volumes, of which 21 were concerned with toxicology and detailed 26 exhibits, as well as 5 volumes concerned with Human Studies, detailing 11 studies.

Provisional clearance was given in 1980 and final clearance embodied in a 'Certificate of Free Sale' in 1985.

Acknowledgement. My thanks to my colleague, D. G. Edwards, for his valuable comments on this presentation.

Mechanisms and Models in Toxicology
Arch. Toxicol., Suppl. 11, 194–199 (1987)
© by Springer-Verlag 1987

The Toxicology of the End Products From Biotechnology Processes

A. B. Wilson

Inveresk Research International Ltd., Musselburgh, Scotland, UK

Introduction

In the past 5 or 10 years spectacular advances have been made in the sciences of microbiology and immunology, with the advent of gene cloning and the production of monoclonal antibodies. These developments are presenting questions to toxicologists and regulators: "Is there a range of contaminants of which toxicologists and regulators should be aware?"; "Do the end products from such techniques have any common and unique toxicological properties?"

Of the two, it is the question of contaminants that has been the subject of more discussion, and rightly so. The result has been a number of papers and discussion documents as exemplified by Espeseth et al. (1983), Petricciani (1983), Office of Biologics Research and Review Center for Drugs and Biologicals (1984, 1985), National Institute for Biological Standards and Control (1986), and the Department of Health and Social Security (1982).

In general, the view has been that the active ingredient should be free from viruses and nucleic acids. This philosophy has meant that the toxicologist has not yet had to consider the problem too seriously. After all, if the contaminants have been removed and if production and quality control methods confirm this, there is no need for the toxicologist to investigate their potential effects. Effort has therefore been put into listing viruses and materials to be checked in the product and into protocols for carrying out these investigations (Inveresk Research International 1985).

The issue of the active ingredient also merits attention. Toxicology staff accustomed to investigating the actual or potential adverse effects of industrial chemicals, agricultural products and pharmaceuticals produced by more traditional methods are often unfamiliar with biotechnology and may be uncertain as to whether special factors should be considered. This presentation is intended to be of assistance under such circumstances.

Background

The products of biotechnology derive for the most part from bacteria, yeasts or mammalian cells. None of these is unfamiliar or unusual. Only a small minority of bacteria are pathogenic or produce toxins (Buchanan and Gibbons 1974): the vast majority are harmless, indeed man and animals depend on them in their digestive systems – most obviously in ruminant animals.

Micro-organisms are used in a number of processes, e.g. brewing, breadmaking, other fermentation processes and vaccines. Some novel foods have also been produced – Kesp (a fungal protein from RHM), Pruteen (a bacterial protein from ICI) and Toprina (a yeast protein from BP). These are all products composed of killed cells which have comfortably survived exhaustive toxicology tests. It can therefore be suggested that bacteria and yeasts are not necessarily or fundamentally toxic or harmful.

Mammalian cells, when dead, form much of our protein and when alive need a highly specialised environment to survive. Indeed, a whole technology has been built up to solve the problems of keeping these cells alive. Toxicologists are also aware that to transplant cells requires either an immunodeficient animal, such as the nude mouse, or that the recipient animal be genetically virtually identical to the cells injected. Like micro-organisms, mammalian cells are not necessarily or fundamentally harmful. However, both can pose safety problems: baceria can be pathogenic and produce toxins; mammalian cells can harbour viruses which may be highly dangerous.

End Products of Biotechnological Processes

Biotechnological end products are listed in Table 1 together with their applications. Working from first principles, the most likely toxic effects or safety questions that might be encountered with each will now be discussed.

Live Micro-organisms

Live micro-organisms may be pathogenic or produce a toxin. There are straightforward tests for pathogenicity, often involving the inoculation of rodents (De-

Table 1. Biotechnological end products and their applications

End product	Application
Micro-organisms: alive	Vaccination, fermentation
dead	Foodstuffs, vaccination
Mammalian cells: live	Organ transplants
	Sources of pancreatic enzyme
dead	Killed tumour cells as vaccines
Micro-organism derivatives	Hormones, enzymes, proteins, vitamins
Mammalian cell derivatives	Monoclonal antibodies, hormones, plasminogen activators

partment of Health and Social Security 1982), and sometimes using animals whose defences are deficient (nude mice or steroid-treated rodents). In general, deaths that occur within a few hours of inoculation are associated with toxins, whilst those occurring after a few days are suggestive of a pathogenic effect – this can be elucidated by culturing a range of tissue from the animal and looking for persistence (and multiplication) of the organism injected. It is possible for a non-pathogenic organism to be made pathogenic by insertion of a new piece of DNA. This, however, seems unlikely since only a small part of the total DNA is altered and in a very specific manner, e.g. insertion of the gene for growth hormone into *E. coli.*

The investigation and identification of toxins are fundamental objects of toxicology. The normal battery of tests ranging from acute to chronic is well established and tests can be selected according to the potential hazard, duration of exposure, numbers of people exposed, etc., in conventional ways.

Dead Micro-organisms

A dead micro-organism cannot, of course, be pathogenic, though the manufacturing process cannot avoid presenting at least the potential for the exposure of the workforce and leakage into the environment of the live organism. The method of killing the micro-organism will not necesarily remove toxins, so the possibility of toxins remains, just as for the live organisms.

Live Mammalian Cells

Normally, live mammalian cells are not present as the end product of a manufacturing process for use in (or resulting in exposure of) humans, although Damon Biotech (Boston, USA) are investigating the encapsulation and injection of pancreatic cells. As stated earlier, these would not be expected to present a hazard. However, the very alterations that allow them to survive and potentially multiply in an animal host could conceivably allow them to survive and multiply in humans, or to transfer an altered gene to other cells and cause disturbed growth, cancers, or other effect.

There are no well-established tests available to respond to these questions. Perhaps studies analogous to those for investigating the pathogenicity of micro-organisms or cell culture tests would be appropriate reference (Inveresk Research International 1985). However, it would be important to identify and understand what procedures had been carried out to modify the mammalian cells before deciding on investigations.

Dead Mammalian Cells

When used as the active product, dead mammalian cells would not seem likely to pose many problems. However, if the cells have been genetically engineered it is conceivable that portions of their nucleic acids could become available to and be incorporated into the normal body cells. This would seem to be a particularly remote possibility if the cells were ingested, indeed, enough live and dead cells are eaten to dismiss perhaps this combination of product and route as a hazard.

Products

More widely publicised currently than the micro-organisms and mammalian cells themselves are their products. These include insulin and growth hormone from genetically altered *E. coli* (Flodh et al. 1982; Food and Drug Administration 1984, 1985), growth hormone from mammalian cells, interferons and monoclonal antibodies. Such materials can be considered in precisely the same manner as any product presented for toxicological investigation, omitting, in this instance, consideration of the by-products or contaminants of the manufacturing process; i.e. it is the end product that is of importance rather than the method of production. However, it is interesting to review any characteristics they might have in common, of which there are several. The products are often:

- identical (or allegedly identical) to those produced in the body
- proteins or peptides
- highly potent
- inactive orally and therefore administered parenterally
- of short half-life
- antigenic

Some of the above bear closer scrutiny. Hormones produced by genetically engineered baceria are not necessarily precisely the same as those produced naturally. Growth hormone from *E. coli* (e.g. protropin from Kabi-Vitrum) has an additional *N*-terminal methionine and it is very possible that proteins produced by bacteria will have different secondary structures from those produced in animals, though in the instance of protropin the secondary and tertiary structures are identical to pituitary growth hormone (Jones and O'Connor 1982). Since baceria do not glycosylate a protein that requires glycosylation, immunoglobulins and tissue plasminogen activator, for instance, will not be produced in their active forms by a bacterial process.

It is very unlikely that the different structure will give rise to any activity beyond antigenicity – indeed, it is more likely to reduce the potency of the protein or peptide. In practice, both growth hormone and insulin from bacterial sources have undergone a range of studies up to subchronic duration with no unexpected effect (Food and Drug Administration 1984, 1985).

From the above there are at least two lessons to be learnt. First, that the exact meaning of 'identical', in the context of a natural material, needs to be more carefully defined. Secondly, that consideration must be given as to what toxicity tests are actually necessary if a material is completely identical to the natural product. In reviewing the latter point, the route, frequency and method of administration are also relevant.

A compound such as a hormone is often administered in a different location and sometimes by a different route from the natural one. This raises possibilities of local effects (not just reaction to injection) and, of course, unexpected toxicological effects, since different organs may encounter the product at different concentrations or quantities from normal. The doses may also turn out to be higher than physiological. Thus, it would be foolhardy not to conduct at least 1-month and probably 3-month studies on materials which will be administered repeatedly to an individual, even if they are shown to be entirely identical to natural materials and achieved concentrations are within the physiological ranges. Pulse dosing might not imitate the normal situation and could give rise to untoward effects (e.g. in reproduction), implying that investigations may be necessary.

A possible complicating factor is the antigenicity of a material – and proteins, lipopolysaccharides, etc., are more than likely to be antigenic. Antigenicity is not per se undesirable; indeed, our defence mechanisms depend upon stimulation of antibody production. These antibodies may bind to the product and reduce its activity confonding toxicological investigations. If a material is administered frequently over a prolonged period it is possible that hypersensitivity reactions will occur. There seems to be no way of predictions with any reliability whether an antigen will give rise to allergic reactions in man, or, to be more exact, under what circumstances and with what frequency they will occur. Animals do not provide adequate information (Parish, this volume 1986). The potential use of monoclonal antibodies is a case in point. Those derived from mice will almost certainly be antigenic to humans: administration is likely to cause the development of antibodies to the monoclonals and, following repeated administration, just possibly an allergic reaction of some type. Hence the emphasis on monoclonals from human cells, which are less likely to be antigenic.

Technical Toxicological Aspects

Many of the pharmaceutical products are likely to be highly potent and therefore given in small quantities, micrograms rather than milligrams. This, added to the complexity of the structures and their similarity to chemicals already in the body, can render analysis of the materials difficult.

Parenteral administration is often required. Intramuscular or subcutaneous techniques are generally straightforward in laboratory animals. However, intravenous administration is also likely to be the route of choice for a significant number of materials. Studies with single daily bolus intravenous injections can be readily accomplished but many of the compounds will be administered several times daily or by a continuous infusion, often to achieve a steady state. This has meant that toxicological laboratories have had to familiarise themselves with long-term cannulation techniques in dogs and primates while the compound is administered via an infusion pump, elastomeric balloon (e. g. a Travenol infusor) or an equivalent method. In rats it is possible to implant osmotic pumps (e.g. Alzet mini-pumps from Alza Corp.) subcutaneously and cannulate the jugular vein. Such techniques are technically difficult and require much development and experience before a high success rate can be achieved.

Conclusions

A high proportion of biotechnology products would apparently not present serious or novel problems. However, there are some areas in which traditional techniques or thinking are not satisfactory. These are:

- The possible transfer of an immortalisation factor from a mammalian cell
- Allergic reactions
- Toxicity assessment of natural products

The toxicologist must also be aware that compounds are not necessarily as closely similar or identical to the natural material as might be first thought.

The above questions (apart from immortalisation factors) are relevant to any method of production of these materials, and not just biotechnology.

Technical problems will sometimes be posed in the simulation of the proposed route and method of human exposure.

Until data are accumulated from practical experience in man it will be necessary to rely on first principles and limited (but increasing) animal data. This is an anxious and uncertain situation. It is therefore to be hoped that those conducting human and animal investigations on the products of biotechnology will publish both negative findings and results that show adverse reactions so that present theories may be evaluated against practical experience.

References

Buchanan RE, Gibbons NE (1974) Bergey's manual of determinative bacteriology. Williams and Wilkins, Baltimore

Department of Health and Social Security (1982) Compendium of licensing requirements for the manufacture of certain biological medicinal products. Her Majesty's Stationery Office, London

Espeseth DA, Shibley GP, Joseph PL, van Deusen RA, Whetstone CA (1983) United States Department of Agriculture licensing policy for biologicals produced by r-DNA. Presented at Joint LABS/WHO meeting, 18th Congress on Standardisation and control of biologicals produced by recombinant DNA technology

Flodh H, Johansson H-E, Jonsson M, Ekvarn S (1982) General toxicity in rats of biosynthetic and pituitary human growth hormone. Proceedings of the FDA-USP workshop on drug and reference standards for insulins, somatotropins and thyroid-axis hormones. United States Pharmacopeial Convention

Food and Drug Administration. Summary basis of approval NDA 19-107. Protropin

Food and Drug Administration. Summary basis of approval NDA 18-781. Human Insulin

Inveresk Research International (1985) Biotechnology products for human use – safety testing. Regulatory Affairs Bulletin 21:9–14

Jones AJS, O'Connor JV (1982) Chemical characterization of methionyl human growth hormone. Proceedings of the FDA-USP workshop on drug and reference standards for insulins, somatotropins and thyroid-axis hormones. United States Pharmacopeial Convention

National Institute for Biological Standards and Control (1986) Consideration for the standardization and control of the new generation of biological products (Draft)

Office of Biologics Research and Review Center for Drugs and Biologics, Food and Drug Administration (1984) Points to consider in the manufacture of injectable monoclonal antibody products intended for human use in vivo (draft, November 1984)

Office of Biologics Research and Review Center for Drugs and Biologics, Food and Drug Administration (1985) Points to consider in the production and testing of new drugs and biologics produced by recombinant DNA technology

Parish WE (1986) Predictive tests for occupational allergies. Arch Toxicol Suppl II:177–181

Petricciani JC (1983) An overview of safety and regulatory aspects of the new biotechnology. Regul Toxicol Pharmacol 3:428–433

United States Department of Agriculture (1984) New biotechnology for preparation of animal biological products. (Veterinary Services Memorandum No 800.68)

Mechanisms and Models in Toxicology
Arch. Toxicol., Suppl. 11, 200–205 (1987)
© by Springer-Verlag 1987

Comparison of Three Assays of Picogram Amounts of Residual Cellular DNA in Biological Products from Continuous Cell Lines

B. Barraud-Hadidane [1], R. P. Martin [1], B. Montagnon [2], and G. Dirheimer [1]

[1] Institut de Biologie Moléculaire et Cellulaire du CNRS, Université Louis Pasteur, 15 rue Descartes, Strasbourg, France
[2] Institut Mérieux, Charbonnières-les-Bains, France

Introduction

Cell cultures are increasingly used to prepare biological products. In many instances, the continuous cell lines used show abnormal cytologic and genetic characteristics. The purification process of the biological products must therefore eliminate contaminant cellular DNA. For example, the purification process of inactivated poliomyelitis vaccines (IPV), prepared from Vero cells grown in microcarrier culture (Montagnon et al. 1981), must be shown to reduce the level of cellular DNA from that of the initial virus harvest by a factor of at least 10^8 (WHO Expert Committee on Biological Standardization 1982). This implies that techniques needed to be elaborated which are sensitive enough to assay picogram amounts of DNA in the vaccines. It is obvious that conventional techniques of DNA detection are not sensitive enough to fulfill these requirements. Three molecular DNA–DNA hybridization techniques were therefore adapted, which work on the general principle of isolating the contaminating Vero-cell DNA from the vaccine, denaturing it, and immobilizing the single-stranded DNA on filters. Heat-denatured Vero-cell DNA which has been labeled is then used as the hybridization probe. The probe binds to the filters only if it is able to base-pair with the DNA which was originally adsorbed. The amount of label retained on the filters is proportional to the amount of Vero-cell DNA in the vaccine. The standardization is done by comparison with a scale of Vero DNA.

The labeled Vero-cell DNA can be obtained using different techniques. The first one uses ^{32}P-radiolabeling of the DNA by nick translation (Rigby et al. 1977). The second, based on the technique of Tchen et al. (1984), uses a probe of Vero-cell DNA treated with N-acetoxy-N-acetylamino-7-iodofluorene (AAIF). After hybridization the filters are treated with an anti-guanine-AAIF rabbit serum and subsequently incubated with alkaline phosphatase-conjugated anti-rabbit-IgG serum. The amounts of DNA originally present in the vaccine samples are detected by staining with fast blue. The third technique uses a probe obtained by incorporation into Vero-cell DNA of thymidine monophosphate that contains a biotin molecule linked to the C-5 position of the pyrimidine ring through a linker arm 11 atoms in length (Langer et al. 1981). Biotine-11-dUTP is incorporated into the DNA by nick translation (Brigati et al. 1983). The biotinylated DNA is hybridized to the filters and the amount of hybrids is assayed by interaction of biotine with streptavidin. The complex formed is detected using biotinylated alkaline phosphatase, which is finally measured by a colorimetric test (Leary et al. 1983).

Materials and Methods

Preparation of Vaccine and Extraction of DNA

Poliovirus vaccines were prepared as previously described (Montagnon et al. 1981). Four steps starting from the crude virus harvest allow production of a purified virus. The vaccine was obtained, after dilution, from a formalin-treated virus–Spherodex fraction (FVS fraction). 10 or 20 ml of FVS fraction were dialyzed against water and concentrated 10 times after addition of 1 µg of yeast DNA as a carrier. The samples, brought to 10 mM tris-HCl pH 7.5, were sonicated at 4 °C. They were then treated, first with 10 µg/ml pancreatic RNase, then with 50 µg/ml of proteinase K, each time at 37 °C for 1 h. The DNA was then phenol-extracted. The aqueous solution was treated by the Sevag procedure and the DNA finally precipitated with ethanol in the presence of 20 µg/ml of E. coli tRNA, as a carrier.

Immobilization of DNA on Nitrocellulose Filters

After denaturation by 0.3 M NaOH for 30 min at 20 °C and rapid chilling, the neutralized samples were fixed on nitrocellulose filters (Millipore 0.22-µm pore diameter or Schleicher and Schull BA 85) previously washed with 6 × SSC buffer (1 × SSC is NaCl 0.15 M, sodium citrate pH 7.6, 0.015 M). After rinsing with 6 × SSC, the filters were dried and baked for 2 h at 80 °C in a vacuum oven.

Preparation of the Probes

Vero-cell DNA was prepared as previously described (Montagnon et al. 1985).
1. ^{32}P-labeling was done by nick translation according to Rigby et al. (1977) in the presence of 10 µCi of each of the four α-[^{32}P]-deoxyribonucleoside triphosphates (3000 Ci/mmol; Amersham, Searle, Inc.) for 2 µg of DNA.
2. AAIF labeling was done according to Tchen et al. (1984).
3. Biotine labeling was done according to Brigati et al. (1983) using a nick translation kit (BRL, Inc.).

DNA–DNA Hybridization

Filters were prehybridized in 6 × SSC, 0.1% sodium dodecyl sulfate (SDS) (0.2 ml per cm^2 of filter) at 65 °C for 30 min. This buffer was then replaced by the same volume of hybridization buffer (HB): 6 × SSC, 1% SDS in Denhardt's

Table 1. Comparison of the three methods for measuring the residual Vero-cell DNA content of poliomyelitis vaccines[a]

Vaccine sample no.	^{32}P-labeled probe (pg/ml)	AAIF-labeled probe (pg/ml)	Biotine-labeled probe (pg/ml)
21	10	8	2
22	41	8	8
23	38	540	n.d.[b]
24	452	540	n.d.[b]
25	22	80	110
26	11	80	110
27	6	80	110
28	3	80	110
29	2	80	110
30	3	80	15
31	2	80	72

[a] Results are expressed in pg/ml in the concentrated vaccine preparation, taking into account DNA recovery.
[b] n.d.: not determined.

solution: BSA (fractions V,Sigma, USA), 0.02% Ficoll 400 (Pharmacia, Sweden), 0.02% PVP (Sigma, USA) and incubated for 4 h at 65 °C.

Each filter was then placed in an individual plastic bag containing 50 µl of HB/ cm^2 of filter. The DNA probe, previously denatured by heating at 100 °C for 5 min and rapidly chilling, was added in an amount exceeding the amount of DNA immobilized on the filters by at least 10 times. Hybridization was for 24 h at 65 °C.

For the biotine-labeled DNA, hybridization was as described by Leary et al. (1983), using the BRL DNA research kit.

Assay of the Hybrids

1. In the case of the ^{32}P-labeled probe, the filters were washed 6 times for 10 min with HB at 65 °C, then twice for 30 min with 1 × SSC, 0.1% SDS at 65 °C and finally for 1 h in 1 × SSC at 20 °C. After drying, the radioactivity was determined by scintillation counting.
2. In the case of the AAIF-labeled probe, the filters were treated according to Tchen et al. (1984).
3. In the case of the biotine-labeled probe, the hybrids were visualized according to Leary et al. (1983).

Results and Discussion

In a first series of experiments, the recovery of Vero-cell DNA from the vaccines after the extraction and immobilization processes was determined. For this purpose, ^{3}H-labeled E. coli DNA was added to the FVS samples prior to DNA ex-

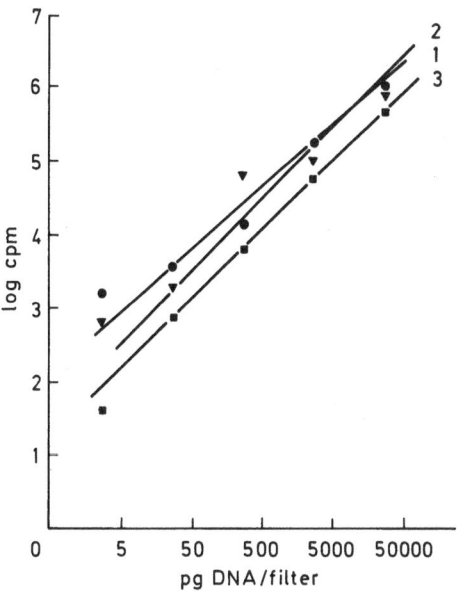

Fig. 1. Three standardization scales of Vero-cell DNA hybridization with [^{32}P]DNA

traction and the amount of [^{3}H]DNA was determined after immobilization on the filters. From these experiments, the recovery of Vero-cell DNA was estimated to be 64% ±4%.

Using [^{32}P]DNA probes of high specific radioactivity (1–2 × 10^8 cpm/μg DNA), the sensitivity and reproducibility of the hybridization method was studied. By dilution of Vero-cell DNA, standardization scales ranging from 5 to 50 000 pg/filter were prepared. As shown in Fig. 1, the values obtained from different series of standardization scales are in a quite good range between 50 and 50 000 pg DNA/filter. However, between 5 and 50 pg/filter, more pronounced variations are observed. The specificity of hybridization was checked by supplementing some of the samples with either purified poliovirus RNA, or yeast DNA, or E. coli tRNA. The results showed that the presence of these molecules did not interfere significantly with the specificity of homologous DNA–DNA hybridization.

To determine the amount of residual Vero-cell DNA in vaccine samples, 14 monovalent FVS batches were tested. The results deduced for the final vaccine preparation (IPV), taking into account the dilution factor and DNA recovery, ranged from 0.025 pg to 1.94 pg DNA/ml vaccine for 10 of the batches (average value of 0.78 pg/ml). The 4 remaining batches contained 2.48, 4.38, 4.95, and 6.31 pg DNA/ml vaccine respectively. Since crude virus harvests contained from 0.6 × 10^7 to 10.3 × 10^7 pg/ml, it was calculated that the process of virus purification used (Montagnon et al. 1985) eliminated residual Vero-cell DNA by an average factor of 1.4 × 10^8.

Hybridization results obtained using a AAIF-labeled Vero-cell DNA probe are shown in Fig. 2 a. The DNA–AAIF method was shown to be sensitive enough to detect 1 pg of DNA. Control experiments performed using either unsubstituted

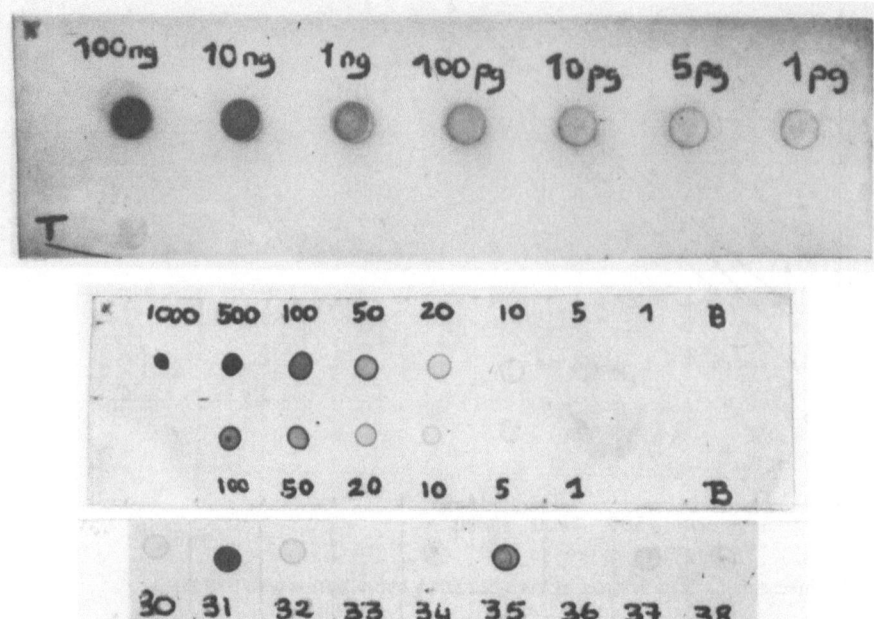

Fig. 2. a Standardization scale of Vero-cell DNA with DNA-AAIF. **b** The same with biotine-labeled DNA and results with vaccine batches 30–38

Vero-cell or yeast DNA, or Vero DNA–AAIF in the absence of guanine-AAIF-specific antibodies, showed very low backgrounds, indicating that the method is specific. With vaccine batches 95, 97 and 98, less than 1 pg DNA/ml FVS was found. As shown in Fig. 2 b, the method which employs a biotinylated DNA probe is also able to detect 1 pg of DNA. The results obtained with batches 30–38 are also shown in Fig. 2 b.

It must be emphasized that the technique which uses ^{32}P-labeling of DNA is able to give numerical hybridization values (scintillation counting), whereas the two other methods depend upon visual appreciation of intensity of coloration by comparison with a standardization scale. Thus results with the latter two methods are only estimates in orders of magnitude. It was even difficult sometimes to visualize a difference between two neighbouring values on the standardization scale, especially for the lower values (5, 10, 50 pg). However, a comparative study on 11 vaccine batches by using the 3 methods of DNA detections in parallel showed that the results deduced from each method are generally concordant for a given batch (Table 1).

In conclusion, the three DNA–DNA hybridization tests which have been developed here permit validation of the purification procedure for preparation of purified IPV produced in Vero-cell microcarrier culture. The weak residual DNA contents of most of the batches demonstrate that the WHO requirements are fulfilled.

References

Brigati DJ, Myerson D, Leary JJ, Spalholz B, Trevis SZ, Fong CKY, Hsiung GD, Ward DC (1983) Detection of viral genomes in cultured cells and paraffin embedded tissue sections using biotin-labeled hybridization probes. Virology 126:32–50

Langer PR, Waldrop AA, Ward DC (1981) Enzymatic synthesis of biotin-labeled polynucleotides; novel nucleic acid affinity probes. Proc Natl Acad Sci USA 78:6633–6637

Leary JJ, Brigati DJ, Ward DC (1983) Rapid and sensitive colorimetric method for visualizing biotin-labeled DNA probes hybridized to DNA or RNA immobilized on nitrocellulose Bio-blots. Proc Natl Acad Sci USA 80:4045–4049

Montagnon BJ, Fanget B, Nicolas AJ (1981) The large scale cultivation of Vero cells in microcarrier culture for virus vaccine production, preliminary results for killed poliovirus vaccine. Dev Biol Stand 47:55–64

Montagnon BJ, Martin R, Barraud B, Bandet R, Fanget B, Paturel J, Mackowiak JF (1985) Residual Vero cell DNA and inactivated polio vaccine; detection by DNA–DNA molecular hybridization. In: Hopps HE, Petriccani JC (eds) In vitro cellular and developmental biology Monograph no 6, pp 82–89

Rigby PWJ, Dieckmann M, Rhodes C, Berg P (1977) Labeling DNA to high specific activity in vitro by nick translation with DNA polymerase I. J Mol Biol 113:237–251

Tchen P, Fuchs RPP, Sage E, Leng M (1984) Chemically modified nucleic acids as immunodetectable probes in hybridization experiments. Proc Natl Acad Sci USA 81:3466–3470

WHO Expert Committee on Biological Standardization (1982) Requirements for poliovirus vaccine (inactivated). WHO, Geneva (Technical report series 673, Annexe 2)

Recent Studies and Technique Developments in Toxicology

Mechanisms and Models in Toxicology
Arch. Toxicol., Suppl. 11, 209–212 (1987)

The Influence of Some Dithiocarbamates on Oxidative Drug Metabolism: Interaction with Cadmium

V. Eybl, D. Kotyzová, J. Koutenský, D. Waitzová, and M. M. Jones[3]

[1] Department of Pharmacology, Faculty of Medicine, Charles University Pilzeň, ČSSR
[2] State Institute for Drug Control, Prague, ČSSR
[3] Vanderbilt University, Nashville, TN, USA

Dithiocarbamates (DCs) have been examined as agents to facilitate the removal of aged cadmium deposits (Gale et al. 1985). Diethyldithiocarbamate (DEDC) has been reported to have an inhibiting effect on microsomal mixed-function oxidation system (Graven et al. 1976; Mayer and Eybl 1973). The present study was undertaken in order to compare this action of DEDC with the effect of some related compounds and to study the interaction of DCs with cadmium. This metal, an important environmental contaminant, inhibits the oxidative drug metabolism (Eybl et al. 1979).

Materials and Methods

The experiments were performed in male ICR mice of 22–24 g body weight, divided into groups as indicated in the figures. The following DCs were used as sodium salts: DEDC, dihydroxyethyl DC (DHDC), N-methyl-D-glucamine DC (MGDC), isonipecotamide DC (INADC).

In the acute experiments the DCs were applied in a single i.p. injection equimolar to 100 mg DEDC/kg, 4 h before injection of pentobarbital, antipyrine, or theophylline. In the experiments with repeated administration of DCs, a dose of DC equimolar to 100 mg DEDC/kg was used in five i.p. injections over a 5-day period, the last injection being 48 h before the administration of pentobarbital. A lower dose equimolar to 25 mg DEDC/kg was used in eight i.p. injections over an 8-day period, the last injection being 24 h before the administration of pentobarbital. Sleep was induced by 50 mg pentobarbital/kg i.p. Duration was registered in minutes, the criterion being the loss of the righting reflex, and calculated as the geometric mean value with 95% confidence limits.

Antipyrine and theophylline were injected at a dose of 20 mg/kg, i.v., always 4 h after the injection of the DCs.

Mice were killed by decapitation and the blood collected 60 min after i.v. injection of antipyrine or 90 min after i.v. injection of theophylline.

Serum concentration of antipyrine and theophylline was determined after extraction by HPLC. The antipyrine levels were estimated by a modification of the method of Danhof et al. (1979). Reverse phase HPLC following serum chloroform–isopropanol (95:5) extraction was used for the estimation of theophylline. Mean values with 95% confidence limits are given.

Results

DC injected i.p. in a single dose equimolar to 100 mg DEDC/kg 4 h before the administration of the drugs lengthened the pentobarbital sleeping time and increased the serum level of antipyrine and theophylline (Figs. 1–3). The influence of DCs on pentobarbital sleeping time and the serum theophylline level was increased after pretreatment with cadmium (Figs. 1, 3). The inhibiting effect of cadmium on oxidative drug metabolism was not abolished but rather was usually enhanced by DC administration.

With the exception of INADC, the influence of DCs on the pentobarbital sleeping time and serum antipyrine level disappeared 24 h after administration. Serum theophylline level was significantly increased only after MGDC.

Pentobarbital sleeping time was shortened significantly after the series of 5 injections of DCs at the higher dosage, on average by 20%. However, the series of

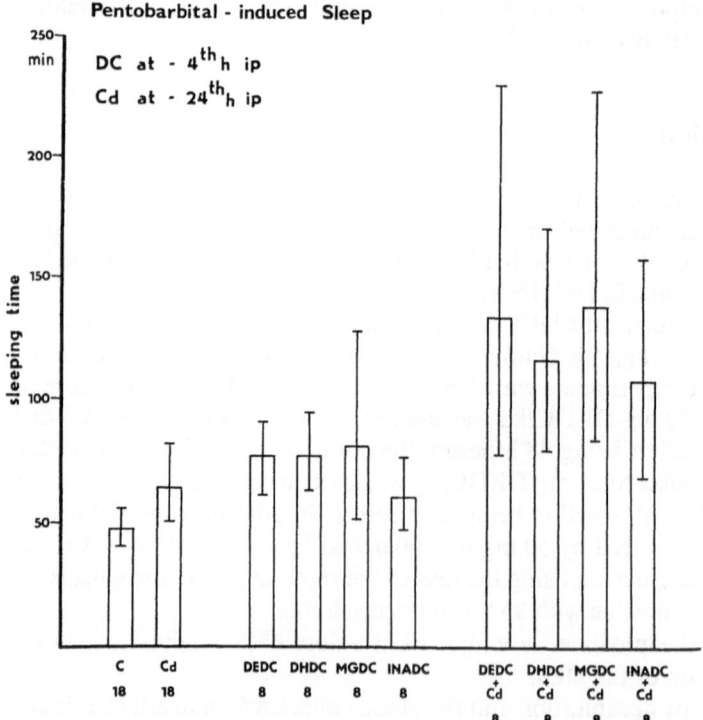

Fig. 1. The influence of cadmium and/or dithiocarbamates (DCs) on pentobarbital-induced sleep in mice. The number of animals in each group is given under the corresponding column; *C*, controls

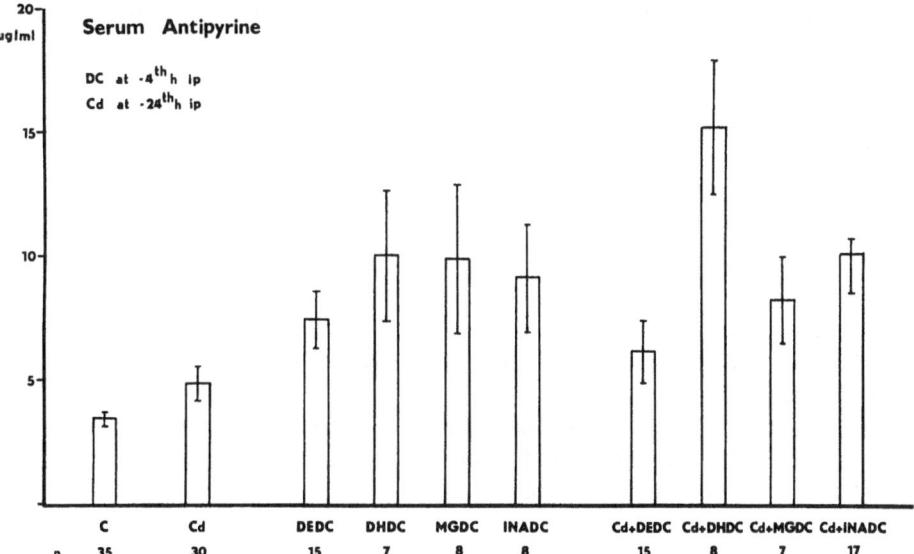

Fig. 2. The influence of cadmium and/or DCs on serum antipyrine levels in mice. The number of animals in each group is given under the corresponding column; *C*, controls

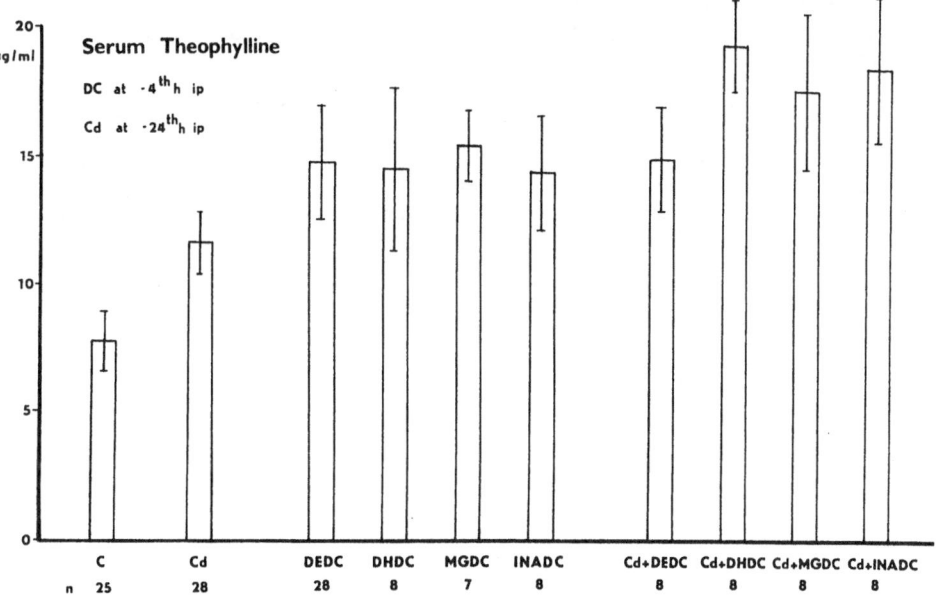

Fig. 3. The influence of cadmium and/or DCs on serum theophylline levels in mice. The number of animals in each group is given under the corresponding column; *C*, controls

8 application of DCs at the lower dosage did not cause any changes in the sleeping time.

Discussion

In the present study it has been shown that not only DEDC but also its derivatives may cause the inhibition of the oxidative drug metabolism. This effect appears to be transient. Some analogues of DEDC are considered to be prospective antidotes in chronic cadmium intoxication. However, these antidotes were not able to diminish the toxic effect of cadmium on oxidative drug metabolism when applied 20 h after the injection of cadmium. Moreover, the action of cadmium was usually increased.

The effect of the repeated administration of higher doses of DCs might be brought about through enzyme induction. However, the possibility of an effect on the central nervous system is not excluded.

References

Danhof M, de Groot-van der Vis E, Breimer DD (1979) Assay of antipyrine and its primary metabolites in plasma, saliva and urine by high-performance liquid chromatography and some preliminary results in man. Pharmacology 18:210–223

Eybl V, Koutenský J, Sýkora J (1979) On the interaction of cadmium and some centrally acting drugs. Cadmium symposium. Schiller University, Jena, pp 44–47

Gale GR, Atkins LM, Smith AB, Jones MM (1985) Effects of diethyldithiocarbamate and selected analogs on cadmium metabolism following chronic cadmium ingestion. Res Commun Chem Pathol Pharmacol 47:107–114

Graven MR, Luscombe DK, Nicholls PJ (1976) Absorption, elimination and duration of action of diethyldithiocarbamate in animals. J Pharm Pharmacol 28:38P

Mayer O, Eybl V (1973) Dithiocarbamate central effects in relation to their possible influence on drug metabolizing enzymes. J Pharm Pharmacol 25:672–676

Mechanisms and Models in Toxicology
Arch. Toxicol., Suppl. 11, 213–215 (1987)

Mechanism of Damage to Liver Cells After Chronic Exposure to Low Doses of Cadmium Chloride

A. F. W. Morselt, W. M. Frederiks, J. H. J. Copius Peereboom-Stegeman, and H. A. van Veen

Laboratory of Histology and Cell Biology, University of Amsterdam, Academic Medical Center, Meibergdreef 15, 1105 AZ Amsterdam, The Netherlands

Introduction

Chronic exposure of rats to low doses of cadmium chloride ($CdCl_2$) results in accumulation of cadmium in the liver, followed by kidney damage (Dudley et al. 1985). It has been proposed that cadmium-metallothionein complexes released from the liver cells provoke kidney damage by lysosomal breakdown of these complexes in the proximal tubule cells of the kidney (Dudley et al. 1985).

The precise mechanism of the release of these complexes from the liver cell is still unknown. In this study, evidence is presented as to the way in which liver cells which accumulate cadmium in the form of metallothionein or other cadmium-binding proteins can be damaged. Specific light microscopical staining was used for different cell and tissue constituents; other techniques employed were membrane enzyme histochemistry and electron microscopy.

Methods

Three times a week, 45 female Wistar rats were injected subcutaneously with either 0.18 or 0.036 mg $CdCl_2$/kg body weight (b.w.) or saline over a period of 72 weeks. After different time intervals pieces of their livers were fixed in Böhm's fixative, embedded in paraffin and cut in to 5-μm sections which were stained for protein-bound disulphides and cadmium thiolate clusters and subsequently by Feulgen staining (Morselt and Van Straalen 1986). On serial sections the picrosirius staining for collagen was performed, followed by a quantitative estimation of fibrosis (Morselt et al. 1978). For electron microscopical examinations, the liver was fixed in 1% glutaraldehyde, followed by postfixation in 1% OsO_4 and embedding in Epon. Ultrathin sections were stained with uranyl acetate and lead citrate. The plasma membrane enzyme 5'-nucleotidase was demonstrated on cryostat liver sections of rats injected subcutaneously daily for 19 days with 0.2, 0.4 or 0.8 mg $CdCl_2$/kg b.w. or with saline (controls) using a method described by Uusitalo (1981).

Results and Discussion

In liver sections of rats treated for 72 weeks with CdCl$_2$ an increased number of loose cell nuclei and cytoplasmic cell constituents were observed in the sinusoidal spaces compared with appropriate controls. If the same locations were observed with electron microscopy (Fig. 1), the loose-lying nuclei showed a similar appearance to the ones in the intact liver cell. The mitochondria observed in the sinusoidal lumen did not show flocculent densities. No cytoplasmic blebs were observed, but holes were visible in the plasma membrane of the liver cells (Fig. 2).

After chronic exposure to low-dose CdCl$_2$, accumulation of cadmium is accompanied by an increase in metallothionein and related cytosolic proteins, which was demonstrated in liver sections using the staining method for protein-bound disulphides and cadmium thiolate clusters (Morselt and Van Straalen 1986). This increase in metallothionein and related cytosolic proteins is large, around 50% per liver cell (Morselt et al. 1985). This large increase, and the electron microscopical picture, showing unchanged nuclei and cell constituents in the sinusoids, gave rise to the idea of a sudden disruption of the liver cell.

A clear and dose-dependent decrease of the liver cell membrane enzyme 5'-nucleotidase was observed after short-term chronic cadmium administration (Fig. 3), indicating a decrease in membrane integrity after cadmium exposure; this agrees with the mechanism proposed. Using quantitative criteria for establishing liver fibrosis, periportal and interlobular fibrosis were established after 50 weeks in rats treated with 0.18 mg CdCl$_2$/kg b.w. Liver fibrosis is known to occur after repeated liver cell damage (Popper 1979), and this indicates that the images shown on Figs. 1 and 2 represent real liver damage and not some kind of artefact. The

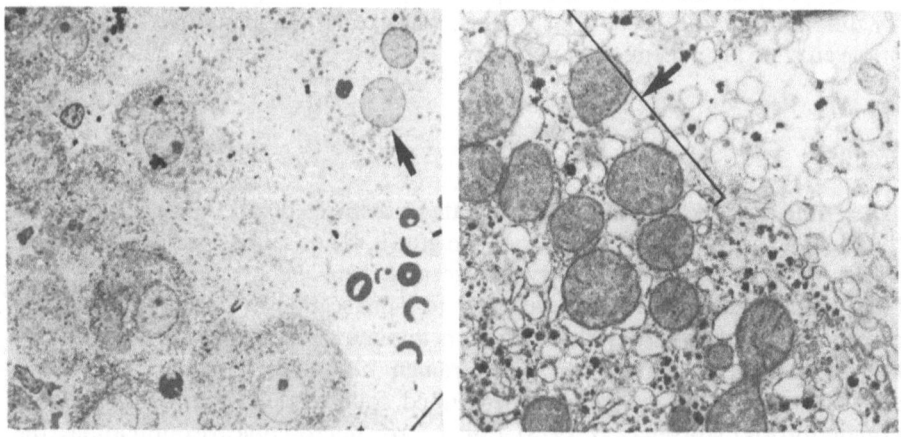

Fig. 1   **Fig. 2**

Fig. 1. Electron micrograph of liver cells from a rat treated for 72 weeks with 0.18 mg CdCl$_2$ per kg b.w. Numerous mitochondria and unchanged liver cell nuclei (*arrow*) can be observed in the sinusoidal lumen. Magnification × 680

Fig. 2. Electron micrograph of the same liver as shown in Fig. 1, showing the hole in the cell membrane (*arrow*) by which mitochondria etc. are leaving the cell. Magnification × 37 200

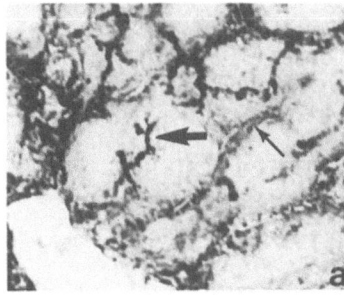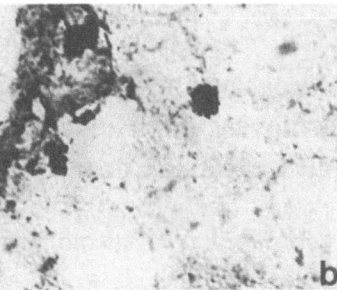

Fig. 3. Microphotographs showing the enzyme histochemical staining on 5′-nucleotidase (bile canalicular and sinusoidal, *thick* and *thin arrow* respectively) on liver sections of rats treated with saline (**a**) or 0.8 mg CdCl₂ per kg b.w. (**b**). Magnification ×480

lack of chromatin condensation in the nuclei excludes a high intracellular cadmium level as the cause of liver cell damage (Puvion and Lange 1980). The nonoccurrence of cytoplasmic blebs and lack of flocculent densities in mitochondria excludes the suggestion of some other noxious influences (Popper 1979). Recently, Dudley et al. (1985) showed a similar type of liver cell damage after chronic cadmium exposure on his microphotographs, which, however, he described differently.

All these facts support the hypothesis regarding the type of liver cell damage after chronic cadmium exposure proposed here, and this might be an important and overlooked type of cellular damage caused by long-term exposure to low doses of cadmium as it occurs in the environment.

References

Dudley RE, Gammel LM, Klaassen CD (1985) Cadmium induced hepatic and renal injury in chronically exposed rats: likely role of hepatic cadmium-metallothionein in nephrotoxicity. Toxicol Appl Pharmacol 77:414–426

Morselt AFW, van Straalen NM (1986) Histochemical staining of cadmium thiolate clusters in livers of rats treated chronically with cadmium. Histochemistry 84:45–47

Morselt AFW, Lesch R, Jöbsis AC, Bosch KS (1978) Histometry of connective tissue in hepatic fibrosis. Acta Histochem [Suppl] XX:331–338

Morselt AFW, van den Hamer CJA, Prinsen L, Jongstra-Spaapen EJ, Copius Peereboom-Stegeman JHJ, Bosch KS (1985) Large increase in disulphide bonds containing cytosol proteins after chronic cadmium administration estimated in isolated rat liver cells. Histochemistry 83:227–229

Popper H (1979) Toxic injury of the liver, 1st edn. Dekker, New York, pp 243–281

Puvion E, Lange M (1980) Functional significance of perichromatin granule accumulation induced by cadmium chloride in isolated liver cells. Exp Cell Res 128:47–58

Uusitalo RJ (1981) ′5 Nucleotidase activity in lymphocytes. Histochem J 13:525–534

Mechanisms and Models in Toxicology
Arch. Toxicol., Suppl. 11, 216–219 (1987)
© by Springer-Verlag 1987

Sex-Related Interactions of Cadmium and Lead in Changing Cardiovascular Homeostasis and Tissue Metal Levels of Chronically Exposed Rats

M. Carmignani[1], V. N. Finelli[2], P. Boscolo[3], and P. Preziosi[4]

[1] Department of Cell Biology and Physiology, University of L'Aquila, I-67100 L'Aquila, Italy,
and Institute of Pharmacology, Catholic University School of Medicine and Surgery, I-00168 Rome,
Italy
[2] Department of Chemistry, Florida Atlantic University, Boca Raton, FL 33431, USA
[3] Chair of Industrial Toxicology, University of Chieti, I-66100 Chieti, Italy
[4] Institute of Pharmacology, Catholic University School of Medicine and Surgery, I-00168 Rome,
Italy

Introduction

The mechanisms by which chronic exposure to lead (Pb), cadmium (Cd) or Pb plus Cd may affect cardiovascular homeostasis are still controversial (Iannaccone et al. 1981; Boscolo et al. 1981; Carmignani et al. 1983). Pb determined sympathetic hyperactivity, baroreflex hyposensitivity, vagal parasympathetic hypofunction, and increased cardiovascular responsiveness to angiotensin II and catecholamines in male Sprague-Dawley rats that received 50 µg/ml of the metal (as acetate) in drinking water for 160–180 days (Iannaccone et al. 1981). Pb also reduced the urinary kallikrein and affected the plasma renin activities of Pb-exposed workers (Boscolo et al. 1978). The mechanisms underlying the cardiac and vascular modifications induced by chronic exposure of both humans and laboratory animals to Cd have been previously reviewed (Carmignani and Boscolo 1984, 1985; Boscolo and Carmignani 1986). Pb and Cd may have additive effects in inducing heart-related diseases or arterial hypertension (Carmignani and Boscolo 1984; Boscolo and Carmignani 1986). However, these additive effects of Pb and Cd were not confirmed in a study carried out on male Sprague-Dawley rats treated with 20 µg/ml of Cd (as acetate) and/or 50 µg/ml of Pb (as acetate) in drinking water for 180–210 days. In this study Cd seemed to act by predominantly peripheral effector mechanisms, while Pb showed central neurogenic actions; both metals altered specifically the levels of zinc (Zn) and copper (Cu) in kidney and brain (Carmignani et al. 1983).

This research was performed to investigate some of the above mechanisms in both male and female rats exposed for the same long-term period to Pb or Pb plus Cd in a 1 : 1 ratio.

Materials and Methods

Male and female Sprague-Dawley rats ($n=8$ in each group) received, for 14 months starting from weaning, deionized drinking water alone (control groups) or containing 20 µg/ml Pb (as acetate) or 20 µg/ml Pb plus 20 µg/ml Cd (both as acetate).

At the end of the treatment, the following cardiovascular indices were monitored polygraphically under thiopental anesthesia (45 mg/kg, i.p.), as previously described (Carmignani and Boscolo 1984): aortic BP, maximum rate of rise of the left ventricular pressure (dp/dt_{max}) and heart rate (HR). The protocol included (a) bilateral carotid occlusion (BCO) and vagotomy and (b) i.v. injection of noradrenaline (NA; 1 µg/kg; Merck), adrenaline (A; 1 µg/kg; Merck), isoprenaline (ISO; 0.625 µg/kg; Merck), acetylcholine (ACH; 2.5 µg/kg; Merck), dopamine (DA; 200 µg/kg; Aldrich), angiotensin I and II (A1, A2; 0.5 µg/kg; Sigma), tyramine (TYR; 250 µg/kg; Merck), papaverine (PAP; 1 mg/kg; Merck), cocaine (COC; 2.5 mg/kg; Angelini) and hexamethonium (HEX; 2.5 mg/kg; Serva Feinbiochemica). All drugs were dissolved in 0.9% saline solution, the doses were expressed in terms of free bases and peak responses were considered. A consecutive test was not performed until all the parameters had spontaneously returned to the values preceding the injection of NA and remained stable.

The levels of Pb, Cd, Zn and Cu in kidney, liver and brain were determined by atomic absorption spectrophotometry, as previously described (Carmignani and Boscolo 1984). The metal levels were referred to the dry weight of the organs.

The paired mean values were tested by the one-way analysis of variance; only a p value below 0.05 was considered to be significant.

Results

Systolic BP was increased and HR reduced in the Pb-plus-Cd-exposed male rats (152 ± 4 mm Hg vs 133 ± 3 mm Hg in the controls, $p < 0.05$; 362 ± 12 beats/min vs 411 ± 28 beats/min in the controls, $p < 0.05$; mean $\pm$ SE); systolic and diastolic BP were increased in the females (144 ± 4 mm Hg and 108 ± 7 mm Hg vs 125 ± 3 mm Hg and 90 ± 4 mm Hg in the controls, $p < 0.05$; mean $\pm$ SE); dP/dt_{max} was unchanged in both groups. Male and female Pb- and Pb-plus-Cd-exposed animals showed no change in cardiovascular responses to BCO, vagotomy, A2, PAP and HEX. In the Pb- and Pb-plus-Cd-treated male rats there was a decrease of the responses to NA, A, ISO, DA and TYR; the responses to ACH were potentiated in the group exposed to Pb plus Cd, while those to A1 and COC were unchanged in both groups (Table 1). The hypertensive effects of A1 and TYR were higher in the Pb-exposed female rats, while those of COC appeared to be reduced in the females exposed to Pb plus Cd (Table 1).

Renal Cd of the rats treated with Pb plus Cd was below the level reported as critical for Cd-exposed workers (300 ± 7 µg/g dry weight in the males and 287 ± 4 µg/g in the females vs 0.2 ± 0.04 µg/g and 0.3 ± 0.35 µg/g, respectively, in the controls; $p < 0.05$; mean $\pm$ SE). Cd was also augmented in the liver (137 ± 7 µg/g in the males and 110 ± 3 µg/g in the females vs 0.3 ± 0.07 µg/g and 0.2 ± 0.07 µg/g, respectively, in the controls; $p < 0.05$; mean $\pm$ SE) but not in the brain of the rats receiving Pb plus Cd. Pb was increased in all the organs of the exposed animals, with mean values ranging from 1.0 µg/g to 3.2 µg/g. Cu and/or Zn were increased in the kidney of the male and female rats treated with Pb plus Cd and of

Table 1. Peak cardiovascular changes following i.v. administration of various substances in male and female rats exposed to Pb or Pb plus Cd (mean ±S.E.)

		Blood pressure ($\pm \Delta$ mm Hg)		dP/dt_{max} ($\pm \Delta$ mm Hg/sec)	Heart rate ($\pm \Delta$ beats/min)
		Systolic	Diastolic		
Male Rats					
Noradrenaline	1	$+36\pm2^*$	$+27\pm2^*$	$+4442\pm440$	$+19\pm3$
(1 µg/kg)		$(+60\pm9)$	$(+43\pm2)$	$(+3959\pm177)$	$(+28\pm6)$
	2	$+29\pm2^*$	$+24\pm1^*$	$+2011\pm342^*$	$+12\pm2^*$
Adrenaline	1	$+24\pm2^*$	$+17\pm3^*$	$+2589\pm432$	$+15\pm3^*$
(1 µg/kg)		$(+52\pm7)$	$(+37\pm6)$	$(+3210\pm378)$	$(+35\pm8)$
	2	$+20\pm3^*$	$+15\pm1^*$	$+1455\pm214^*$	$+11\pm2^*$
Isoprenaline	1	-38 ± 3	-39 ± 4	$+1091\pm73^*$	$+30\pm4^*$
(0.625 µg/kg)		(-40 ± 5)	(-41 ± 1)	$(+2140\pm328)$	$(+60\pm6)$
	2	-43 ± 4	-45 ± 3	$+1178\pm94^*$	$+18\pm3^*$
Acetylcholine	1	-55 ± 7	-42 ± 4	-2040 ± 52	-26 ± 5
(2.5 µg/kg)		(-49 ± 5)	(-43 ± 2)	(-2140 ± 270)	(-19 ± 4)
	2	$-75\pm4^*$	$-57\pm4^*$	$-3458\pm102^*$	-25 ± 6
Dopamine	1	$+52\pm4^*$	$+46\pm3^*$	$+2138\pm148^*$	$+40\pm5$
(200 µg/kg)		$(+70\pm6)$	$(+63\pm7)$	$(+3424\pm274)$	$(+30\pm6)$
	2	$+51\pm5^*$	$+44\pm4^*$	$+1926\pm84^*$	$+32\pm3$
Tyramine	1	$+36\pm5^*$	$+32\pm5^*$	$+1572\pm104^*$	$+24\pm3^*$
(250 µg/kg)		$(+69\pm1)$	$(+50\pm2)$	$(+3424\pm388)$	$(+54\pm9)$
	2	$+32\pm3^*$	$+29\pm2^*$	$+1096\pm48^*$	$+14\pm3^*$
Female Rats					
Angiotensin I	1	$+49\pm6^*$	$+39\pm1^*$	-1712 ± 56	-14 ± 4
(0.5 µg/kg)		$(+24\pm2)$	$(+23\pm2)$	(-1605 ± 48)	(-9 ± 3)
	2	$+22\pm3$	$+22\pm2$	-1412 ± 39	-13 ± 4
Tyramine	1	$+64\pm8^*$	$+43\pm2^*$	$+1494\pm362$	$+21\pm4$
(250 µg/kg)		$(+34\pm5)$	$(+31\pm2)$	$(+1699\pm122)$	$(+19\pm3)$
	2	$+39\pm4$	$+36\pm4$	$+1471\pm104$	$+16\pm3$
Cocaine	1	$+26\pm7$	$+29\pm8$	$+2312\pm188$	-22 ± 4
(2.5 mg/kg)		$(+42\pm6)$	$(+35\pm2)$	$(+1924\pm202)$	(-25 ± 8)
	2	$+20\pm2^*$	$+18\pm3^*$	$+2247\pm248$	-38 ± 9

The cardiovascular responses of the control rats are indicated in brackets. In the exposed rats, only the cardiovascular responses significantly different from those of the control rats are reported (see text). 1, Pb-exposed rats; 2, Pb-plus-Cd-exposed rats
* $p<0.05$.

the female rats treated with Pb, in the liver of the female rats treated with Pb plus Cd and in the brain of the male and female rats treated with Pb or Pb plus Cd. Kidney Cu was higher in the females exposed to Pb plus Cd than in males (126 ± 3 µg/g and 67 ± 2 µg/g vs 26 ± 1 µg/g and 20 ± 2 µg/g, respectively, in the controls; $p<0.05$; mean $\pm$ SE). Zn was reduced in the liver of the male rats receiving Pb (13.2 ± 0.1 µg/g vs 17.5 ± 0.7 µg/g in the controls, $p<0.05$; mean $\pm$ SE).

Discussion

Pb did not affect systemic haemodynamics, although it increased the vascular reactivity to A1 and to TYR-released NA in the female rats. Higher levels of exposure to this metal are required for modifying either central neurogenic or peripheral neurohumoral mechanisms leading to arterial hypertension (Carmignani et al. 1983). Cd did not oppose the Pb-induced cardiovascular hyporeactivity to both α- and β-adrenoceptor stimulation of the male rats; however, in these animals it determined arterial hypertension (with reflex bradycardia), possibly related to the observed myocardial hypersensitivity to stimulation of the cholinergic receptors by ACH but not to neurogenic nor baroreflex mechanisms (Carmignani and Boscolo 1984; Boscolo and Carmignani 1986). On the other hand, Cd evidenced a cocaine-like mechanism at the vascular sympathtic junction in the female rats; this mechanism might mask the above vascular effects of Pb observed in the females treated with Pb alone.

The similarities and differences among the levels of Pb, Cd, Zn and Cu in various organs of the exposed rats were in part previously described in Cd-exposed male rats and rabbits (Carmignani and Boscolo 1984, 1985; Boscolo and Carmignani 1986).

This research confirms that sex may be a significant variable for functional interactions between Pb and Cd at the cardiovascular level.

Acknowledgements: This work was supported by grants from the Italian CNR, No. 85.00721.56, and the Commission of the European Communities, No. ENV-567-I(S).

References

Boscolo P, Carmignani M (1986) Mechanisms of cardiovascular regulation in male rabbits chronically exposed to cadmium. Br J Ind Med 43:605–610

Boscolo P, Porcelli G, Cecchetti G, Salimei E, Iannaccone A (1978) Urinary kallikrein activity of workers exposed to lead. Br J Ind Med 35:226–230

Boscolo P, Porcelli G, Carmignani M, Finelli VN (1981) Urinary kallikrein and hypertension in cadmium-exposed rats. Toxicol Lett 7:189–194

Carmignani M, Boscolo P (1984) Cardiovascular responsiveness to physiological agonists of male rats made hypertensive by long-term exposure to cadmium. Sci Total Environ 34:19–33

Carmignani M, Boscolo P (1985) Long-term exposure to cadmium and cardiovascular alterations in the rabbit. Arch Toxicol [Suppl] 8:322–326

Carmignani M, Boscolo P, Ripanti G, Finelli VN (1983) Effects of chronic exposure to cadmium and/or lead on some neurohumoral mechanisms regulating cardiovascular function in the rat. In: Proceedings of the international conference on heavy metals in the environment (German; Müller, Ed.) Heidelberg, September 1983. CEP, Edinburgh, pp 557–560

Iannaccone A, Carmignani M, Boscolo P (1981) Neurogenic and humoral mechanisms in arterial hypertension of chronically lead-exposed rats. Med Lav 1:13–21

Mechanisms and Models in Toxicology
Arch. Toxicol., Suppl. 11, 220–222 (1987)

Cytotoxic, Irritant and Fibrogenic Effects
of Metal-Fume Particulate Materials Investigated
by Intramuscular Injection in the Rat and Guinea Pig

R. Hicks, R. O. Oshodi, and M. J. Pedrick

Metal Fume Research Group, Postgraduate School of Pharmacology, University of Bradford, Bradford, West Yorkshire, BD7 1DP, UK

Introduction

Fume products from metal-working processes are complex mixtures of metals and other elements, often potentially toxic and inhalable, e.g. fumes from welding ferrochromium steels. Previous investigations (Hicks et al. 1983) indicated that the toxic effects most usually exercised by such fumes when inhaled were irritancy, fibrogenicity and cytotoxicity. For simple comparative purposes, intramuscular administration was used as a means of producing particle deposits, being precise in dosage and location and not subject to aggressive translocation mechanisms. Toxic effects of ferrochromium metal products were compared, in particular, fume particles from manual metal-arc welding of stainless steel. Such fumes are rich in chromium in the hexavalent, highly reactive form. Fume particles from an innovative 'low-fume' electrode, welding product were also tested.

Methods and Materials

Female albino guinea pigs (Dunkin-Hartley strain; Bradford University breeding colony) weighing 400–500 g were used, or male albino rats (CSE strain) weighing 200–250 g. Test or control materials, in solution or suspension, were injected into the vastus lateralis muscle in dose volumes of 0.1 ml. After intervals ranging from 2 days to 8 weeks, the animals were killed and the injected muscles removed. The lesion was assessed visually and microscopically. Welding fumes were produced and the particles collected by a system described by Hicks et al. (1983). Electric-arc welding was performed, using either metal inert gas (MIG) or manual metal-arc (MMA) processes, consuming electrodes of stainless (SS) or mild steel (MS) with various fluxes or unfluxed welding wire. For fume contents, see Table 1.

Table 1. Elemental constituents of welding fumes (% w/w)

Fume type	Fe	Ni	Mn	Cr	Cr^{6+} (% of total Cr)
Manual metal-arc fumes (MMA)					
Stainless steel (Nicrex-1; MMA-SS)	4.3	0.9	6.7	4.7	82.2
Mild steel (Satinex; MMA-MS)	31.5	0.1	9.5	0.1	–
Stainless steel, "low fume"[a] (LF 308L)	17.2	1.0	8.2	10.4	1.8
Metal inert gas Fumes (MIG)					
Stainless steel (Bostrand 316; MIG-SS)	35.2	6.4	7.4	12.5	4.1

Other steel constituents, e.g. Mo, Co, are also present in various concentrations and, in MMA fumes so are flux constituents such as Na, K, Ca, Al, and Ti. Most elements are present as mixtures of metal, oxide or mixed-oxide spinels. MMA fluxed rod fumes also contained silica, approximately 20%–25% w/w.
[a] Fume formation rate from "low-fume" electrodes in normal manual welding is approximately one-tenth of corresponding conventional stainless steel rods.

Results

Lesions and tissues were from groups of five animals, rats or guinea pigs, treated with injections of solutions or suspensions of test materials in concentrations of 1, 10 or 100 mg/ml, for periods of 2, 4 or 7 days or 2, 4, 6 or 8 weeks. A general assessment of the effects is shown in Table 2. There were no important differences between effects in the tissues of the rat or guinea pig. Few qualitative differences were discernible between lesions produced by injections of different doses; only the extent of the lesions increased with high dosage.

Table 2. Local intramuscular toxic effects of welding-fume particles or components

Material	Irritancy	Fibrogenicity	Cytotoxicity
MMA-SS	+ + +	+ + + +	+ + +
MMA-MS	+	+ + +	+
MMA-SS "low fume"	+	+ +	–
MIG-SS	+	±	–
Silica-fumed	+ +	+ +	+
Silica-quartz	+ +	+ + + +	–
Manganese dioxide	+ +	+ + +	±
Fe_2O_3 Fe_3O_4 Cr_2O_3 TiO_2	0	0	0
$K_2Cr_2O_7$ K_2CrO_4 CrO_3	+ + +	Delayed scarring	+ + + +
Saline	0	0	0

Discussion

Irritant or fibrogenic effects were readily revealed, as the skeletal muscle would normally be devoid of macrophages or inflammatory cells and only sparsely provided with fibrous connective tissue elements. Any significant developments of macrophage granulomata or fibrotic granulation tissue are thus clearly displayed.

In the intramuscular milieu one of the test materials, manual metal-arc stainless steel (MMA-SS) fume particles, clearly caused severe local inflammation, provoked vigorous development of collagenous granulation tissue and killed muscle fibres. The other two types of manual metal-arc particle were less toxic and less irritant. However, they provoked formation of granulomatous nodules. They were less fibrogenic. Injection of the insoluble metal oxides of iron, chromium or titanium proved to be benign. No irritant, fibrogenic or toxic effects were revealed and phagocytosis was very effective. The test was therefore shown to be discriminating. Very little irritancy or toxicity was shown by the flux-free, metal inert gas, stainless steel (MIG-SS) sample. The tests conducted with other fume constituents indicated that fibrogenesis, irritancy and toxicity were associated with the hexavalent form of chromium or possibly flux components like alkaline oxides or silica.

References

Hicks R, Al-Shamma KJ, Lam HF, Hewitt PJ (1983) An investigation of fibrogenic and other toxic effects of arc-welding fume particles deposited in the rat lung. J Appl Toxicol 3:297–306

Mechanisms and Models in Toxicology
Arch. Toxicol., Suppl. 11, 223–226 (1987)

Intrapulmonary Pretreatment by Metal-Fume Components Causing Inhibition of Delayed Hypersensitivity

L. Q. de A. Caldas and R. Hicks

Metal-Fume Research Group, School of Studies in Pharmacology, University of Bradford, Richmond Road, Bradford, West Yorkshire, BD7 1DP, UK

Introduction

Earlier experiments have demonstrated that cutaneous hypersensitivity evoked by components from stainless steel welding fumes, such as chromium or nickel, may be inhibited by treatment with these haptens, given by intratracheal, intrapulmonary or oral administration prior to the sensitization procedure (Hicks and Caldas 1985). The inhibitory effects were interpreted as manifestations of tolerance. Further investigations were performed to decide which component of the welding-fume particles contributes most to such tolerance. These properties have previously been tested using potassium dichromate. However, the form of chromium in stainless steel metal fumes is predominantly as the chromate, which interacts with protein by a tanning-like process differing from that of dichromate. It was therefore desirable to verify that chromate could also induce tolerance. It was desirable also to investigate nickel, as this did not appear to produce consistent effects.

Materials and Methods

Groups of five guinea pigs, Dunkin-Hartley strain, weighing 250–300 gm, were used in all experiments. A water-soluble, extractable fraction was prepared from particles produced by manual metal-arc welding of stainless steel electrodes, Nicrex-1 (Murex, UK), giving fumes rich in chromium and nickel. Particles were suspended and shaken in normal saline (150 µg/ml) for 8 h.

'Tolerizing' and Sensitizing Procedures

One, two or three sets of intrapulmonary injections were given, each set comprising 1, 3, 5 or 6 injections at daily or alternate daily intervals, and with intervals of 3, 7, 9, 14 or 24 days between the sets or preceding the cutaneous sensitization procedure.

Animals were sensitized using the method of Polak et al. (1973). Sensitizations used a 1% aqueous solution, and elicitation a 0.1% solution. The water-soluble, extractable components were used in a 10% dilution for sensitization and 1% dilution for elicitation.

Results

Tolerization pretreatments, employing 2 or 3 sets of 3–5 intrapulmonary injections of potassium chromate solution (total dose of 42 mg/kg), all produced significant reductions in subsequently evoked cutaneous hypersensitivity to chro-

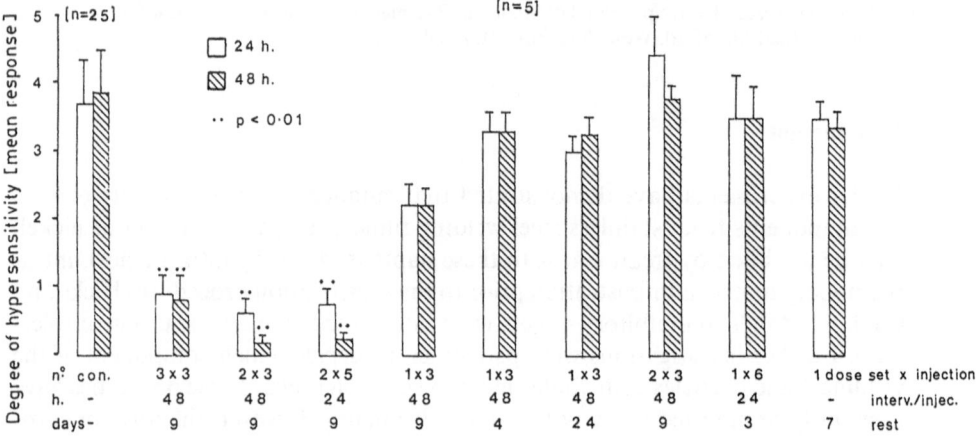

Fig. 1. Tolerance due to K_2CrO_4 pretreatment

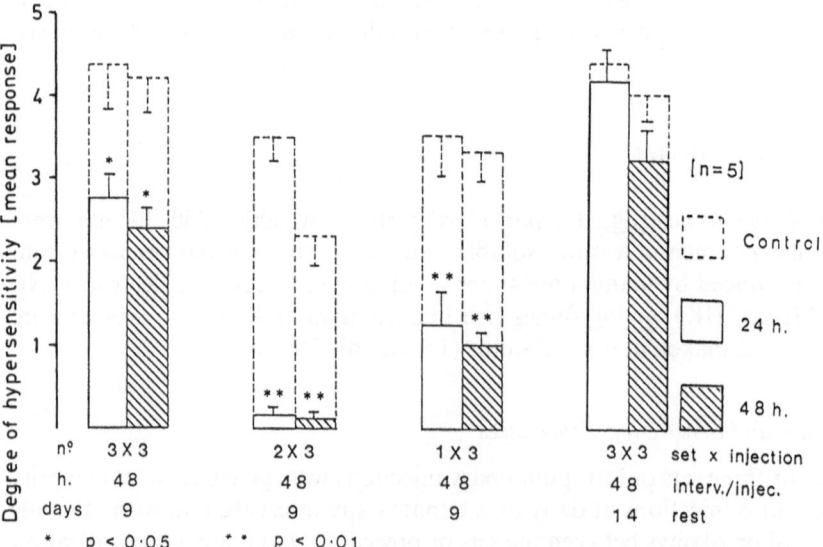

Fig. 2. Tolerance due to welding-fume components

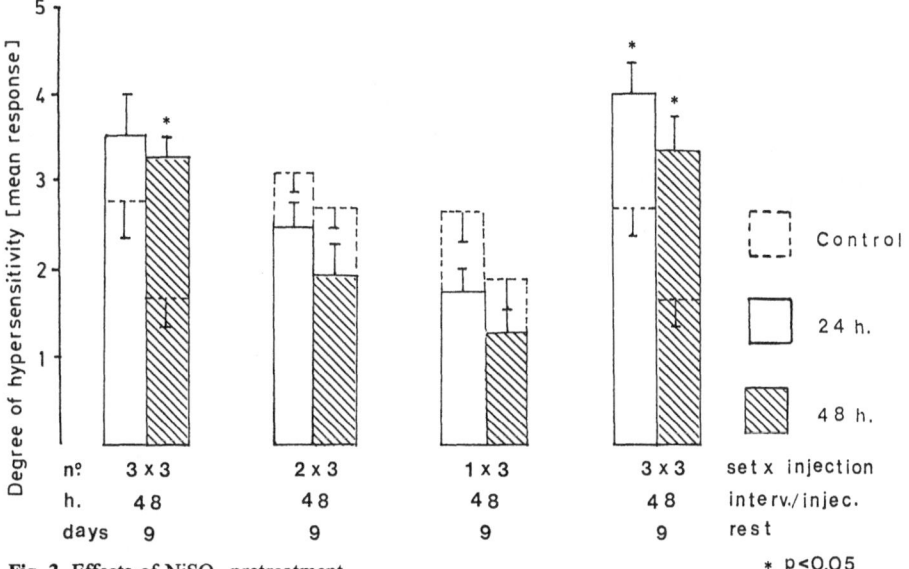

Fig. 3. Effects of NiSO$_4$ pretreatment

mate (Fig. 1). Pretreatments administering single sets of 3 injections were ineffective. Pretreatment sequences of 2 or 3 sets of 3 intrapulmonary injections of the solution of welding-fume components (total doses equivalent to 100 mg/kg of original fume particles) significantly inhibited the subsequent sensitization-elicitation procedures (Fig. 2). Only one set of 3 injections was ineffective. In animals given 3 sets of 3 injections of nickel sulphate (total dose 42 mg/kg), followed by sensitization, cutaneous reactions were significantly potentiated (Fig. 3). Single or double sets of pretreatments were not effective. Pretreatment with potassium chromate did not alter hypersensitivity provoked by nickel sulphate and the reverse was also true, i.e. no cross-tolerance was revealed. However, in animals pretreated using the mixture of chromate and nickel, subsequent sensitization and challenge procedures indicated cross-inhibition. Sensitization to potassium chromate and nickel was significantly inhibited.

Discussion

These experiments confirm that, as with dichromate, intrapulmonary pretreatment with potassium chromate produced a specific inhibition of cutaneously-induced hypersensitivity. Thus, the overall 'tolerizing' effect of the water-soluble welding-fume component mixture is explicable in terms of its major component. However, rather than exerting an inhibitory action, pretreatments with the nickel salt caused some potentiation. On the other hand, the very strong inhibitory effects of the mixtures of chromate and nickel salts suggest that the higher concentration of chromate exerted the predominant effect, masking any specific potentiation due to nickel. This may well be the result of antigenic competition, e.g. on presenting or suppressor cells (Polak 1985).

References

Hicks R, Caldas LQA (1986) Immunologic unresponsiveness to chromium or nickel in the guinea-pig induced by stainless steel welding fume components. Arch Toxicol Suppl. 9, 421–422

Polak L (1985) Antigenic competition in the induction of contact sensitivity in the guinea pig. Int Archs Allergy Appl Immunol 76:275–281

Polak L, Turk JL, Frey JR (1973) Studies on contact hypersensitivity to chromium compounds. Prog Allergy 17:145–226

Mechanisms and Models in Toxicology
Arch. Toxicol., Suppl. 11, 227–230 (1987)

The Effect of Lead and Aluminium
on Rat Dihydropteridine Reductase

P. Cutler and J. A. Blair

Molecular Sciences Department, Aston University, Birmingham, B4 7ET, UK

Methods

Assay of brain and liver dihydropteridine reductase (DHPR) activity was that of
Craine et al. (1972). A 30% homogenate (w/v) was prepared in 0.5 M tris-maleate
buffer, pH 6.8; cytosolic fraction was isolated by centrifugation at 40000 rpm,
45 min. DHPR activity was assayed by the decrease in absorbance of nicotinamide adenine dinucleotide reduced (NADH), at 340 nm, 37 °C. Quininoid dihy-
drobiopterin (qBH$_2$) was generated with peroxidase and H$_2$O$_2$. The standard assay contained the following in a final volume of 1 ml: 0.05 M Tris-maleate buffer,
pH 6.8; 2.5×10^{-4} M sodium azide; 10^{-3} M H$_2$O$_2$; 8 µg horseradish peroxidase;
10^{-4} M dimethyltetrahydropteridine (DMPH$_4$): 10^{-4} M NADH and 0.2 ml
DHPR source. The activity was determined as nanomoles NADH oxidised/
min · mg protein.

Assay of DHPR activity in blood was a modification of the method used by
Hasegawa et al. (1978) based on the nonenzymatic reaction of tetrahydrobiopterin (THB) with ferrocytochrome c to form qBH$_2$ and ferrocytochrome c. qBH$_2$
is reduced back by DHPR to THB in the presence of NADH. A sample of whole
blood was diluted approximately 25-fold for haemolysis with distilled water. The
components of the assay system in a total volume of 1 ml were 0.05 M Tris-maleate buffer, pH 6.8, 5×10^{-5} M ferricytochrome c, 10^{-4} M NADH, 10^{-5} M
DMPH$_4$ and 0.1 ml DHPR source. The reduction of ferricytochrome c was followed by measurement of the increase in absorbance at 550 nm. The activity was
determined as nanomoles of cytochrome c reduced/min per · mg of protein.

Results

Subchronic exposure to lead significantly reduces DHPR activity in rat brain and
blood. Aluminium, scandium and gallium all significantly reduce blood DHPR
activity and scandium and gallium significantly reduce brain DHPR activity
(Table 1).

Table 1. DHPR activity in rats dosed intraperitoneally with heavy metals

		n	Mean	S.D.	Probability
Brain	Control	12	275	44.1	
	Lead	11	212	46.4	0.003
	Control	6	210	42.5	
	Aluminium	5	166	37.6	0.099
	Control	6	173	17.5	
	Gallium	6	144	14.8	0.044
	Scandium	6	139	32.0	0.012
Liver	Control	6	359	70.1	
	Aluminium	5	159	62.5	0.001
Blood	Control	12	0.31	0.08	
	Lead	11	0.16	0.08	<0.0005
	Control	6	0.40	0.04	
	Aluminium	5	0.27	0.07	0.002
	Control	6	0.52	0.23	
	Gallium	6	0.21	0.07	0.009
	Scandium	6	0.21	0.07	0.009

Animals dosed intraperitoneally every 12 h for 3 days with either 0.759 mg/kg lead acetate, 0.75 mg/kg aluminium acetate, 0.512 mg/ kg gallium nitrate hydrate, or 0.302 mg/kg scandium-111 chloride nitrate in isotonic saline. Controls received isotonic saline. Specific activity in the brain and liver was measured as nmoles NADH oxidized/min per mg protein. Specific activity in blood was measured as nmoles cytochrome c reduced/min per mg protein.

Table 2. The effect of a subchronic intraperitoneal dose of lead on plasma, brain and liver phenylalanine and tyrosine levels

		Phenylalanine μmol/l (SΔ)	Tyrosine μmol/l (SΔ)
Brain	Control	6.04 (0.95)	5.21 (0.57)
	Lead	4.99 (0.97)	10.63 (2.92)
	Probability	0.086	0.002
Liver	Control	9.07 (1.37)	7.54 (0.76)
	Lead	14.74 (5.40)	20.70 (7.81)
	Probability	0.030	0.002
Plasma	Control	35.65 (8.57)	44.18 (8.90)
	Lead	29.81 (3.94)	34.11 (9.49)
	Probability	> 0.10	0.085

Animals were dosed intraperitoneally every 12 h for 3 days with 0.759 mg/kg lead acetate in isotonic saline. Controls received isotonic saline. Levels are determined as μmol/l of a 20% tissue preparation or μmol/l plasma. $n=6$ in all cases.

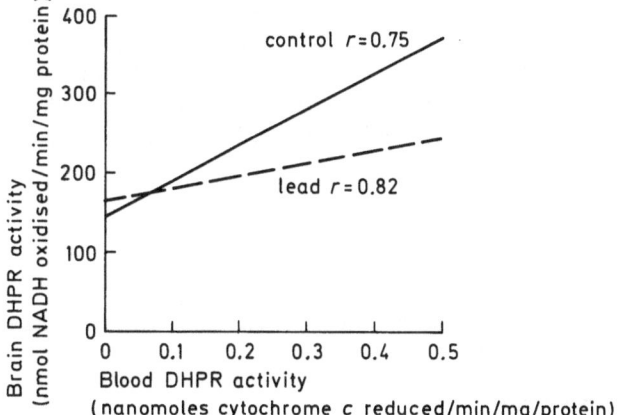

Fig. 1. Correlation between blood and brain DHPR activity in rats. The animals were dosed intraperitoneally every 12 h with 0.759 mg/kg lead acetate isotonic saline for 3 days before death

The lead-induced reduction in DHPR activity results in decreased hydroxylation of phenylalanine and tyrosine. This is illustrated by the rise in brain tyrosine and liver phenylalanine, the tissue sites of the respective hydroxylases (Table 2). There is a correlation between blood and brain DHPR activity both in control and lead-treated animals (Fig. 1).

Discussion

Lead exposure reduced DHPR activity. The reduction is greatest in the blood and least in the brain. This is attributed to the presence of the blood-brain barrier. Aluminium, gallium and scandium inhibit blood DHPR activity. Gallium and scandium significantly inhibit brain DHPR activity. It is thought that the lack of inhibition of brain DHPR activity by aluminium is due to the presence of the blood-brain barrier. Reduced DHPR activity resulting from subchronic lead and aluminium loading produces a reduction in the hydroxylation of the aromatic amino acids and a subsequent loss of catecholamine neurotransmitter biosynthesis. Lead is a well-known neurotoxin (Rutter and Russell Jones 1983) which dramatically alters adrenergic and cholinergic nervous transmission (Hrdina et al. 1980). The results shown suggest a possible mechanism for the neurological dysfunction following lead poisoning.

Aluminium toxicity has been implicated in several disorders of the central nervous system including senile dementia of the Alzheimer type, parkinsonism dementia, dialysis dementia and some forms of epilepsy (Liss 1980; Wisniewski et al. 1985). The reduction in DHPR activity observed suggests a possible mechanism for the neurotoxicity of aluminium. Further study of aluminium toxicity is hindered by the lack of a suitable radioisotope. Scandium and gallium, congeners of aluminium, are both good inhibitors of DHPR activity, and preliminary studies suggest that they represent good models for aluminium.

There is a correlation between blood and brain DHPR activity. This exists for control animals ($r = 0.75$, $p < 0.005$) and lead-treated animals ($r = 0.82$, $p < 0.004$). Similar correlations have been obtained for animals loaded with aluminium ($r = 0.81$, $p < 0.006$), scandium ($r = 0.62$, $p < 0.006$) and gallium ($r = 0.63$, $p < 0.006$). This makes possible a rapid and convenient estimation of brain DHPR activity from blood samples.

References

Craine JE, Hall ES, Kaufman S (1972) The isolation and characterisation of dihydropteridine reductase from sheep liver. J Biol Chem 247:6082–6091

Hasegawa H, Nakanishi N, Akino M (1978) Stoichiometric studies on the oxidation of tetrahydrobiopterin with ferricytochrome c. J Biochem 84:499–506

Hrdina PD, Hanin I, Dubas TC (1980) Neurochemical correlates in lead toxicity. In: Shingal RA, Thomas JH (eds) Lead toxicity. Urban and Schwarzenberg, pp 273–300, Baltimore

Liss L (1980) Aluminium neurotoxicity. Pathotox Publishers Inc., Illinois

Rutter M, Russell Jones R (1983) Lead versus health. Wiley, Chichester

Wisniewski HM, Sturman JA, Shek JW, Iqbal K (1985) Aluminium and the central nervous system. J Environ Pathol Toxicol Oncol 6:1–8

Mechanisms and Models in Toxicology
Arch. Toxicol., Suppl. 11, 231–235 (1987)
© by Springer-Verlag 1987

Intestinal Absorption of Aluminium in Rats: Effect of Sodium

G. B. van der Voet and F. A. de Wolff

Laboratorium voor Toxicologie, Academisch Ziekenhuis, Rijnsburgerweg 10, 2333 AA Leiden, The Netherlands

Introduction

Aluminium (Al) is no longer known as a non-toxic element. Al is the cause of several dialysis-related diseases (microcytic anaemia, vitamin D-resistant osteomalacia, dialysis encephalopathy) and plays a possible role in various other disorders (Alzheimer's disease, amyotrophic lateral sclerosis) (Flendrig et al. 1976; Alfrey et al. 1976; Wills and Savory 1983). The Al uptake from the intestine may be one of the main sources of Al in the body and, therefore, of Al toxicity, especially in renal patients on oral Al hydroxide therapy (Clarkson et al. 1972; Cam et al. 1980; Griswold et al. 1983; Randall 1983; Kaye 1983; Cannata et al. 1983a).

Since no physiological functions of Al are known as yet, Al absorption may take place along pathways for essential metals. Interactions between intestinal absorption of Al and such metals may be predisposed to by analogies in their respective charge, mass, hydration or complexation characteristics. Recent observations speak for an interaction between metabolic pathways of Al and iron (Fe) or Al and calcium (Ca) (Bommer et al. 1983; Touam et al. 1983; Trapp 1983; Blaehr et al. 1985; van der Voet and de Wolff 1985; Cannata et al. 1983b).

Observations on Al entering metabolic pathways of sodium (Na) led us to study a possible interaction between the intestinal absorption of Al and Na (Witters et al. 1984; Muniz and Leivestad 1980a; Muniz and Leivestad 1980b). The investigation was performed with an in vivo perfusion system of rat small intestine combined with systemic blood sampling previously described by van der Voet and de Wolff (1984).

Materials and Methods

Perfusion of Rat Small Intestine

Experiments were performed with Wistar rats (females, weighing between 200–230 g) which were fed on a standard diet (Hope Farms, Linschoten, The Netherlands) with tap water ad libitum (<10 µg/l Al). The rats had fasted 24–48 h at the start of each experiment. Anticoagulation was carried out with 300 IU heparin i.v. (Thromboliquine, Organon Teknika, Oss, The Netherlands) and the animals were anaesthetized with 45 mg/kg pentobarbital sodium i.p. (Nembutal, Ceval s.a. International Division, Neuilly-sur-Seine, France).

Perfusion media contained 20 mmol/l Al ($AlCl_3 \cdot 6H_2O$), made isosmotic with 120 mmol/l Na(NaCl) or choline chloride (120 mmol/l). The pH of all media was established at 3.0 with 6 N HCl. The media (50 ml each) were recirculated for 60 min through the small intestine, between the Treitz ligament and the ileocoecal valve, at a perfusion rate of 10 ml/min. Six rats were perfused with each type of perfusion medium. Samples of 100 µl were collected from the perfusion medium before the start and at the end of the perfusion period, while 20-µl samples were collected from the systemic (tail) blood at the same time. The zero-time samples were collected immediately after saturating the tube system with metal(s) containing perfusate, just before perfusion. Samples were diluted in 0.2% Triton X-100 before analysis.

Analysis of Al and Na in Perfusate and Blood

Al in perfusate and blood was analyzed with flameless atomic absorption spectrophotometry (Perkin-Elmer PE 2380 and HGA 500, Norwalk, Conn., USA). Graphite tubes were pyrolitically coated (PE 091504). A Perkin-Elmer hollow cathode lamp was operated at 25 mA at 309.3 nm with a spectral bandwidth of 0.7 nm. The furnace programme has been described elsewhere (van der Voet et al. 1985). Standards were prepared to a concentration of 0, 0.74, 1.85 and 3.70 µmol Al/l (0, 20, 50, and 100 µg/l) in 0.2% Triton X-100.

Na in perfusate and blood was analyzed with a routine flame photometric method. Na-containing standards were prepared to a concentration of 130 and 150 mmol/l for both the analyses. All analyses were performed in duplicate. No interference between Al and Na was observed.

Results

Intestinal Retention and Absorption of Al

The retention of Al by the mucosal wall, which can be calculated as the difference between the Al concentration in the perfusate at zero-time and the Al concentration after 60 min perfusion, amounted to about 6 mmol Al/l (300 µmol per rat), and did not differ significantly when the intestine was perfused with a Na-containing medium or a choline-containing medium (Fig. 1 A).

The actual intestinal absorption of Al after 60 min perfusion, i.e. the difference between the Al concentration in the blood at 60 min and the Al concentration in the blood at zero-time, amounted to about 2 µmol Al/l in the presence of Na, but rose above 100 µmol Al/l in the absence of sodium (Fig. 1 B).

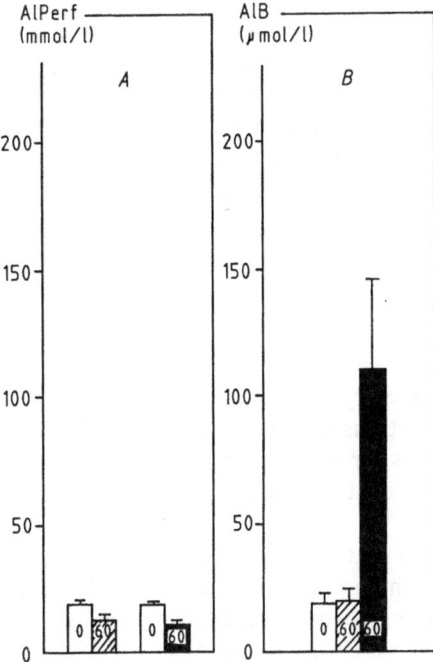

Fig. 1. Concentration of Al in (**A**) the perfusate (AlPerf) and (**B**) systemic blood (AlB) at zero-time (□) and after 60 min perfusion with a Na-containing medium (▨) and a choline-containing medium (■). Each column represents the mean of the Al concentration in six perfusates or in the blood of six rats. Standard errors of the mean are indicated on top of each column

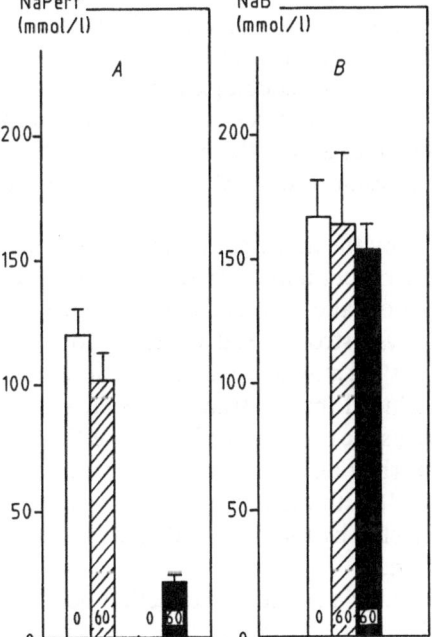

Fig. 2. Concentration of Na in (**A**) the perfusate (NaPerf) and (**B**) systemic blood at zero-time (□) and after 60 min perfusion with a Na-containing medium (▨) and a choline-containing medium (■). Each column represents the mean Na concentration in six perfusates or in the blood of six rats. Standard errors of the mean are indicated on top of each column

Intestinal Retention and Absorption of Na

The amount of Na retained by the intestinal wall amounted to 20 mmol/l in the course of 60 min perfusion. An amount of about 20 mmol/l appeared into the Na-free choline-containing medium after 60 min perfusion (Fig. 2A). No significant rise of Na was seen in the blood after perfusion with a sodium-containing medium. The level of Al was reduced, though insignificantly $(0.50 > p > 0.25)$, when the intestine was perfused with a choline-containing medium (Fig. 2B).

Discussion

Intestinal absorption of Al may be the main entry of Al into the body leading to systemic toxicity. Since no physiological functions are yet described for Al it may well be that Al makes use of transport routes for other, essential, metals such as Fe or Na, i.e. determined by analogy in charge, atomic size, hydration characteristics, etc.

So far, clinical and animal studies indicate that the intestinal absorption of Al is concentration-dependent and pH-dependent, and that Fe may either inhibit or promote absorption of Al, and that citric acid strongly enhances intestinal absorption of Al (Clarkson et al. 1972; Cam et al. 1980; Griswold et al. 1983; Randall 1983; Kaye 1983; Cannata et al. 1983a, b; Blaehr et al. 1985; van der Voet and de Wolff 1985; van der Voet and de Wolff 1984; Slanina et al. 1984; van der Voet and de Wolff 1986). The absorption of Al may be biphasic, as for Fe and Ca (Manis and Schachter 1962). Apparently, no data are as yet available for interactions between Na and Al at intestinal absorption, while the molecular size and hydrations heat may predict an interaction. Ecotoxicological data, however, are available on a negative interaction between Al and Na influx into the adult waterbug *Corixa punctata* living in acid bog lakes and in the brown trout *Salmo trutta* L. (Witters et al. 1984; Muniz and Leivestad 1980a; Muniz and Leivestad 1980b).

The amount of Al retained and absorbed by the intestinal wall is comparable with data from our previous studies (van der Voet and de Wolff 1984; van der Voet et al. 1985; Slanina et al. 1984; van der Voet and de Wolff 1986). Absorption of Al from a choline-containing medium shows a strong negative interaction with the intestinal absorption of Na, suggesting that Al may share the absorption route for Na. On the other hand, it cannot be excluded that Al transport is facilitated by choline. The actual Na absorption as well as the exorption of Na in the Na-free choline-containing medium appears undisturbed and confirms data from other investigators (de Wolff 1977; Pandjaitan 1984), although an inhibition of the Na absorption by Al may be present but undetected by the thousand-fold quantitative difference between Na and Al absorption.

It may be concluded that there is evidence for a negative interaction between Al and Na during intestinal absorption. Further analysis of this phenomenon may be performed by studying absorption of Al from other isosmotic salt solutions. The clinical implications may be apparent, especially in renal patients taking phosphate binders containing Al, who are often kept on a Na-free diet.

References

Alfrey AC, Legendre GR, Kaehny WD (1976) The dialysis encephalopathy syndrome. Possible aluminium intoxication. N Engl J Med 294:184–188

Blaehr H, Madsen S, Andersen J, Ladefoged J (1985) Effect of iron-loading on intestinal aluminum – absorption in chronic renal insufficiency. Trace Element Med 2:105

Bommer J, Waldherr R, Wieser PH, Ritz E (1983) Concomitant lysosomal storage of iron and aluminium in dialysis patients. Lancet I:1390

Cam JM, Luck VA, Eastwood JB, DeWardener HE (1980) The effect of aluminium hydroxide orally on calcium, phosphorus and aluminium metabolism in normal subjects. Acta Paediatr Scand 69:793–796

Cannata JB, Briggs JD, Junor BJR, Fell GS (1983 a) Aluminium hydroxide intake: real risk of aluminium toxicity. Br Med J 286:1937–1938

Cannata JB, Briggs JD, Junor BJR, Fell GS, Beastall G (1983 b) Effect of acute aluminium overload on calcium and parathyroid-hormone metabolism. Lancet I:501–503

Clarkson EM, Luck VA, Hynson WV, Bailey RR, Eastwood JB, Woodhead JS, Clements VR, O'Riordan JLH, DeWardener HE (1972) The effect of aluminium hydroxide on calcium, phosphorus and aluminium balances, the serum parathyroid hormone concentration and the aluminium content of bone in patients with chronic renal failure. Clin Sci 43:519–531

de Wolff FA (1977) Drug effects on intestinal epithelium. PhD Thesis, University of Leiden

Flendrig JA, Kruis H, Das HA (1976) Aluminium and dialysis dementia. Lancet I:1235

Griswold WR, Reznik V, Mendoza SA, Trauner D, Alfrey AC (1983) Accumulation of aluminium in a nondialysed uremic child receiving aluminium hydroxide. Pediatrics 71:56–58

Kaye M (1983) Oral aluminium toxicity in a non-dialysed patient with renal failure. Clin Nephrol 20:208–211

Manis JG, Schachter D (1962) Active transport of iron by intestine: features of a two step mechanism. Am J Physiol 203:73–80

Muniz TP, Leivestad H (1980 a) Toxic effects of aluminium on the brown trout, Salmo trutta L. In: Drablos D, Tollan A (eds) Proceedings of the international conference on ecological impact of acid precipitation. OSCO SNSF, pp 320–321

Muniz TP, Leivestad H (1980 b) Acidification-effects on fresh fish. In: Drablos D, Tollan A (eds) Proceedings of the international conference on ecological impact of acid precipitation. OSCO SNSF, pp 84–92

Pandjaitan P (1984) Effects of drugs and electrolytes on intestinal absorption of glucose and glycine. An in vivo study in the rat. PhD Thesis, University of Leiden

Randall ME (1983) Aluminium toxicity in an infant not on dialysis. Lancet I:1327–1328

Slanina P, Falkeborn Y, Frech W, Cedergren A (1984) Aluminium concentration in the brain and bone of rats fed citric acid, aluminium citrate or aluminium hydroxide. Food Chem Toxic 22:391–397

Touam M, Martinez F, Lacour B, Bourdon R, Tingraff J, DiGiulio S, Drüeke T (1983) Aluminium-induced, reversible microcytic anemia in chronic renal failure: clinical and experimental studies. Clin Nephrol 19:299–308

Trapp GA (1983) Plasma aluminum is bound to transferrin. Life Sci 33:311–316

van der Voet GB, de Wolff FA (1984) A method of studying the intestinal absorption of aluminium in the rat. Arch Toxicol 55:168–172

van der Voet GB, de Wolff FA (1985) The effect of iron on the intestinal absorption of aluminium in rats. Trace Element Med 2:134–135

van der Voet GB, de Wolff FA (1986) Intestinal absorption of aluminium in rats, effect of intraluminal pH and aluminium concentration. J Appl Toxicol 6:37–41

van der Voet GB, de Haas EJM, de Wolff FA (1985) Monitoring of aluminium in whole blood, plasma, serum, and water by a single procedure using flameless atomic absorption spectrophotometry. J Anal Toxicol 9:97–100

Wills MR, Savory J (1983) Aluminium poisoning: dialysis encephalopathy, osteomalacia and anaemia. Lancet II:29–34

Witters H, Vangenechten JHD, van Puymbroeck S, Vanderborght OLJ (1984) Interference of aluminium and pH on the Na-influx in an aquatic insect Corixa punctata (Illig). Bull Environ Contam Toxicol 32:575–579

Mechanisms and Models in Toxicology
Arch. Toxicol., Suppl. 11, 236–239 (1987)
© by Springer-Verlag 1987

Neurotoxicity of a Spent Phosphoric Acid Catalyst

N. J. Sarginson [1], N. L. Roberts [2], C. J. Fish [2], and M. K. Johnson [3]

[1] Essochem Europe Inc., Mechelsesteenweg 363, 1950 Kraainem, Belgium
[2] Huntingdon Research Centre, Huntingdon, Cambs., UK
[3] MRC Toxicology Unit, Woodmansterne Road, Carshalton, Surrey, UK

Introduction

Analytical investigations carried out on a spent phosphoric catalyst used in the production of higher olefins (octenes, nonenes, decenes) had shown the presence of percentage levels of organophosphorus compounds. In view of the known acute and delayed neurotoxicity of organophosphorus compounds, and the potential for human exposure during the removal of the catalyst from the reactors, it was decided to investigate the neurotoxicity of the spent catalyst.

Methods

The protocol followed was based on guidelines published by the OECD (Organisation for Economic Co-operation and Development), final draft 418, *Acute Delayed Neurotoxicity of Organophosphorus Substances,* adopted on May 30, 1983.

The test species chosen was the domestic hen (*Gallus gallus domesticus*) in view of its known sensitivity to organophosphorus compounds. Birds were 12 months old at the start of the study. They were group-housed according to treatment group in a poultry building designed to provide suitable environmental conditions, with temperature (range 15–22 °C), relative humidity (range 36–57%), and lighting (12 h light/dark cycle) regulated. Standard Huntingdon Research Centre layer rations in pellet form were provided ad libitum throughout the study, except for an overnight starvation period prior to dosing.

The test material, spent phosphoric acid catalyst, consisted of a grey-black powder, and was a mixture of several reactor batches. Tri-*o*-cresyl phosphate (TOCP) was used as the positive control material.

Preliminary range-finding studies using 3 birds established that the test material could be administered at 5000 mg/kg body wt., as a 30% suspension in corn oil.

Birds were allocated to treatment groups 7 days before dosing, as follows:

Group	No. of birds	Treatment	Dose level (mg/kg)	Dose volume (ml/kg)
1	10	Corn oil	–	16.7
2	5	TOCP	500	4
3	15	Catalyst	5000	16.7

After the 7-day acclimatisation period, birds were dosed once by oral intubation according to the above schedule. Dosing was followed by a 21-day observation period, at the end of which all group 2 birds (TOCP) were killed. All negative control and test birds were redosed at the end of day 21. A further 21-day observation period followed the second dose.

The following observations were made: mortalities (daily); bird health (daily); ataxia assessment [daily, according to a point award system similar to that described by Cavanagh et al. (1961). The scale ranges from 0 to 8, with the highest score representing the greatest degree of ataxia]; body weights (weekly).

Macroscopic post-mortem examinations were carried out on all birds killed on day 21 and all birds surviving until termination of the study on day 42. Birds which died during the study were also examined.

After perfusion through the heart with fixative, the brain, spinal column and sciatic nerves were taken from each bird and stored in 10% buffered formalin. Samples of these were taken for histology. Histological sections were cut at 8 μm and stained with haematoxylin and oesin. Additional sections were stained by the Glees and Marsland method (Marsland et al. 1954) for axons and with solochrome cyanin for myelin (Page 1970).

The neuropathological grading system employed has five grades, ranging from grade I (no lesions), to grade V (most severe changes). In general, grades III and above indicate significant degeneration.

In order to provide additional information on the neurotoxicity of the spend catalyst, neuropathy target esterase (NTE, formerly neurotoxic esterase) assays were carried out on an additional two negative control, two positive control, and four test compound birds, which were dosed according to a similar procedure to that used in the main study. The NTE assays were carried out at 24 and 48 h after dosing, and were carried out 'blind' according to the method of Johnson (1977). Inhibition of NTE is thought to be the initial biochemical lesion which eventually leads to delayed neurotoxicity.

Results

General bird health was good throughout the study. Two mortalities occurred in group 1, one on day 2 and one on day 8. One bird in group 3 (spent catalyst) was found dead on day 7. These deaths were unrelated to vehicle or test compound administration.

No signs of toxicity (including neurotoxicity) were observed in any test or negative control birds following dosing. Four out of five birds dosed with TOCP developed signs of ataxia following dosing, the first signs occurring at day 12.

Table 1. Results of NTE assays

Bird no.	Treatment	Brain	Spinal cord
		nmol/min/g	
AT 24 h			
83	Corn oil	3160	606
81	TOCP	203	78
82	Catalyst	2890	619
84	Catalyst	2920	649
AT 48 h			
85	Corn oil	2990	511
87	TOCP	304	100
86	Catalyst	2270	462
88	Catalyst	2680	549

Body weight changes were considered to be within normal limits in groups 1 and 3. In group 2 a marked body-weight loss occurred between days 14 and 21. Food consumption corresponded with the body-weight changes.

No macroscopic abnormalities which could be related to treatment were detected at post mortem.

Detailed histopathological evaluation revealed no evidence of any treatment-related changes in the nerve tissue of negative control or test group birds. However, significant axonal degeneration occurred in birds dosed with TOCP.

The results of the NTE assay are shown in Table 1. NTE inhibition was profound in both the brain and spinal cord of birds dosed with TOCP. Birds nos. 82, 83 and 84 were indistinguishable in NTE content of brain and spinal cord 24 h after the second dose. At 48 h after the second dose, bird no. 86 had lower activities than birds nos. 85 and 88 for both brain and spinal cord. The depression of NTE activity compared to the negative control was 24% in the brain and 10% in the spinal cord. These values are at the edge of biological variation and were seen in only one bird dosed with test compound.

Conclusions

Unter the conditions of this test, oral administration of a single dose of spent phosphoric acid catalyst at 5000 mg/kg body wt., followed by a repeat dose after 21 days, did not produce any clinical signs of neurotoxicity. This absence of neurotoxicity was confirmed by histopathological investigations and NTE assays.

The positive control material, TOCP, produced clinical and histopathological effects, and profoundly inhibited NTE activity. A correlation between clinical, histopathological and biochemical findings was thus demonstrated. NTE assays provided useful additional information. More widespread use of this sensitive biochemical marker could eventually lead to a reduced requirement for animals in neurotoxicity testing, the rapid provision of results, and a better understanding of the mechanisms of neurotoxic effects.

References

Cavanagh JB, Davies DR, Holland P, Lancaster M (1961) Comparison of the functional effects of dyflos, tri-*o*-cresyl phosphate and tri-*p*-ethylphenyl phosphate in chickens. Br J Pharmacol 17:21–27

Johnson MK (1977) Improved assay of neurotoxic esterase for screening organophosphates for delayed neurotoxicity potential. Arch Toxicol 37:113–115

Marsland TA, Glees P, Erikson LB (1954) Modification of Glees Silver impregnation for paraffin sections. J Neuropathol Exp Neurol 14:587–591

Page KM (1970) Histological methods for peripheral nerves. J Med Lab Tech 27:1–17

Mechanisms and Models in Toxicology
Arch. Toxicol., Suppl. 11, 240–242 (1987)
© by Springer-Verlag 1987

The Effect of Solvents on the Toxicity of DDT to Fish Cells

C. Parkinson and C. Agius

Department of Analytical and Biological Chemistry, Kingston Polytechnic,
Penrhyn Road, Kingston-upon-Thames, Surrey, KT1 2EE, UK

Introduction

Water-insoluble compounds such as 1,1,1-trichloro-2,2-*bis*-(*p*-chlorophenyl) ethane (DDT) usually require the use of a suitable solvent for introduction into in vitro testing systems, and in this experiment the effect of acetone and dimethyl sulfoxide (DMSO) on the toxicity of DDT was investigated. The in vitro system used was a recently established cell line from tilapia (*Oreochromis spilurus*) brain called TSB cells. LC_{50} values for DDT to tilapia in vivo are 0.50, 0.23 and 0.06 mg/l at 24, 48 and 96 h respectively (unpublished data).

Methods

TSB cells, pass number 22, were trypsinized to obtain a single cell suspension in Leibovitz medium supplemented with 10% v/v fetal calf serum, antibiotics and 20 mM N-2-hydroxyethylpiperazine-N'2-ethane-sulfonic acid (HEPES) (Gibco Ltd.). The cells were seeded into 24-well plates at a density of 3.5×10^5 cells per well, maintained at 30 ± 1 °C and allowed to grow untreated for 48 h. Acetone (BP Chemicals Ltd., minimum 99.5% by mass) or DMSO (BDH Chemicals Ltd., minimum 98% by mass) was used to dissolve DDT and was added to the media at 0.3%, 1% or 3% v/v. DDT (BDH Chemicals Ltd., minimum 98% by mass) was applied at a concentration of 0, 2, 4 or 8 µg/ml in the media containing the three levels of each solvent. All treatments were performed in triplicate. The effects on the cells were monitored over a 96-h period by microscopy and by protein determination as an indication of cell number. The protein content of each well was determined by digesting the washed monolayer with 0.1 ml of 1 N NaOH and assaying by the method of Ohnishi and Barr (1978).

Results

Following a 96-h exposure to solvent alone, cell necrosis occurred in cultures exposed to 3% acetone, 3% DMSO and 1% DMSO. After 96 h, all cultures exposed to DDT in DMSO and 8 µg DDT/ml in acetone showed cell necrosis; the degree of necrosis increased with increasing DDT and solvent concentration. However, 2 or 4 µg DDT/ml with acetone as the solvent did not cause any signs of cell necrosis. Protein determinations (Fig. 1) gave graphically estimated LC_{50} values for DDT as shown in Table 1.

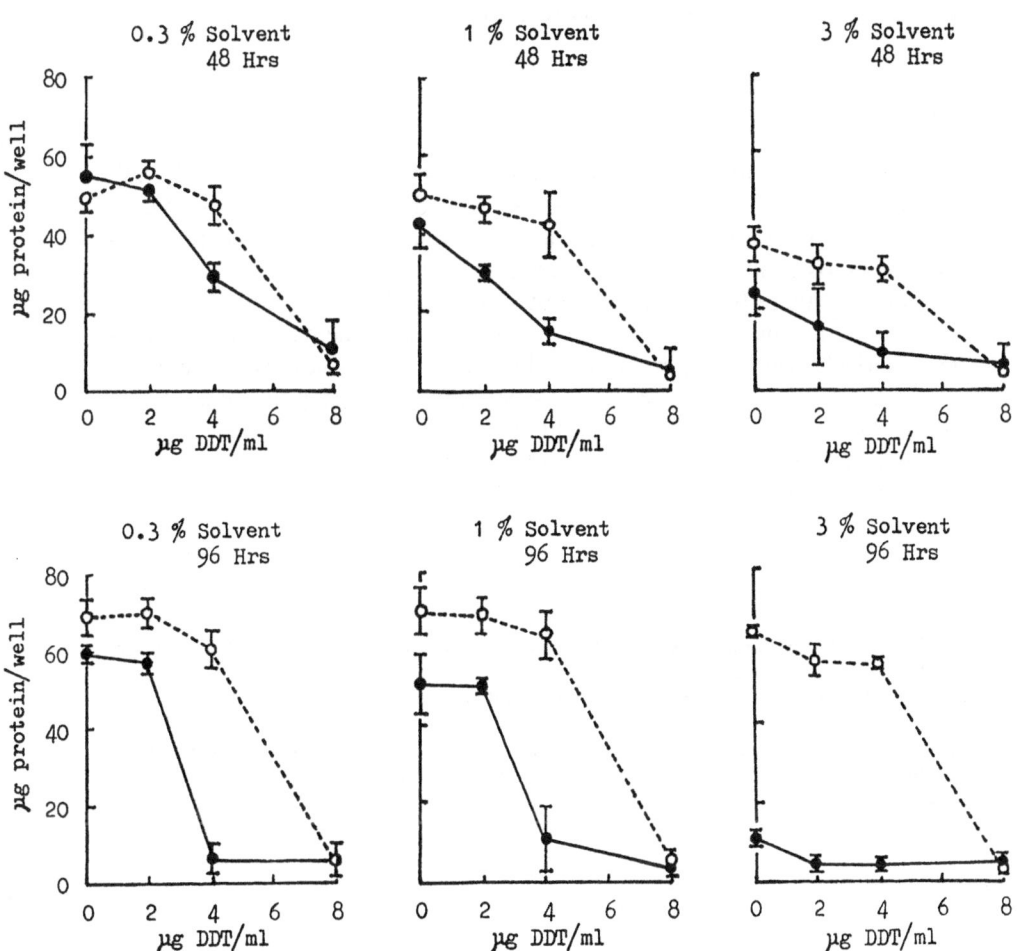

Fig. 1. Well protein content following 48- or 96-h exposure to DDT dissolved in acetone or DMSO. --o--, Acetone; —•— DMSO

Table 1. LC_{50} values for DDT estimated from protein determinations

	48-h LC_{50} (μg/ml)	96-h LC_{50} (μg/ml)
Acetone 0.3%	6.2	5.9
1%	5.7	5.9
3%	5.7	5.7
DMSO 0.3%	4.7	3.1
1%	3.2	3.2
3%[a]	3.4	1.7

[a] Cultures showed severe cell necrosis due to solvent alone.

Discussion

At the 0.3% level of either solvent there was a no-effect level of 2 μg DDT/ml. 4 μg/ml with DMSO as the solvent caused near total destruction of the monolayer after 96 h, while at 4 μg/ml with acetone as the solvent there were no signs of toxicity and no statistically significant reduction in well protein content. Three possible reasons for these findings are suggested: (a) DMSO, being more persistent in the medium, may increase DDT solubility, with a subsequent increase in access to the cells; (b) DMSO, being more toxic than acetone, may have sublethal toxic effects on the cells that increase their susceptibility to DDT poisoning; (c) the membrane binding of DMSO and the alteration in membrane dynamics may result in easier access of DDT to the cell and promote DDT toxicity (Pribor 1975; Tapiero et al. 1983).

References

Ohnishi ST, Barr J (1978) A simplified method of quantitating protein using the biuret and phenol reagents. Anal Biochem 86:193–200
Pribor DB (1975) Biological interactions between cell membranes and glycerol or DMSO. Cryobiology 12:309–320
Tapiero H, Zwingelstein G, Fourcade A, Portoukalian J (1983) The effect of dimethyl sulfoxide on the membrane dynamics and the phospholipid composition of two different cell lines. Ann NY Acad Sci 411:383–388

Mechanisms and Models in Toxicology
Arch. Toxicol., Suppl. 11, 243–246 (1987)

The Effect of the Cholinergic Neurotoxin ECMA on Neural Function in Brain Reaggregate Cultures

A. M. Pillar [1], A. K. Prince [1], and C. K. Atterwill [2]

[1] Department of Pharmacology, King's College, Strand, London, WC2R 2LS, UK
[2] Department of is Specialised Toxicology, Smith Kline and French Research Ltd., The Frythe, Welwyn, Herts., AL6 9AR, UK

Introduction

Alzheimer's disease appears to be associated with the loss of the cholinergic innervation to cortical and limbic areas of the brain. In attempting to produce an in vitro model for studying Alzheimer's disease, therefore, one feature must be the presence of a deficit in cholinergic neuronal function.

Ethylcholine mustard aziridinium ion (ECMA) has been postulated to be a relatively specific cholinergic neurotoxin on the basis of in vivo experiments where reductions in choline transport and choline acetyltransferase (ChAT) activity in rat brain are seen (Mantione et al. 1983). These changes are accompanied by alterations in cognitive function, including the impairment of performance on the passive avoidance test (Walsh et al. 1984). ECMA has also been shown to affect cholinergic function in vitro, causing the inhibition of choline transport and ChAT activity in rat brain synaptosomes (Pedder and Prince 1985). The work reported on here, therefore, was undertaken to investigate the effect of ECMA in vitro, using fetal rat brain reaggregate cultures. These are organotypic cultures which acquire and retain the characteristics of the differentiated brain while in culture.

Materials and Methods

Fetal rat brain reaggregate cultures were grown as previously described (Atterwill et al. 1984a), in S+ culture medium. This consists of Dulbecco's modified Eagle's medium (Gibco Bio-cult, Europe) plus 10% fetal calf serum (Gibco) plus extra glutamine. ECMA was freshly prepared before use from the precursor acetylethylcholine mustard (Research Biochemicals Inc.) by cyclisation to form the aziridinium moiety and hydrolysis to remove the acetyl grouping. The conversion to the aziridinium was monitored by thiosulphate titration.

ECMA was added to the cultures on either the 9th or the 12th day in vitro (9 or 12 DIV), in concentrations ranging from 12.5–100 μM. In some experiments, hemicholinium-3 (HC-3; Sigma; final concentration 40 μM, sufficient to inhibit both high- and low-affinity choline transport) was added to the cultures 30 min before ECMA.

ChAT activity, muscarinic receptor binding and Na^+, K^+-ATPase activity were determined as previously described (Atterwill et al. 1984a, b). All other chemicals used were of the highest purity available and obtained from either Sigma Chemical, BDH or Amersham International.

Results

The exposure of the reaggregate cultures to 12.5, 25 and 50 μM ECMA from 9–14 DIV resulted in a significant reduction in ChAT activity in all cases. The inhibition seen was in the range 55%–80% and there was no apparent dose-response relationship (Fig. 1 a). The effect of ECMA (25, 50 and 100 μM) added to the cultures at 12 DIV was examined over a period of 48 h after addition. In these circumstances, the inhibition of ChAT activity was seen to be rapid in onset, being initiated within 2 h, except in the case of 25 μM ECMA, when inhibition was slower but reached the same value as 50 and 100 μM after 48 h (Fig. 1 b). The extent of the inhibition was essentially constant over the 48 h, averaging 38%.

It appears, therefore, that there may be a difference in the results of short- (2–48 h) and long-term (2–120 h) exposure to ECMA. Treatment of the cultures with 50 μM ECMA at 9 DIV also resulted in the onset of the inhibition of ChAT activity within 2 h. However, this effect was prevented by pretreatment with HC-3. The long-term result of exposure to ECMA, however, was not preventable by HC-3 pretreatment.

The effect of ECMA exposure (12.5–50 μM) between 9 and 14 DIV on muscarinic cholinergic receptors, as measured by [³H]-quinuclidinyl benzilate binding, was also examined. Significant inhibition of muscarinic receptor binding was seen only with 50 and 25 μM ECMA, with some form of dose-response relationship present (results not presented).

This was also seen when the activity of the more general cell (plasma-membrane) marker Na^+, K^+-ATPase was examined in the same batch of cultures. In the case of both muscarinic receptors and ATPase the extent of inhibition was less marked at 12.5 than at 25–100 μM ECMA.

Discussion

ECMA appears to have a two-stage effect on the cholinergic neurons in these cultures, as determined by its effects on ChAT activity. The initial response, which is established within 2 h and is preventable by pretreatment with HC-3, would appear to be mediated via the choline transport system and may represent a functional 'shut-down' in response to ChAT inhibition. The loss of ChAT activity over the longer time interval, which is not preventable by HC-3, may reflect a more progressive cellular toxicity response.

The difference between the effect of ECMA at 12.5 μM on ChAT activity and its effects on muscarinic receptor binding and Na^+, K^+-ATPase activity may

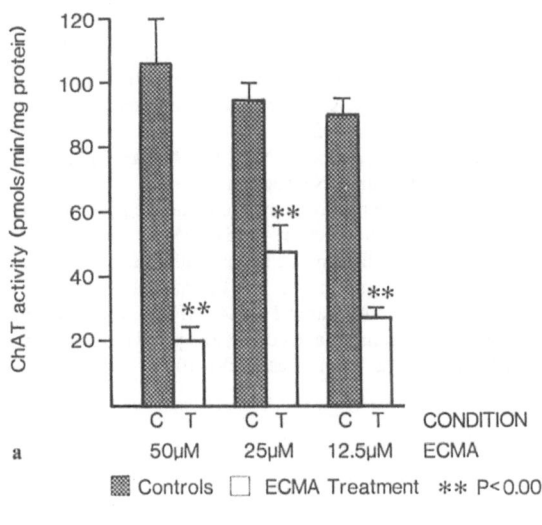

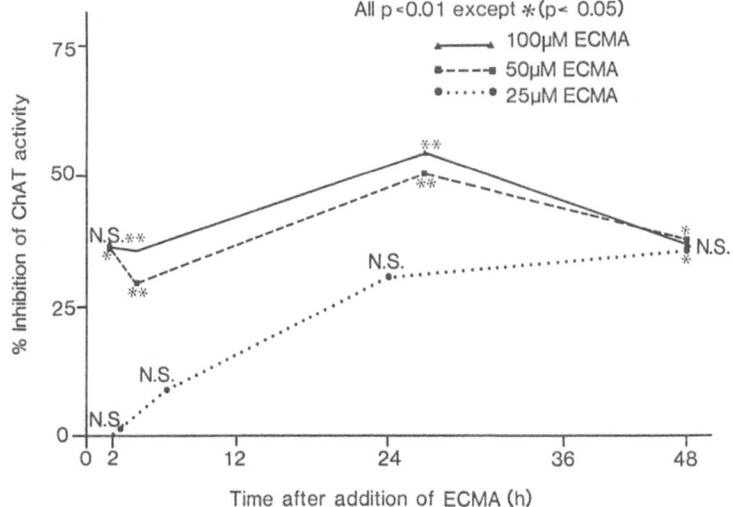

Fig. 1. a ChAT activity in the reaggregate cultures at 14 DIV following treatment with different concentrations of ECMA from 9–14 DIV. Results represent the mean of 6–8 determinations. Vertical lines indicate SEM. **b** The inhibition of ChAT activity over a 48-h period following exposure to different concentrations of ECMA at 12 DIV. The results are expressed as % inhibition of ChAT activity when compared to matched controls. Each point represents a minimum of four determinations. (Statistics were performed using Student's *t*-test.)

indicate a degree of neural specificity in this agent, in that a dose of ECMA which maximally inhibited ChAT activity did not affect muscarinic receptor binding and only slightly reduced Na^+, K^+-ATPase activity.

Low doses of ECMA, therefore, may be suitable for producing a cholinergic neuronal 'lesion' in whole-brain reaggregate cultures. The exact degree of specific of this lesion is currently under further investigation.

References

Atterwill CK, Kingsbury A, Nicholls J, Prince AK (1984a) Development of markers for cholinergic neurones in reaggregate cultures of foetal rat whole brain in serum-containing and serum-free media: effects of triiodothyronine (T_3). Br J Pharmacol 83:89–102

Atterwill CK, Cunningham VJ, Balazs R (1984b) Characterisation of Na^+, K^+-ATPase in cultured and separated neuronal and glial cells from rat cerebellum. J Neurochem 43:8–18

Mantione CR, Zigmond MJ, Fisher A, Hanin I (1983) Selective presynaptic cholinergic neurotoxicity following intrahippocampal AF64A injection in rats. J Neurochem 41:251–255

Pedder EK, Prince AK (1985) Ethylcholine mustard aziridinium (ECMA): inhibition of rat brain synaptosome choline uptake and choline acetyltransferase (ChAT). Br J Pharmacol 84:114P

Walsh TJ, Tilson HA, DeHaven DL, Mailman RB, Fisher A, Hanin I (1984) AF64A, a cholinergic neurotoxin, selectively depletes acetylcholine in hippocampus and cortex, and produces long-term passive avoidance and radial-arm maze deficits in the rat. Brain Res 321:91–102

Mechanisms and Models in Toxicology
Arch. Toxicol., Suppl. 11, 247–249 (1987)

Interactions of Thyroid Hormone and Tricyclic Antidepressants on Rat Brain β-Adrenoceptor Function

L. C. Catto, D. M. Lee, and C. K. Atterwill

Department of Toxicology, Smith Kline & French Research Ltd., The Frythe, Welwyn, Herts., AL6 9AR, UK

Introduction

L-triiodothyronine (T_3) and desipramine (DMI) are known separately to affect β-adrenoceptor numbers in rat brain (Atterwill et al. 1984; Crews et al. 1981), and it is thought that the decrease in number produced by DMI correlates with its therapeutic actions (Racagni and Brunello 1984). Since a single administration of T_3 can be useful as an adjunct to tricyclic antidepressant (TCA) therapy (Prange et al. 1984), the following study examined the interaction between T_3 and DMI in inducing changes in rat brain β-adrenoceptors, in the hope of identifying a possible mechanism to explain the clinical observations.

Materials and Methods

Male Sprague-Dawley rats weighing 60–70 g (Charles River UK Ltd.) were injected twice daily, at 08.30 and 16.30 h, with DMI (5 mg/kg, i.p.) plus either T_3 (100 µg/kg, s.c.) on day 1 only or vehicle. Animals were killed by thoracic blow followed by decapitation 18 h after the final dose of DMI was administered on either day 1, 3 or 14. The cerebral cortex and corpus striatum were dissected, frozen in liquid nitrogen, then stored at $-40\,°C$. On thawing, the tissue was homogenised in 25 times its own volume of 50 mM tris-HCl (pH 7.8 at $0°-5\,°C$) using a motor-driven homogeniser with a polytetrafluoroethylene pestle end and glass body. The subsequent membrane fractionation procedure and binding estimations using [³H]dihydroalprenolol ([³H]DHA) were performed according to Atterwill et al. (1984), with the exception that all membrane fractions were stored at $-40\,°C$ prior to binding estimations. The scintillation cocktail used was Instagel (Packard Ltd.) acidified to 0.1% v/v with concentrated HCl. In the case of cerebral cortex a detailed kinetic analysis was performed at six different [³H]DHA concentrations (0.5–4 nM). Data were analysed by Scatchard analysis to obtain values for the maximal number of binding sites (B_{max}) and the equilibrium dissociation constant (K_D). Binding in the corpus striatum was determined at one 'saturating' ligand concentration (2 nM) only.

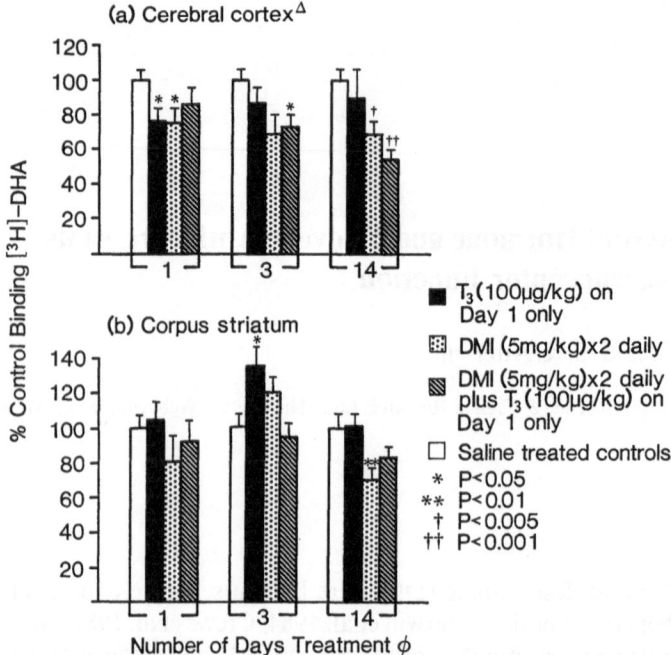

Fig. 1. Effect of T_3 and DMI on [³H]DHA binding in rat brain. (a) Binding is expressed as % control B_{max} value obtained from Scatchard analysis. ᐃData taken from previously published work (Atterwill et al. 1986) (b) Binding is expressed as % control binding measured at ligand concentration $= 2$ nM. *Note:* $\theta =$ except T_3 alone, when abscissa represents days after receiving a single injection of T_3

DMI HCl (as Pertofran) was kindly donated by Ciba-Geigy Pharmaceuticals, Horsham, W. Sussex. L-3,3′,5-triiodothyronine (sodium salt) and –isoprenaline (bitartrate salt) were obtained from Sigma Chemical Co. [³H]DHA 77–82 Ci/ mmol was obtained from Amersham International plc.

Results

DMI caused a rapid down-regulation of β-adrenoceptors in the cerebral cortex after only 1 day's treatment, but in the corpus striatum not until 14 days. Co-administration of a single injection of T_3 with DMI failed to accelerate or enhance, but tended to attenuate, the initial DMI-induced down-regulation observed in both brain regions. T_3 given alone resulted in a rapid down-regulation in the cerebral cortex by day 1 but an increase in β-adrenoceptor number in the corpus striatum by day 3. These responses were transient and returned to control levels by 14 days (Fig. 1).

Discussion

In both cerebral cortex and corpus striatum a single injection of T_3 failed to accelerate the onset of the DMI-induced down-regulation in β-adrenoceptors, but tended to reduce (by 45%) the magnitude of the initial down-regulation observed. In the cortex this was expected since the DMI-induced response was near-maximal and more rapid than others have previously reported (Crews et al. 1981). In contrast, a single injection of T$_3$ caused a 25% down-regulation in cortical β-adrenoceptor number. This observation may be of importance to an understanding of the usefulness of T$_3$ in the treatment of depression, although the precise level of this interaction is still unknown. Such changes were not seen by Atterwill et al. (1984) following 14 days treatment with the same dose of T$_3$, indicating possible adaptation. In the corpus striatum the increase in β-adrenoceptor number observed in the present study is consistent with the findings of Atterwill et al. (1984) where chronic T$_3$ treatment elevated striatal [^{3}H]DHA binding and may help to explain why T$_3$ failed to accelerate the onset of the DMI-induced down-regulation.

It is probable, therefore, that the interaction of T$_3$ with TCAs to enhance their clinical efficacy is not primarily related to effects on β-adrenoceptors but more likely to be an interaction at the α-adrenoceptor level. Atterwill et al. (1986) showed that a single injection of T$_3$ (100 µg/kg, s.c.) accelerated DMI-induced inhibition of pre-synaptic α-adrenoceptor function.

Other neurotransmitter systems are also affected by thyroid status (Atterwill 1981) and together with the results of the present study highlight the toxicological significance of interactions between hormones and centrally acting drugs.

References

Atterwill CK (1981) Effect of acute and chronic tri-iodothyronine (T$_3$) administration to rats on central 5-HT and dopamine-mediated behavioural responses and related brain biochemistry. Neuropharmacology 20:131–144

Atterwill CK, Bunn SJ, Atkinson DJ, Smith SL, Heal DJ (1984) Effects of thyroid status on presynaptic α_2-adrenoceptor function and β-adrenoceptor binding in the rat brain. J Neural Transm 59:43–55

Atterwill CK, Bloomfield J, Bristow LJ, Catto LC, Elliot JM, Heal DJ (1986) The influence of thyroid hormone (T$_3$) on the effects of desipramine on α_2- and β-adrenoceptor function in rat brain. Br J Pharmacol 87:221

Crews FT, Paul SM, Goodwin FK (1981) Acceleration of β-receptor desensitisation in combined administration of antidepressants and phenoxybenzamine. Nature 290:787–789

Prange AJ, Loosen PT, Wilson IC, Lipton MA (1984) The therapeutic uses of hormones of the thyroid axis in depression. In: Post RM, Ballenger JC (eds) Neurobiology of mood disorders. Williams and Wilkins, Baltimore, p 311

Racagni G, Brunello N (1984) Transynaptic mechanisms in the action of antidepressant drugs. Trends in Pharmalogical Sciences 5:527–530

Mechanisms and Models in Toxicology
Arch. Toxicol., Suppl. 11, 250–252 (1987)
© by Springer-Verlag 1987

Thyroid Toxicity and Iodothyronine Deiodination

C. A. Jones, C. G. Brown, and C. K. Atterwill

Department of Toxicology, Smith Kline and French Research Ltd, The Frythe, Welwyn, Herts., AL6 9AR, UK

Introduction

Long-term administration to rats of high doses (up to 1000 mg kg^{-1} daily, p.o.) of SKF 93479 (2-(2-(5-(dimethylaminomethyl)furan-2-ylmethylthio)-ethyl-amino)-5-(6-methylpyrid-3-ylmethyl)-pyrimidin-4-one trihydrochloride), a novel histamine H$_2$ receptor antagonist, resulted in marked changes in thyroid gland morphology. Even after administration of the highest dose for only 3 days, colloid depletion, follicular cell hyperplasia and hypertrophy were seen. These changes indicate increased activity of the thyroid gland, which was confirmed by an increased uptake of ^{125}I (Brown et al. 1987). Further studies showed that this was not due to a direct effect on the thyroid gland, but to a rapidly enhanced plasma clearance of thyroxine (T$_4$) (Brown et al. 1987).

As deiodination is the major route of clearance of thyroid hormones (see Cavalieri and Pitt-Rivers 1981), studies were performed to examine the hypothesis that the increase in T$_4$ clearance seen after administration of SKF 93479 to rats could be due to an increase in peripheral 5′-deiodinase activity. Changes in the activity of this enzyme were investigated in liver and kidney from rats treated with SKF 93479. These results were compared to activity in liver after treatment with triio-dothyronine (T$_3$) or propylthiouracil (PTU), agents known to modulate deiodinase activity (Kaplan and Utiger 1978; Cavalieri and Pitt-Rivers 1981).

Method

In the positive control studies six male SKF Wistar rats were treated with T$_3$ 100 µg kg^{-1} s.c., PTU 50 mg p.o. (four rats), or control solutions daily for 14 days. SKF Wistar rats of both sexes received SKF 93479 1000 mg kg^{-1} or control solution p.o. daily for 6 h, 1, 4, 7 or 14 days.

Deiodinase activity was estimated by a method based on that of Hufner et al. (1977). Formation of T$_3$ was measured after addition of T$_4$ to 10% homogenates of tissue in the presence of 27 mmol l^{-1} phosphate buffer, 23 mmol l^{-1} Tris,

114 mmol l^{-1} sucrose and 3 mmol l^{-1} dithiothreitol at pH 7.5 and 37 °C. After 10 min, reactions were terminated by addition of 2 volumes ice-cold ethanol. After removal of the protein precipitate and solvents, T$_3$ was measured in the residue using Amerlex T$_3$ RIA kits (Amersham International). Results were calculated as the amount of T$_3$ formed in 10 min per unit of protein in the reaction mixture. Effects of treatments are expressed as percentage of the activity in homogenates from control animals.

Results

In the positive control study PTU, a known inhibitor of peripheral 5'-deiodinase, almost completely abolished activity of this enzyme in male liver homogenates, whereas T$_3$, which stimulates activity of this enzyme, produced an increase to 160±12% of control values.

Treatment with SKF 93479 did not significantly increase 5'-deiodinase in liver or kidney homogenates at any of the time points studied. However, decreases in activity were seen in the male livers at 7 days (53% of control activity), the female livers at 1 day (59%) and 7 days (57%) and in the female kidneys at 6 h (70%) and 1 day (64%) (see Table 1).

Discussion

It is concluded that the increased clearance of T$_4$ seen after administration of SKF 93479 to rats is not due to an increase in 5'-deiodinase activity in liver or kidney. In contrast, a decrease in activity of this enzyme would tend to decrease clearance of the thyroid hormones. As conjugation reactions also play an important role in the metabolism of T$_4$, the effect of SKF 93479 treatment on the activity of the enzyme uridine diphosphate glucuronyl transferase is now being investigated.

Table 1. Effect of pretreatment with SKF 93479 on deiodinase activity in liver and kidney homogenates. Results are expressed as a percentage of control values, mean ±SEM of six animals

Duration of treatment	Liver		Kidney	
	Males	Females	Males	Females
6 h	102±11	206±64	91± 8	70± 7[a]
1 d	102±11	59±10[b]	82± 3	64± 7[b]
4 d	104±15	86± 6	110± 5	106± 9
7 d	53± 4[a]	57± 8[b]	83± 9	126±10
14 d	68± 9	100±19	138±14	81±11

Significant differences from controls, Student's t test.
[a] $p > 0.05$, [b] $p < 0.01$.

References

Brown CG, Harland RF, Atterwill CK (1987) Increased thyroxine clearance in rats treated with high
    doses of a histamine H_2-antagonist SK & F 93479. Arch Tox [Suppl] 11:253–256
Cavalieri RR, Pitt-Rivers R (1981) The effects of drugs on the distribution and metabolism of thyroid
    hormones. Pharmacol Rev 33:55–80
Hufner M, Grussendorf M, Ntokalou M (1977) Properties of the thyroxine (T_4) monodeiodinating sys-
    tem in rat liver homogenate. Clin Chim Acta 58:251–259
Kaplan MM, Utiger RD (1978) Iodothyronine metabolism in liver and kidney homogenates from hy-
    perthyroid and hypothyroid rats. Endocrinology 103:156–161

Mechanisms and Models in Toxicology
Arch. Toxicol., Suppl. 11, 253–256 (1987)

Increased Thyroxine Clearance in Rats Treated with High Doses of a Histamine H_2-Antagonist, SKF 93479

C. G. Brown, R. F. Harland, and C. K. Atterwill

Department of Toxicology, Smith Kline and French Research Ltd., The Frythe, Welwyn, Herts, AL6 9AR, UK

Introduction

Treatment of rats with high doses (200–1000 mg/kg) of a histamine H_2-antagonist, SKF 93479 (2-(2-(5-(dimethylaminomethyl)furan-2-ylmethylthio)- ethyl-amino)-5-(6-methylpyrid-3-ylmethyl)pyrimidin-4-one trihydrochloride), is associated with histological changes in the thyroid glands. These changes were observed as early as 3 days after the start of treatment, and include follicular cell hypertrophy and colloid depletion, which are indicative of increased thyroid activity. Similar thyroid histological changes have previously been observed in rats following treatment with classical antithyroid compounds such as methimazole (Owen et al. 1973). Several investigations were carried out in order to determine the mechanism of the effect of SKF 93479 on thyroid activity. In particular, the possibility of a direct or indirect effect of the compound (the latter via alterations in the pituitary feedback mechanism) was examined by studying plasma thyroxine (T_4) and thyroid stimulating hormone (TSH) concentrations, thyroidal iodide-[125] uptake and T_4 clearance in rats treated with SKF 93479.

Methods

Male SKF Wistar rats (8–10 weeks of age) were used throughout these studies.

Thyroid ^{125}I-Uptake

Groups of five rats were dosed orally with SKF 93479 (1000 mg/kg) or control solution for 1 and 10 days. Twenty-four hours after the final dose, each rat was given an intraperitoneal injection of 0.1 ml containing 1 μCi Na[125]I (Amersham). Three hours later, rats were killed and the thyroid glands removed on the trachea, rinsed in saline and γ-emission (cpm) monitored. [125]I uptake is expressed as a percentage of the γ-emission (cpm) administered.

Thyroid ^{125}I uptake was also studied in groups of hypophysectomised (Charles River Ltd.) rats pretreated with T_4 (250 µg/kg, s.c., 4 days) and given either control solution or 1000 mg/kg SKF 93479 for 10 days.

T_4 and TSH Measurements

Groups of five rats were dosed orally with SKF 93479 (1000 mg/kg) or control solution for 14 days. On days 1, 3, 7 and 14, blood samples were taken from a lateral tail vein 6 h after dosing and plasma or serum prepared and stored at $-20\,°C$ until assayed. Total T_4 was measured using Amerlex RIA kits (Amersham). TSH was measured by RIA using specific reagents supplied by the Pituitary Hormones and Antisera Center, University of California.

$[^{125}I]T_4$ Clearance Measurements

Groups of six rats which had been dosed with either one oral dose of 1000 mg/kg SKF 93479 or control solution were given approximately 10 µCi/kg $[^{125}I]T_4$ (specific activity > 1200 µCi/µg, Amersham) intravenously into a lateral tail vein 4 h later. Rats also received 1 mg NaI (2 ml/kg in saline, i.p.) twice daily in order to prevent thyroidal accumulation of free ^{125}I. Blood samples (50 µl) were collected from a cut tail vein at specified intervals for up to 30 h later. Protein-bound radioactivity $[^{125}I]T_4$) was precipitated with 10% trichloroacetic acid solution and the γ-emission of the precipitate measured. $[^{125}I]T_4$ disappearance curves were plotted and clearance values estimated using the method described by Chiou (1979).

Results

Thyroid ^{125}I Uptake

After treatment with SKF 93479 for 1 and 10 days, ^{125}I uptake into the thyroid glands was significantly increased (Table 1). This effect of SKF 93479 was not seen following treatment for 10 days of rats which had been either hypophysectomised or pretreated with T_4, although the absolute ^{125}I uptake had decreased markedly (results not shown).

Table 1. Effect of treatment with SKF 93479 on thyroid iodide-125 uptake (expressed as a percentage of iodide-125 administered). Results are mean $\pm$SEM of five animals

Days of treatment[a]	Control	SKF 93479, 1000 mg/kg
1	6.3 ± 0.4	9.3 ± 0.6[b]
10	7.0 ± 0.4	13.1 ± 0.9[c]

[a] Measurement made 24 h following dosing.
Results were compared with control values using Student's t test.
[b] $p < 0.05$, [c] $p < 0.001$.

Table 2. Effect of treatment with SKF 93479 on plasma thyroxine (T_4) concentrations and serum thyroid stimulating hormone (TSH). Results are mean $\pm$ SEM of five animals

Days of treatment[a]	T_4		TSH	
	Control	SKF 93479, 1000 mg/kg	Control	SKF 93479, 1000 mg/kg
1	9.44 ± 0.65	7.88 ± 0.47[b]	1.12 ± 0.09	1.60 ± 0.25
3	8.10 ± 0.29	6.10 ± 0.19[b]	1.23 ± 0.13	2.51 ± 0.25[c]
7	6.96 ± 0.23	5.54 ± 0.41[c]	1.02 ± 0.08	2.75 ± 0.42[c]
14	9.05 ± 0.46	6.08 ± 0.41[c]	0.98 ± 0.11	1.37 ± 0.19

[a] Samples taken 6 h after dosing.
Results were compared with control values using Student's t test.
[b] $p < 0.05$, [c] $p < 0.01$.

T_4 and TSH Measurements

Total T_4 concentrations were significantly reduced on days 1, 3, 7 and 14, 6 h following dosing with SKF 93479 (Table 2). This was generally paralleled by increased TSH concentrations, which were significantly different from control on days 3 and 7 of treatment with SKF 93479 (see Table 2).

$[^{125}I]T_4$ Clearance Measurements

Treatment with one oral dose of 1000 mg/kg SKF 93479 was associated with an approximate doubling in T_4 clearance (control: 1.67 ± 0.14 ml/h; 1000 mg/kg SKF 93479: 2.96 ± 0.41 ml/h).

Discussion

Following treatment with SKF 93479, the thyroid histopathological changes suggested increased thyroid activity. This was confirmed in this study by observing increased ^{125}I uptake into the thyroid glands after treatment with SKF 93479. Since the effect of SKF 93479 on iodide uptake was not seen in rats which had been either hypophysectomised or pretreated with T_4, this suggested that the effect was TSH-dependent and was not a result of a direct thyroid stimulation.

Increased serum TSH concentrations were observed after 3 and 7 days of treatment with SKF 93479 as well as decreased plasma T_4 concentrations at 1, 3, 7 and 14 days of treatment. These results indicate that the increased TSH concentrations may be secondary to the reduction in T_4 concentrations.

Although the thyroid histopathological and biochemical changes appear similar to those following administration of methimazole, there are important differences. First, methimazole reduces iodide uptake (Tsukui et al. 1978), an effect which arises due to a primary inhibitory effect on iodide organification in the thyroid gland, whereas SKF 93479 increased iodide uptake. Secondly, the time course of the reduction in plasma T_4 suggests an effect of SKF 93479 on T_4 metabolism rather than on thyroidal T_4 synthesis, since the first decrease in T_4 concentrations occurred as early as 6 h after dosing.

[^{125}I]T_4 clearance studies confirmed that SKF 93479 reduces plasma T_4 concentrations by increasing T_4 clearance. Other studies in our laboratory have confirmed the lack of a direct effect of SKF 93479 on iodide metabolism in vivo (Atterwill et al., this volume) and in thyroid cells maintained in vitro (Brown et al. 1986).

References

Brown CG, Fowler K, Nicholls PJ, Atterwill CK (1986) Assessment of thyrotoxicity using *in vitro* cell culture systems. Food Chem Toxicol 24:557–562
Chiou WL (1979) Critical evaluation of the potential error in pharmacokinetic studies of using the linear trapezoidal rule method for the calculation of the area under the plasma level-time curve. J Pharmacokin Biopharm 6:539–546
Owen NV, Worth HM, Kiplinger GF (1973) The effects of long-term ingestion of methimazole on the thyroids of rats. Food Cosmet Toxicol 11:649–653
Tsukui T, Aizawa T, Yamada T, Kawabe T (1978) Studies on the mechanisms of goitrogenic action of diphenylhydantoin. Endocrinology 102:1662–1669

Mechanisms and Models in Toxicology
Arch. Toxicol., Suppl. 11, 257–260 (1987)
© by Springer-Verlag 1987

Enzymic Deglycosylation of Ricin Lowers its Uptake by Rat Liver Non-Parenchymal Cells

D. N. Skilleter[1] and B. M. J. Foxwell[2]

[1] MRC Toxicology Unit, Woodmansterne Road, Carshalton, Surrey, SM5 4EF, UK
[2] Cellular Pharmacology Laboratory, ICRF, London, WC2A 3PX, UK

Introduction

The toxic glycoprotein ricin from castor beans (*Ricinus communis*) is a potent inhibitor of protein synthesis in eukaryote cells (Olsnes et al. 1974). This property has rendered it of considerable interest recently as a candidate antineoplastic agent in cancer chemotherapy, based on the rationale that conjugation of ricin with various 'address' molecules, usually antibodies, should direct the toxin to specific tumour cells (Olsnes 1981; Vitetta and Uhr 1985). A major problem with this approach has been that in vivo ricin is rapidly removed from the blood, mainly to the liver (Fodstad et al. 1976), as a result of recognition by hepatic non-parenchymal cells of mannose-containing oligosaccharide side chains present in the toxin (Skilleter et al. 1981, 1985).

Each molecule of ricin comprises two disulphide bond linked glycoprotein subunits; the A chain, which is the protein synthesis inhibitor component, and the B chain, generally regarded as necessary for both binding to galactosyl sites on cells and transfer of the A chain to its site of action in the cytosol (Olsnes and Pihl 1982). The A chain carbohydrate is heterogeneous, comprising a single complex structure of composition (*N*-acetyl-D-glucosamine)$_2$-(D-xylose)-(L-fucose)- (D-mannose)$_{3-4}$ [(GlcNAc)$_2$-(Xyl)-(Fuc)-(Man)$_{3-4}$] in addition to a mannose-rich oligosaccharide, whilst the B chain contains two high mannose oligosaccharides of composition (GlcNAc)$_2$-(Man)$_{4-6}$ (Foxwell et al. 1985). Not all of the oligosaccharides may be exposed in intact ricin, but their alteration or removal might avoid recognition of the toxin by the reticuloendothelial system, thus improving the therapeutic value of ricin immunotoxins. An earlier report described how after separation of the ricin A and B chains their carbohydrate can be removed using α-mannosidase and endoglycosidase H treatments (Foxwell et al. 1985). The present study examines the effect of enzymic deglycosylation of ricin on its hepatic clearance from the blood and recognition and uptake by rat liver non-parenchymal cells in vitro.

Materials and Methods

Ricin isolated by the method of Nicolson and Blaustein (1972) was split into its constituent chains by reduction with 2-mercaptoethanol followed by ion exchange on DEAE-Sepharose (Pharmacia). Contaminating ricin was removed from the A chain by twice-over passage through aisalofetuin-Sepharose and the B chain by ion-exchange chromatography on CM-Sepharose (Pharmacia) as described previously (Foxwell et al. 1985). Deglycosylated A chain in which the molecular weight was decreased by about 2000 was prepared by α-mannosidase (Sigma) treatment at room temperature for 2 days in 0.2 M citrate buffer pH 5.5, as described elsewhere (Foxwell et al. 1985). Deglycosylation of B chain (M_r <1200–1500) was achieved by treatment with endoglycosidase H (Miles Labs) in 0.1 M citrate buffer pH 5.5 containing 0.2 M D-galactose for 2 days, followed by additions of α-mannosidase for a further 24 h and purification on ConA Sepharose (Foxwell et al. 1985). Ricin A and B chains (untreated and deglycosylated) were recombined to form the hollotoxin, essentially according to the method of Uchida et al. (1978). The untreated toxin possessed electrophoretic and haemagglutination properties similar to that of native ricin, and deglycosylation had no detrimental effect on the ability of the toxin to inhibit protein synthesis in the reticulocyte lysate assay (Thorpe et al. 1981). Recombined ricin solutions were labelled with ^{125}I using the Iodo-Gen reagent (Pierce Chemicals) adjusted to a specific activity of 4×10^6 dpm/μg by adding unlabelled homologue and stored at 20 μg/ml in phospate-buffered saline (137 mM NaCl, 2.7 mM KCl, 8.1 mM Na$_2$ HPO$_4$, 1.5 mM KH$_2$PO$_4$, pH 7.3) containing 5 mg/ml bovine serum albumin.

The ^{125}I-labelled toxin was administered to adult male Wistar rats (LACP) via a tail vein. After 15 min the animals were killed, a blood sample was taken and the major body organs were removed. Tissue distribution of ricin was determined from the radioactivity present in the organs after correction for blood ^{125}I content (Wish et al. 1950). Rat liver cells were isolated from adult rats by collagenase liver perfusion and cultured as monolayers on plastic dishes for toxin uptake measurements as described in detail previously (Skilleter et al. 1985).

Results and Discussion

Untreated recombined ricin was rapidly cleared from the bloodstream after intravenous injection into rats and the liver was the major site of clearance. After 15 min nearly 30% of the injected material was present in the liver, with much smaller amounts (4%–9%) in the spleen, kidneys and lungs (Table 1). Deglycosylated ricin was removed from the blood much more slowly than untreated ricin. Approximately 40% of the injected dose remained in the blood after 15 min and only half as much (15%) was accumulated by the liver. Uptake of ricin by the other major tissues was essentially unaffected by enzymic deglycosylation of the toxin (see Table 1).

Untreated ricin was only poorly accumulated in vitro by parenchymal cells (3–5 ng/10^6 cells in 20 min) but was actively taken up by non-parenchymal cells.

Table 1. Tissue distribution of untreated and deglycosylated ricin after intravenous administration to rats

Organ/tissue	Tissue distribution			
	Untreated ricin (ng/g tissue)	% Injected dose	Deglycosylated ricin (ng/g tissue)	% Injected dose
Blood	64.2 ± 2.1	25%	100.7 ±11.4	40%
Liver	133.5 ±12.9	30%	64.4 ± 4.6	15%
Spleen	433.5 ±47.8	8%	490.2 ±68.4[a]	9%
Kidneys	6.72± 3.4	4%	8.96± 3.3[a]	5%
Heart	13.7 ± 2.0	1%	20.3 ± 0.8[a]	1%
Lungs	125.5 ± 3.2	4%	139.5 ± 3.1	4%

Adult male Wistar (LACP) rats (200 g) were injected intravenously with 4 µg ^{125}I-labelled untreated or deglycosylated ricin and after 15 min tissue and organ samples were taken from terminally anaesthetised animals. Toxin present in each of the tissues was determined after correction for blood ^{125}I content as detailed in Materials and Methods. Values are quoted as mean ±SD five separate determinations.
[a] Not significantly different from values for untreated ricin.

Table 2. Uptake of untreated and deglycosylated ricin by rat liver non-parenchymal cells in vitro

Ricin	Uptake (ng/10⁶ cells)	% Inhibition in the presence of				
		D-mannose (100 mM)	L-fructose (100 mM)	D-galactose (100 mM)	D-xylose (100 mM)	Ovalbumin (1 mg/ml)
Ricin	14.8±3.1	72	75	32	24[b]	68
Deglycosylated ricin	10.5±1.9[a]	39	46	58	26[b]	22

Toxin uptake was measured in monolayer cultures of 2×10^6 non-parenchymal cells which were incubated for 20 min at 37 °C in 3 ml serum-free culture medium (GMEM, Gibco-Europe) containing 0.1 µg/ml ^{125}I-labelled ricin in the presence and absence of the additions indicated in the Table. Uptake values are quoted as mean ±SD for five separate determinations.
[a] Significantly different from uptake of ricin ($p < 0.005$) on the basis of a two-way analysis of variance of the data from replicate assays using separate non-parenchymal cell preparations.
[b] Similar values obtained in the presence of other irrelevant sugars (cf. Skilleter et al. 1985).

Ricin uptake by non-parenchymal cells was strongly inhibited by D-mannose, L-fucose and the mannose-terminating glycoprotein ovalbumin, but inhibited only slightly by D-galactose and non-specifically by D-xylose (Table 2). These results are consistent with previous reports (Skilleter et al. 1981, 1985) and illustrate the importance of mannose receptor-mediated uptake of the toxin by hepatic non-parenchymal cells. Deglycosylation of ricin resulted in a consistent 30% decrease in its uptake by non-parenchymal cells in vitro, although the absolute values of uptake for both forms of the toxin varied within 15%–20% of mean values between replicate assays carried out using separate non-parenchymal cell preparations. Uptake of deglycosylated ricin was also much less sensitive to inhibition by D-mannose, L-fucose or ovalbumin but more sensitive to D-galactose (see Table 2).

These are similar characteristics to those observed for the uptake by non-parenchymal cells of enzymatically deglycosylated ricin B chain (Skilleter and Foxwell 1986) or ricin chemically modified by $IO_4^-/CNBH_3^-$ treatment (Skilleter et al. 1985), and in each case probably reflects an enhanced interaction of the modified toxin with galactosyl binding sites on the cells.

In summary, the present findings show that enzymic removal of the high mannose oligosaccharides from ricin impedes its hepatic clearance from the bloodstream and diminishes mannose-dependent uptake of the toxin by cultured liver non-parenchymal cells. This suggests therefore that antibody-ricin conjugates prepared from deglycosylated ricin should prove to be more successful antineoplastic reagents in vivo, by virtue of allowing more of the immunotoxin to reach its target tissue.

References

Fodstad O, Olsnes S, Pihl A (1976) Toxicity distribution and elimination of the cancerostatic lectins abrin and ricin after parenteral injection into mice. B J Cancer 34:318–425

Foxwell BMJ, Donovan TA, Thorpe PE, Wilson G (1985) The removal of carbohydrates from ricin with endoglycosidases H, F and D and α-mannosidase. Biochim Biophys Acta 840:193–203

Nicolson GL, Blaustein J (1972) The interaction of *Ricinus communis* agglutinin with normal and tumor cell surfaces. Biochim Biophys Acta 266:543–547

Olsnes S (1981) Directing toxins to cancer cells. Nature 290:84

Olsnes S, Pihl A (1982) Toxic lectins and related proteins. In: Cohen P, van Hegningen S (eds) Molecular actions of toxins and viruses. Elsevier, New York, pp 51–105

Olsnes S, Refsnes K, Pihl A (1974) Mechanism of action of the toxic lectins abrin and ricin. Nature 249:627–631

Skilleter DN, Foxwell BMJ (1986) Selective uptake of Ricin A-chain by hepatic non parenchymal cells in vitro: importance of mannose oligosaccharides in the toxin. FEBS Lett 196:344–348

Skilleter DN, Paine AJ, Stirpe F (1981) A comparison of the accumulation of ricin by hepatic parenchymal and non parenchymal cells and its inhibition of protein synthesis. Biochim Biophys Acta 677:495–500

Skilleter DN, Price RJ, Thorpe PE (1985) Modification of the carbohydrate in ricin with meta-periodate and cyanoborohydride mixtures: effect on binding uptake and toxicity to parenchymal and non parenchymal cells of rat liver. Biochim Biophys Acta 842:12–21

Thorpe PE, Brown ANF, Ross WCJ, Cumber AJ, Detre SI, Edwards DC, Davies AJS, Stirpe F (1981) Cytotoxicity acquired by conjugation of an anti-Thy 1 : 1 monoclonal antibody and the ribosome-inactivating protein gelonin. Eur J Biochem 116:447–454

Uchida T, Yamaizumi M, Mekada E, Okada Y, Tsuda M, Kurukawa T, Sagino Y (1978) Reconstitution of hybrid toxin from fragment A of diphtheria toxin and sub unit of *Wistaria floribunda* lectin. J Biol Chem 253:6307–6310

Vitetta E, Uhr JW (1985) Immunotoxins: redirecting nature's poisons cell. Cell 41:653–654

Wish L, Furth J, Storey RH (1950) Direct determination of plasma cell and organ blood volumes in normal and hypervolemic mice. Proc Soc Exp Biol Med 74:644–648

Mechanisms and Models in Toxicology
Arch. Toxicol., Suppl. 11, 261–263 (1987)
© by Springer-Verlag 1987

Mutagen Activation by Hepatic Fractions from Conventional, Germfree and Monoassociated Rats

I. R. Rowland[1], A. K. Mallett[1], C. B. Cole[2], and R. Fuller[2]

[1] British Industrial Biological Research Association,
   Woodmansterne Road, Carshalton, Surrey, SM5 4DS, UK
[2] AFRC Institute of Food Research, Reading Laboratory, Shinfield, Reading, Berks., RG2 9AT,
   UK

Introduction

The presence of a microbial population in the gut is known to influence metabolism not only within the intestinal tract but also at other sites in the body, particularly the liver (Wostmann 1984). It is possible, therefore, that the gut microflora may affect the activities of hepatic drug-metabolising enzymes, some of which are involved in the activation of foreign compounds to carcinogenic or mutagenic derivatives.

Methods

Chemicals: Aflatoxin B_1 (AFB$_1$; purity $>98\%$) was bought from Sigma Chemical Co., 3-amino-1-methyl-5H-pyrido[4,3-b]indole (Trp-P-2) from Wako Chemical Co., and 2-amino-3,4-dimethylimidazo[4,5-f]quinoline (MeIQ) was a gift of Dr S. Grivas. On analysis by HPLC, Trp-P-2 and MeIQ yielded single peaks.

In Vitro Mutagenicity Assay

Hepatic S9 fractions were prepared from IFR-Lister Hooded rats, aged 4 weeks (Ames et al. 1975). Four groups of six rats were used, whose gut microflora was, respectively, germfree (GF), conventional (CV), *E. coli*-associated and *Bacteroides sp.*-associated. The S9 fractions were incubated for 45 min in a final volume of 0.5 ml with mutagen, *Salmonella typhimurium* and cofactors, before addition of top agar and layering onto Vogel Bonner agar. Plates were incubated for 40 h and revertant colonies counted.

In Vivo Mutagenicity Assay

Following Arni et al. (1977), a suspension of *S. typhimurium* TA98 (4–6 × 10^9 cells) was given i.v. to GF or CV Balb/c mice (7–10 weeks old), immediately before a p.o. dose of DMSO (control) or AFB_1 (10 mg/kg body wt.). After 1 h the mice were killed and the bacteria recovered from the liver and plated on Vogel Bonner agar to determine numbers of revertants.

Results

The optimal concentration of S9 in the activation system (10% v/v for MeIQ and IQ, 5% for AFB_1 and Trp-P-2) was used in all experiments. Hepatic S9 from GF rats showed in general a greater capacity to activate MeIQ and Trp-P-2 to mutagens than that from CV rats. By contrast, S9 from CV animals was markedly more efficient than GF S9 in its activation of AFB_1 (Table 1, Fig. 1). Contamination of GF rats with *E. coli* or *Bacteroides sp.* had little effect on the activating

Table 1. Activation of mutagens by hepatic S9 from CV, GF and monoassociated rats

Microbiological status	Solvent control	His^+ revertants per plate (mean $\pm$ SE: $n=4$)			
		MeIQ		Trp-P-2	
		10 ng	30 ng	10 ng	30 ng
CV	22 ± 2	954 ± 74	1154 ± 50	96 ± 5	247 ± 6
E. coli	34 ± 6	1081 ± 120	$1478^a \pm 62$	$178^c \pm 6$	$357^a \pm 16$
Bacteroides sp.	27 ± 3	955 ± 110	$1498^a \pm 153$	$145^b \pm 8$	337 ± 24
GF	23 ± 4	1085 ± 51	$1532^a \pm 76$	$171^c \pm 13$	$432^b \pm 61$

Mutagen, S9 mix and bacteria (*Salmonella typhimurium* TA98) were incubated for 45 min at 37 °C before addition of top agar for overlay of Vogel Bonner agar.
Statistical significance relative to CV group: ^{a} $P<0.05$; ^{b} $P<0.01$; ^{c} $P<0.001$ (analysis of variance).

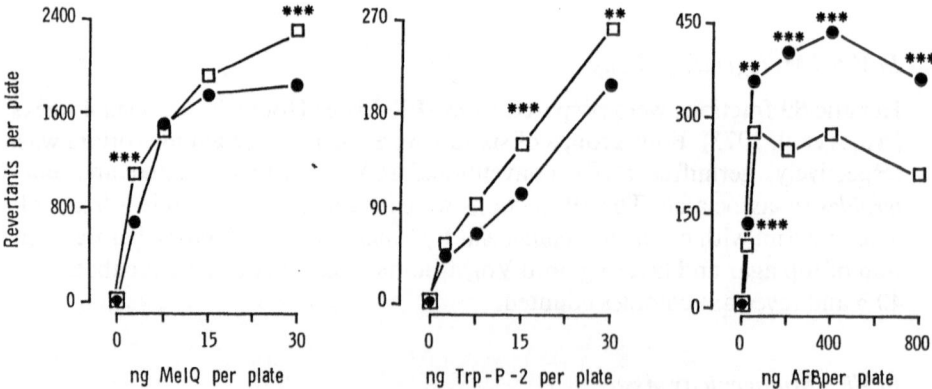

Fig. 1. Activation of mutagens by hepatic S9 from GF and CV rats. Each point is the mean of six rats and asterisks indicate that the results for GF (□) and CV (●) rats were significantly different: *$p<0.05$; **$p<0.01$; ***$p<0.001$

capacity of the S9 fractions towards MeIQ and Trp-P-2. In general, the decreased activation of the mutagens seen in S9 from CV animals was not observed in S9 from the monocontaminated rats (see Table 1).

The relevance of the in vitro results to activation of mutagens in the intact animal was investigated in GF and CV Balb/c mice. AFB_1 (10 mg/kg body wt.; p.o.) given to mice induced mutations in *S. typhimurium* TA 98 recovered from the liver. Significantly greater ($p < 0.001$) numbers of revertants were induced by AFB_1 in CV mice (142 ± 26 revertants per plate) than in GF animals (68 ± 16 revertants per plate).

Discussion

The results indicate that gross qualitative differences in the gut microflora can influence sites of metabolism remote from the gut itself. With some mutagens (MeIQ and Trp-P-2) the presence of the gut flora decreases the activation capacity of the liver, with others (AFB_1) the capacity is increased by the presence of the flora. Experiments with rats monoassociated with *E. coli* or *Bacteroides sp.* suggest that these organisms are not responsible for the differences in mutagen activation ability of GF and CV rats.

Acknowledgements. We thank the United Kingdom Ministry of Agriculture, Fisheries and Food for financial support, and the MRC Laboratories, Carshalton, for the germfree mice.

References

Ames BN, McCann J, Yamasaki E (1975) Methods for detecting carcinogens and mutagens with the *Salmonella*/mammalian microsome mutagenicity test. Mutat Res 31:347–364

Arni P, Mantel Th, Deparade E, Muller D (1977) Intrasanguine host-mediated assay with *Salmonella typhimurium*. Mutat Res 45:291–307

Wostmann BS (1984) Other organs. In: Coates ME, Gusstafsson BE (eds) The germ-free animal in biomedical research. Laboratory Animals, London, pp 215–231

Mechanisms and Models in Toxicology
Arch. Toxicol., Suppl. 11, 264–269 (1987)
© by Springer-Verlag 1987

Effects of Metronidazole, Azanidazole, and Azathioprine on Cytochrome P_{450} and Various Mono-Oxygenase Activities in Hepatic Microsomes from Control and Induced Mice

G. Cantelli-Forti, M. Paolini, P. Hrelia, E. Sapigni, and G. L. Biagi

Istituto di Farmacologia dell'Università, Via Irnerio, 48-40126 Bologna, Italy

Introduction

Drugs containing the imidazole ring have been reported to exert a potent inhibitory effect on microsomal mixed function mono-oxygenase (MFO) activity in man and experimental animals (Wilkinson et al. 1972; Pelkonen and Puurunen 1980; Murray 1984; Kapetanovic and Kupferberg 1984; Koop and Coon 1984; Kadderis and Rickert 1985; Horai et al. 1985). Such effects, mainly found in the liver and, recently, also in gonad and adrenal tissues (Mason et al. 1985), depend upon many factors. Species- and age-related differences have been established (Tu et al. 1981; Hajek and Novak 1982; Reinke et al. 1985). However, single or repeated administration of some imidazole derivatives was shown to result in an inhibition or an induction of MFO activity (Hajek and Novak 1982). By considering the multiplicity of cytochrome (Cyt) P_{450} isoenzymes in microsomes, these conflicting results become understandable.

Metronidazole (ME)-, azanidazole (AZN)-, and azathioprine (AZT)-related drugs are nitroimidazole derivatives widely used as chemotherapeutic agents and more recently as sensitizers of hypoxic cell tumors for supporting radiotherapy (Warkman 1980). Although results on their genotoxicity are available (Biagi et al. 1983; Cantelli-Forti et al. 1983, 1985), little is known about their effect on MFO activity. In the present work, the changes in the Cyt P_{450} content and aminopyrine N-demethylase (APD), p-nitroanisole O-demethylase (p-NAD), dinemorphan N-demethylase (DND), 7-ethoxycoumarin O-deethylase (ECD), and 7-ethoxyresorufin O-deethylase (ERD) activities in hepatic microsomes from uninduced and induced mice, injected daily with three i.p. doses of ME, AZN, or AZT, were studied.

Materials and Methods

Male and female Swiss albino mice, CD_1 strain (b.w. 30–40 g) in the basal state or induced for 3 consecutive days i.p. before the experiments with 100 mg/kg b.w. phenobarbital (PB) or with a single i.p. injection of 80 mg/kg b.w. β-naphthoflavone (β-NF; 48 h before), were treated for 3 consecutive days with i.p. metronidazole (ME; 45 and 90 mg/kg b.w.), azanidazole (AZN; 62.5 and 125 mg/kg b.w.), or azathioprine (AZT; 125 and 250 mg/kg b.w.). They were starved the night before being killed by cervical dislocation. S9 fractions were prepared (Cantelli-Forti et al. 1984). The supernatant was poured into clear centrifuge tubes and centrifuged at $105,000 \times g$ for 60 min. The resultant microsomal pellet was resuspended in 0.01 M Na$^+$/K$^+$ phosphate buffer (pH 7.45) containing KCl 1.15% (w/v) using a hand-driven Potter-Elvehjem homogenizer. The resuspended pellet was centrifuged at $105,000 \times g$ for 60 min. The resultant washed microsomes were resuspended as before and stored at $-80\,°C$. The APD, p-NAD, ECD, and protein concentration methods used were as previously reported (Cantelli-Forti et al. 1984). The DND, ERD, and cytochrome P_{450} assays were carried out as reported by Gervasi et al. (1984), Klotz et al. (1984), and Omura and Sato (1964), respectively. Statistical analysis was made using the Wilcoxon rank method.

Results and Discussion

The in vivo effects on Cyt P_{450} and various phase-I enzyme activities of the drug metabolism in uninduced animals are summarized in Table 1. The pattern and extent of enzyme inhibition of these drugs differed markedly. DND activity, specifically catalyzed by the PB-Cyt P_{450} isoenzymes, was significantly inhibited by ME in male mice ($P < 0.01$) and to a lesser extent by AZN and AZT. In contrast, ERD activity specifically catalyzed by β-NF-Cyt P_{448} isoenzymes, was preferentially inhibited by AZN ($P < 0.05$ and $P < 0.01$ in females and males, respectively) and AZT ($p < 0.01$ in male animals).

In order to add more information to the above results, additional experiments were carried out on hepatic microsomal preparations from PB- or β-NF-pretreated mice, in which the amounts of Cyt P_{450} and P_{448} were enhanced. Table 2 shows that the DND activity was markedly inhibited by ME ($p < 0.01$ and $p < 0.05$ in females and males, respectively), but not by AZN and AZT in PB-induced microsomes. As reported in Table 3, the ERD activity, catalyzed by β-NF-induced microsomes, was indeed markedly inhibited by both AZN and AZT ($p < 0.05$ and $p < 0.01$ in females and males, respectively). The ME shows an inhibitory effect only in males at the highest dose. Changes in Cyt P_{450} content were not observed in all situations. These findings showed a predominant inhibition by the drugs under study towards specific forms of Cyt P_{450}. However, an unspecific inhibitory effect is present, as indicated by APD, p-NAD, and ECD changes, both in uninduced and induced animals. Sex-related differences probably reflect the contributions of sex-specific Cyt P_{450} isoenzymes to overall microsomal metabolism. Therefore, in order to understand these differences, experiments on purified Cyt P_{450} isoenzymes are to be carried out.

Conclusions

This work shows that imidazole-related drugs may affect the metabolism of other chemicals. Thus, pharmacokinetic interactions may be a consequence of the co-

Table 1. Effects of metronidazole, azanidazole, and azathioprine on mouse microsomal mono-oxygenase system. The values are the means ±S.D. of results obtained from 5 animals

Treatment[a]	APD[b]		p-NAD[b]		DND[b]		ECD[b]		ERD[b]		Cyt P$_{450}$[c]	
	♀	♂	♀	♂	♀	♂	♀	♂	♀	♂	♀	♂
Control	1.62± 0.30	1.71± 0.39	0.62± 0.17	0.59± 0.21	1.25± 0.34	1.30± 0.33	0.80± 0.21	0.78± 0.32	0.33± 0.13	0.41± 0.14	0.51± 0.11	0.55± 0.16
Metronidazole (45 mg/kg b.w.; daily × 3)	1.68± 0.30	1.73± 0.39	1.48± 0.22	0.55± 0.19	1.34± 0.28	0.96± 0.20[d]	0.81± 0.29	0.70± 0.35	0.37± 0.11	0.38± 0.09	0.58± 0.17	0.44± 0.15
Metronidazole (90 mg/kg b.w.; daily × 3)	1.54± 0.29	1.60± 0.21	0.50± 0.12[d]	0.62± 0.12	1.09± 0.27	0.74± 0.19[e]	0.64± 0.30	0.62± 0.35	0.24± 0.08	0.19± 0.09[d]	0.48± 0.16	0.53± 0.06
Azanidazole (62.5 mg/kg b.w.; daily × 3)	1.66± 0.28	1.69± 0.35	0.56± 0.12	0.49± 0.31	1.18± 0.23	1.33± 0.35	0.73± 0.26	0.84± 0.30	0.17± 0.09[d]	0.22± 0.07[d]	0.53± 0.16	0.46± 0.19
Azanidazole (125 mg/kg b.w.; daily × 3)	1.33± 0.19[d]	1.58± 0.28	0.66± 0.10	0.44± 0.27	0.92± 0.15[d]	1.23± 0.26	0.67± 0.23	0.64± 0.29	0.15± 0.05[d]	0.19± 0.08[e]	0.46± 0.18	0.31± 0.32
Azathioprine (125 mg/kg b.w.; daily × 3)	1.56± 0.25	1.79± 0.27	0.58± 0.16	0.46± 0.17	1.34± 0.39	1.16± 0.28	0.92± 0.22	0.70± 0.15	0.40± 0.16	0.21± 0.10[d]	0.44± 0.10	0.30± 0.18
Azathioprine (250 mg/kg b.w.; daily × 3)	1.29± 0.19[d]	1.58± 0.33	0.40± 0.15	0.33± 0.11[d]	1.16± 0.20	0.91± 0.25[d]	0.55± 0.16[d]	0.64± 0.27	0.25± 0.08	0.18± 0.08[e]	0.43± 0.15	0.49± 0.13

[a] Uninduced animals.
[b] nmol × mg^{-1} × min^{-1}.
[c] nmol × mg^{-1}.
[d] $P < 0.05$, [e] $P < 0.01$ when compared with control.

Table 2. Effects of metronidazole, azanidazole, and azathioprine on mouse microsomal mono-oxygenase system. The values are the means ±S.D. of results obtained from 5 animals

Treatment[a]	APD[b]		p-NAD[b]		DND[b]		ECD[b]		ERD[b]		Cyt P_{450}[c]	
	♀	♂	♀	♂	♀	♂	♀	♂	♀	♂	♀	♂
Control	3.67 ± 0.48	3.49 ± 0.36	2.28 ± 0.27	2.50 ± 0.47	2.74 ± 0.31	2.85 ± 0.34	2.11 ± 0.25	1.97 ± 0.38	0.45 ± 0.12	0.39 ± 0.08	1.32 ± 0.26	1.41 ± 0.23
Metronidazole (45 mg/kg b.w.; daily ×3)	3.29 ± 0.52	2.95 ± 0.32	2.34 ± 0.35	2.44 ± 0.38	2.58 ± 0.31	2.65 ± 0.39	2.31 ± 0.36	2.10 ± 0.27	0.35 ± 0.15	0.33 ± 0.14	1.29 ± 0.18	1.35 ± 0.24
Metronidazole (90 mg/kg b.w.; daily ×3)	2.96 ± 0.32	2.88 ± 0.27[d]	2.11 ± 0.22	2.37 ± 0.31	2.18 ± 0.39[e]	2.48 ± 0.23[d]	2.24 ± 0.30	1.89 ± 0.36	0.30 ± 0.08[d]	0.31 ± 0.13	1.18 ± 0.29	1.30 ± 0.31
Azanidazole (62.5 mg/kg b.w.; daily ×3)	3.39 ± 0.27	3.27 ± 0.20	2.33 ± 0.35	2.44 ± 0.38	2.66 ± 0.45	2.70 ± 0.29	2.24 ± 0.26	2.07 ± 0.25	0.30 ± 0.21	0.24 ± 0.09[d]	1.38 ± 0.25	1.41 ± 0.32
Azanidazole (125 mg/kg b.w.; daily ×3)	3.50 ± 0.52	3.07 ± 0.21[d]	2.19 ± 0.25	2.35 ± 0.29	2.68 ± 0.33	2.56 ± 0.20	1.85 ± 0.36	2.01 ± 0.25	0.21 ± 0.08[e]	0.19 ± 0.10[e]	1.30 ± 0.21	1.22 ± 0.25
Azathioprine (125 mg/kg b.w.; daily ×3)	3.59 ± 0.55	3.41 ± 0.35	2.31 ± 0.37	2.44 ± 0.30	2.70 ± 0.47	2.68 ± 0.42	2.24 ± 0.26	2.15 ± 0.27	0.40 ± 0.16	0.30 ± 0.12	1.15 ± 0.20	1.27 ± 0.18
Azathioprine (250 mg/kg b.w.; daily ×3)	3.32 ± 0.34	2.11 ± 0.24[d]	2.15 ± 0.32	2.29 ± 0.41	2.52 ± 0.36	2.55 ± 0.40	1.95 ± 0.36	1.74 ± 0.18[d]	0.32 ± 0.14	0.21 ± 0.07[e]	1.24 ± 0.26	1.50 ± 0.39

[a] The animals were previously induced with PB.
[b] $nmol \times mg^{-1} \times min^{-1}$.
[c] $nmol \times mg^{-1}$.
[d] $P < 0.05$, [e] $P < 0.01$ when compared with control.

Table 3. Effects of metronidazole, azanidazole, and azathioprine on mouse microsomal mono-oxygenase system. The values are the means ±S.D. of results obtained from 5 animals

Treatment[a]	APD[b]		p-NAD[b]		DND[b]		ECD[b]		ERD[b]		Cyt P$_{450}$[c]	
	♀	♂	♀	♂	♀	♂	♀	♂	♀	♂	♀	♂
Control	2.27±0.31	2.11±0.26	1.33±0.20	1.45±0.26	1.12±0.22	0.99±0.27	1.21±0.19	1.09±0.17	2.35±0.34	2.60±0.39	0.81±0.20	0.73±0.17
Metronidazole (45 mg/kg b.w.; daily ×3)	1.96±0.45	2.22±0.28	1.10±0.23	1.30±0.31	0.93±0.24	0.68±0.12[d]	1.29±0.28	1.18±0.22	2.10±0.29	2.30±0.19	0.93±0.19	0.85±0.12
Metronidazole (90 mg/kg b.w.; daily ×3)	2.16±0.25	1.94±0.37	1.09±0.29	1.23±0.35	0.97±0.25	0.55±0.13[e]	1.06±0.27	0.89±0.18	2.15±0.23	2.06±0.21[d]	0.76±0.12	0.89±0.15
Azanidazole (62.5 mg/kg b.w.; daily ×3)	2.25±0.36	2.24±0.25	1.19±0.30	1.37±0.29	1.19±0.17	0.86±0.18	1.33±0.31	1.20±0.24	1.93±0.21[d]	1.61±0.32[e]	1.91±0.11	0.95±0.09
Azanidazole (125 mg/kg b.w.; daily ×3)	1.83±0.44	1.86±0.41	1.15±0.27	1.26±0.30	1.01±0.22	0.70±0.12[d]	1.16±0.22	0.99±0.20	1.98±0.19[d]	1.40±0.26[e]	0.80±0.08	0.72±0.19
Azathioprine (125 mg/kg b.w.; daily ×3)	2.34±0.39	2.20±0.28	1.39±0.31	1.21±0.33	1.26±0.30	1.17±0.31	1.17±0.34	1.15±0.26	2.20±0.26	2.15±0.29[d]	0.74±0.13	0.79±0.10
Azathioprine (250 mg/kg b.w.; daily ×3)	2.16±0.19	1.83±0.25[d]	1.25±0.32	1.13±0.27[d]	1.19±0.24	0.92±0.23	0.97±0.34	0.85±0.22[d]	1.97±0.26[d]	1.88±0.23[e]	0.78±0.15	0.84±0.13

[a] The animals were previously induced with β-NF.
[b] nmol × mg^{-1} × min^{-1}.
[c] nmol × mg^{-1}.
[d] $P<0.05$, [e] $P<0.01$ when compared with control.

administration of ME, AZN, and AZT with another drug which is biotransformed by the MFO system. The general picture emerging from the data available suggests that considerable caution should be exercised in the interpretation of imidazole-derivative modulation in microsomal metabolism.

Acknowledgement. This work was supported by CNR (National Research Council of Italy) target project "Oncology" (contract no. 85.02070.44).

References

Biagi GL, Barbaro AM, Guerra MC, Cantelli-Forti G, Aicardi G, Borea PA (1983) Quantitative relationship between structure and mutagenic activity in a series of 5-nitroimidazoles. Teratogen Carcin Mut 3:429–438

Cantelli-Forti G, Aicardi G, Guerra MC, Barbaro AM, Biagi GL (1983) Mutagenicity of a series of 25 nitroimidazoles and two nitrothiazoles in *Salmonella typhimurium.* Teratogen Carc Mut 3:51–63

Cantelli-Forti G, Paolini M, Hrelia P, Corsi C, Biagi GL, Bronzetti G (1984) NADPH-generating system: influences on microsomal mono-oxygenase stability during incubations for the liver microsomal assay with rat and mouse S9 fractions. Mutat Res 129:291–297

Cantelli-Forti G, Hrelia P, Paolini M, Bronzetti G, Biagi GL (1985) The organo-specific activity of metronidazole and azanidazole in the intrasanguinous host-mediated assay. Drug Exp Clin Res 11:755–759

Gervasi PG, Benedetti D, Citti L, Del Monte M, Turchi G (1984) Dinemorphan N-demethylation by mouse liver microsomes. Experientia 40:180–182

Hajek KK, Novak RF (1982) Spectral and metabolic properties of liver microsomes from imidazole-pretreated rabbit. Biochem Biophys Res Commun 108:664–672

Horai Y, White PF, Trevor AY (1985) The effect of etomidate on rabbit liver microsomal drug metabolism in vitro. Drug Metab Dispos 13:364–367

Kapetanovic IM, Kupferberg HJ (1984) Nafimidone and imidazole anticonvulsant and its metabolite as potent inhibitors of microsomal metabolism of phenytoin and carbamazepine. Drug Metab Dispos 12:560–563

Kadderis GL, Rickert DE (1985) Loss of rat liver microsomal cytochrome P-450 during methimazole and metabolism. Drug Metab Dispos 13:58–61

Klotz AV, Stageman VV, Walsh C (1984) An alternative 7-ethoxycoumarin O-deethylase activity assay: a continuous visible spectrophotometric method for measurement of cytochrome P-450 mono-oxygenase activity. Anal Biochem 140:138–145

Koop DR, Coon MJ (1984) Purification of liver microsomal cytochrome P-450 isoenzymes 3a and 6 from imidazole treated rabbits. Mol Pharmacol 25:494–501

Mason JI, Murray BA, Olcott M, Sheets JJ (1985) Imidazole antimycotics: inhibitors of steroid aromatase. Biochem Pharmacol 34:1087–1092

Murray M (1984) In vitro effects of quinoline derivatives on cytochrome P-450 and aminopyrine N-demethylase activity in rat hepatic microsomes. Biochem Pharmacol 33:3277–3281

Omura T, Sato R (1964) The carbon monoxide-binding pigment of liver microsomes. I. Evidence for its hemoprotein nature. J Biol Chem 239:2370–2378

Pelkonen O, Puurunen J (1980) The effect of cimetidine on in vitro and in vivo microsomal drug metabolism in the rat. Biochem Pharmacol 29:3075–3080

Reinke LA, Sexter SH, Rikans LE (1985) Comparison of ethanol and imidazole pretreatments on hepatic mono-oxygenase activities in the rat. Res Commun Chem Pathol Pharmacol 47:97–105

Tu YY, Sonnenberg J, Lewis KF, Yang CS (1981) Pyrazole-induced cytochrome P-450 in rat liver microsomes: an isozyme with high affinity for dimethylnitrosamine. Biochem Biophys Res Commun 103:905–912

Warkman P (1980) Pharmacokinetics of hypoxic cell radiosensitizers. Cancer Clin Trials 3:237–241

Wilkinson CF, Hetnarski CF, Yellin TO (1972) Imidazole-derivatives. A new class of microsomal enzyme inhibitors. 21:3187–3192

Mechanisms and Models in Toxicology
Arch. Toxicol., Suppl. 11, 270–272 (1987)

An Animal Model of Cisplatin-Induced Magnesium Deficiency

T. Ormond, M. P. Ryan, and I. S. Pratt

Department of Pharmacology, University College Dublin, Fosters Avenue, Blackrock, Co. Dublin, Ireland

Introduction

Cisplatin (*cis*-diamminedichloroplatinum) is an inorganic metal complex which has major antitumour activity against many solid cancers including testicular, ovarian, bladder and lung (Rosencweig et al. 1977). Cisplatin has relatively little effect on the bone marrow, but it can induce significant renal dysfunction (Dentino et al. 1978). Clinical use of the drug is limited by the dose-related nephrotoxicity.

The development of hypomagnesaemia with cisplatin therapy has been noted by a number of investigators in recent years (Schilsky and Anderson 1979; Vega et al. 1983; Teeling et al. 1985). The hypomagnesaemia is thought to result from a cisplatin-induced defect in renal tubular magnesium conservation leading to urinary magnesium wasting. However, the sites and mechanisms of the cisplatin-induced renal tubular damage leading to renal magnesium wasting remain to be established.

The aims of the present studies were:

1. To develop animal models of cisplatin nephrotoxicity
2. To assess enzymuria, in particular urinary excretion of the lysosomal enzyme β-N-acetylglucosaminidase (β-NAG) as a means of detecting early nephrotoxic effects of cisplatin
3. To investigate the relationship between nephrotoxicity assessed by either traditional methods such as blood urea nitrogen and creatinine, or by urinary excretion of β-NAG and the magnesium wasting caused by the drug

Methods

The effects of multiple cisplatin administration (28-day studies involving 4 doses of 3.0 mg cisplatin/kg each week) on magnesium status and other indices of nephrotoxicity were investigated in male Wistar rats fed either standard laboratory rat diet (study series A), or synthetic diet with low magnesium content (5 mmol Mg/kg; study series B).

Cisplatin (Sigma Chemical, UK) was administered intraperitoneally in normal saline once a week for 4 weeks. Appropriate control groups were used in both series of studies. In series A, all rats were allowed free access to normal laboratory rat chow and tap water. In series B, animals were pair-fed the synthetic diet containing 5 mmol Mg/kg and given free access to deionized water.

Urine samples were collected at intervals throughout the experiments. Urinary magnesium (using atomic absorption spectrophotometry) and β-NAG (using a fluorimetric assay) excretions were monitored.

Animals were killed by anaesthetic overdose at the end of week 4 in both series A and B. Kidneys were removed and the kidney to body weight ratio was noted. Blood was taken and plasma separated. Blood urea nitrogen, plasma creatinine and plasma magnesium were determined.

Results and Discussion

The results for rats fed normal diet are shown in Table 1. Urinary excretion of β-NAG was increased significantly following cisplatin treatment. Peak excretion of β-NAG tended to occur in the early phase of the study and the results for day 3 are shown in Table 1. The results suggest lysosomal labilization resulting from nephrotoxic damage induced by cisplatin. Renal wasting of magnesium was detected in the later phases of the study and results for day 13 are shown in Table 1. Other indices of nephrotoxicity including increased blood urea nitrogen and plasma creatinine were significantly elevated following cisplatin administration. These results are shown in Table 1. However, it is notable that despite significant nephrotoxicity and renal wasting of magnesium, hypomagnesaemia was not detected in this series. The lack of hypomagnesaemia may be due to mobilization from body stores such as bone or enhanced absorption of magnesium from the gastrointestinal tract.

The effects of cisplatin were therefore investigated in rats fed a diet marginal in magnesium content. A synthetic diet containing 5 mmol Mg/kg was prepared and control and cisplatin-treated rats were pair-fed this diet; experiments were

Table 1. Indices of nephrotoxicity following cisplatin administration (3 mg/kg each week) for 4 weeks in rats fed normal diet

Group	Urinary excretion		Plasma		
	β-N-acetyl-glucosaminidase (units/24 h; day 3)	Magnesium (mmol/24 h; day 13)	Blood urea nitrogen (mg/dl)	Creatinine (mg/dl)	Magnesium (mmol/l)
Control ($n=5$)	47± 29	6.2±2.3	16.5±2.2	0.55±0.34	0.96±0.10
Cisplatin ($n=4$)	4139±1665	58.3±6.0	49.1±9.9	1.42±0.22	0.97±0.05
p value	<0.05	<0.001	<0.02	<0.01	N.S.

Table 2. Indices of nephrotoxicity following cisplatin administration (3 mg/kg each week) for 4 weeks in rats fed a magnesium-deficient diet (5 mmol/kg)

Group	Urinary excretion		Plasma		
	β-N-acetyl-glucosaminidase (units/mg creatinine; day 11)	Magnesium (mmol/mg creatinine; day 15)	Blood urea nitrogen (mg/dl)	Creatinine (mg/dl)	Magnesium (mmol/l)
Control ($n=6$)	352± 60	0.44±0.18	21.8± 1.5	0.48±0.02	0.79±0.05
Cisplatin ($n=6$)	1170±434	1.79±0.32	65.5±14.4	0.85±0.11	0.48±0.09
p value	<0.05	<0.01	<0.01	<0.005	<0.02

carried out for the same time period as in the previous series where rats were fed a normal diet.

The indices of nephrotoxicity following cisplatin treatment in rats fed a diet low in magnesium are shown in Table 2. Following cisplatin treatment, urinary excretion of β-NAG increased significantly. The results for day 11 are shown in Table 2. Cisplatin-treated animals showed significantly increased urinary excretion of magnesium. In this series of experiments, the magnesium wasting resulted in the development of significant hypomagnesaemia. Blood urea nitrogen and plasma creatinine were also increased following cisplatin treatment.

In summary, animal models of chronic cisplatin (3 mg/kg each week for 4 weeks) nephrotoxicity were established in male Wistar rats. Urinary excretion of β-NAG tended to peak in the early phases of the studies, whereas urinary excretion of magnesium tended to peak in the later phases – suggesting that damage resulting in magnesium wasting may be dissociated from damage resulting in leakage of β-NAG. Rats fed a low-magnesium diet and treated with cisplatin development significant hypomagnesaemia. This represents a useful model of cisplatin-induced magnesium deficiency. Further studies are required to elucidate the mechanisms involved in cisplatin-induced magnesium deficiency.

Acknowledgement. This work was supported by the Medical Research Council of Ireland

References

Dentino M, Luft FC, Yumm MN (1978) Long-term effect of cisdiammine dichloride platinum (CDDP) on renal function and structure in man. Cancer 41:1274–1281

Rosencweig U, Von Hoff D, Slank M (1977) Cis DDP (II) – a new anti-cancer drug. Ann Intern Med 86:803–812

Schilsky RL, Anderson T (1979) Hypomagnesaemia and renal magnesium wasting in patients receiving cisplatin. Ann Intern Med 90:929–931

Teeling M, Conlon D, Pratt I, Carney D, Ryan MP (1985) Prospective investigation of cisplatin-induced nephrotoxicity including renal magnesium wasting in cancer patients. J Am Coll Nutr 4:389

Vega F, Suarez F, Panizo A (1983) Hypomagnesaemia – a usual manifestation of cisplatin nephrotoxicity. Kidney Int 24:130

Mechanisms and Models in Toxicology
Arch. Toxicol., Suppl. 11, 273–276 (1987)
© by Springer-Verlag 1987

Quantitative Methods for Assessing the Effects of Some Anticancer Drugs on Mouse Spermatogenesis

I. Wahed [1], M. C. Bibby [2], and T. G. Baker [1]

[1] School of Biomedical Sciences, University of Bradford, Bradford BD7 1DP, UK
[2] School of Clinical Oncology, University of Bradford, Bradford BD7 1DP, UK

Introduction

In order to evaluate the survival of stem cells, after treatment with some anti-cancer drugs, two assays were carried out based on the ability of the stem cells to produce spermatocytes, spermatids and spermatozoa. These assays comprise the measurement of the levels of the enzyme LDH-X and the number of sperm heads in testicular homogenates. LDH-X is the X isozyme of lactate dehydrogenase which in mammals is found only in testis and spermatozoa (Wheat and Goldberg 1975). LDH enzyme levels provide a "fingerprint" in the study of spermatogenesis (Bishop 1968).

Materials and Methods

Pure strain male NMRI mice (aged 8–12 weeks) from an inbred colony were used. Three standard drugs, 5-fluorouracil (5-FU), thioTEPA, methyl CCNU (MeCCNU) and a new investigational drug 8 carbamoyl-3-(2-chloroethyl-imid-azo (5,i–d))-1,2,3,5 tetrazin-4(3H)-one (mitozolomide, NSC353451 M & B 39565) were used at maximum tolerated single doses. Groups of 5 mice were killed at 5, 22, 32, 42 and 53 days after injection and the testes were removed and placed into distilled water (1 testis/ml). The samples were then homogenized for 5 s, sonicated for 30 s and an aliquot was removed for sperm head count. The remainder of the sample was heated to 55 °C for 5 min to destroy activity of other enzymes without affecting LDH-X. The supernatant obtained after centrifugation at 27 000 g for 10 min was assayed at room temperature (24 ± 1 °C) by measuring the oxidation of nicotinamide adenine dinucleotide, reduced (NADH) at 340 nm. The assay was performed in 0.05 M sodium phosphate buffer at pH 7.4 containing as a substrate 3×10^{-5} M α-ketovalerate and 1.5×10^{-4} M NADH (Meistrich et al. 1978).

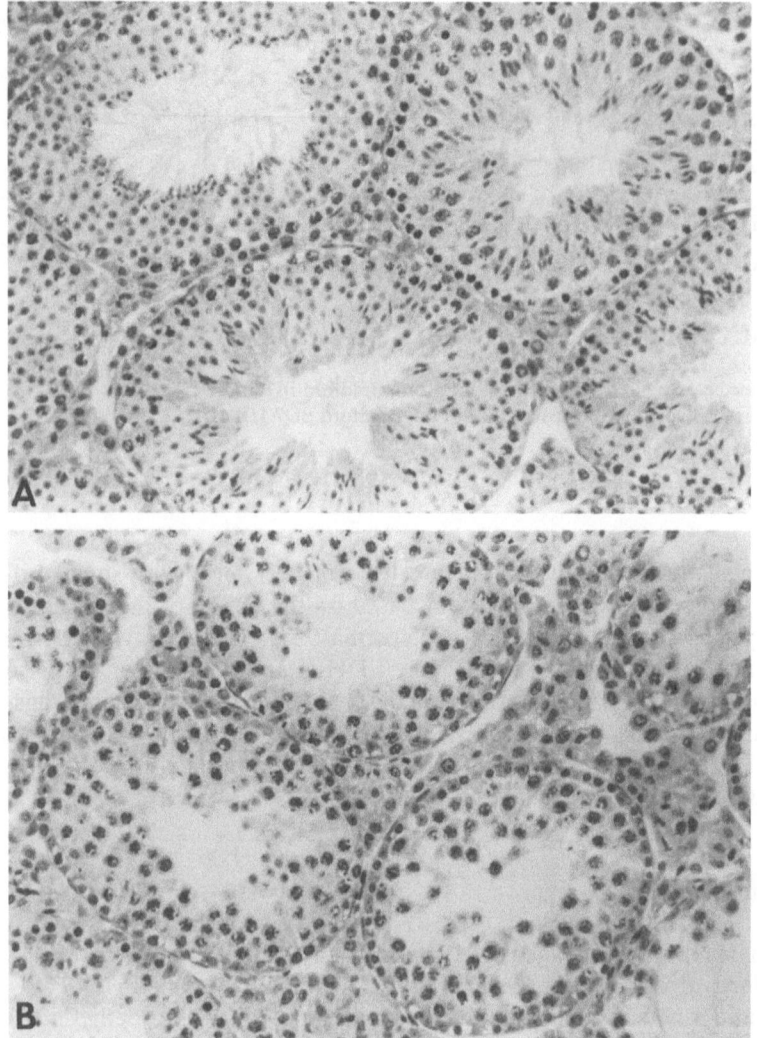

Fig. 1. Cross section of mouse testis (haematoxylin and eosin). **a** Control, × 500. **b** Mitozolomide, × 700

Results

Following i.p. injection of mitozolomide (Fig. 1) and thioTepa, the number of sperm heads was depressed from day 22 to day 32, while with 5-FU there was a small depression at 22 days after injection. There was no significant damage with MeCCNU (Fig. 2). The activity of LDH-X declined at 22 days after injection, with all drugs, but this depression was not statistically significant when compared with controls. At 32 days after injection there was a significant decline in the levels of LDH-X in testes treated with mitozolomide and thioTepa, while in the testes

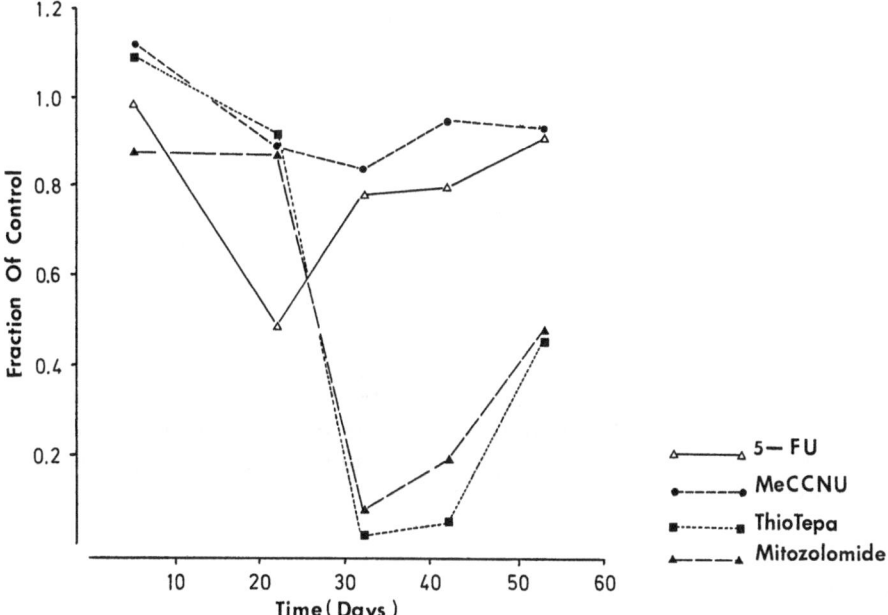

Fig. 2. Effects of mitozolomide (40 mg/kg), thioTepa (20 mg/kg), 5-FU (120 mg/kg) and MeCCNU (15 mg/kg) on sperm head counts in mouse testes

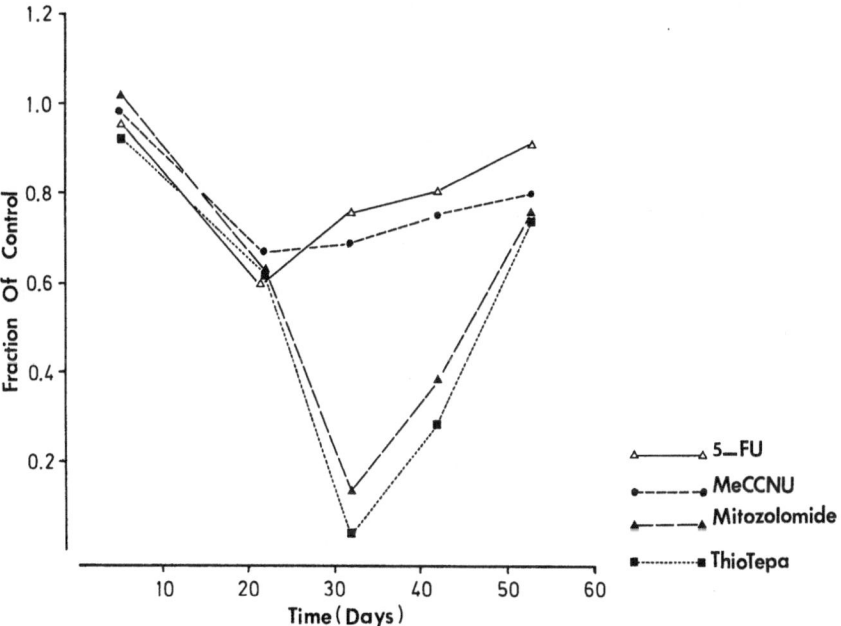

Fig. 3. Effects of mitozolomide (40 mg/kg), thioTepa (20 mg/kg), 5-FU (120 mg/kg) and MeCCNU (15 mg/kg) on LDX-X activity (i.v./g tissue) in mouse testes

treated with 5-FU and MeCCNU the levels of LDH-X started to return to normal at 32 days after injection (Fig. 3).

Discussion

Other authors have demonstrated sperm count depression in patients treated with anticancer drugs (Fukutani et al. 1981; Berthelsen 1984) and in mice exposed to irradiation (Meistrich et al. 1978). The present study shows similar results in mice following treatment with cytotoxic agents. ThioTepa and mitozolomide cause the most significant depression in sperm head count, and the same result is seen with LDH-X levels. The sperm head count (Searle and Beechey 1974) and LDH-X levels (Erickson et al. 1975; Goldberg and Hawtrey 1970) provide good quantitative markers of the effects of anticancer drugs on spermatogenesis, and a rapid method for assessing potential testicular toxicity of new drugs which complement the histological assessment of testicular damage.

References

Berthelsen J (1984) Sperm count and serum follicle-stimulating hormone levels before and after radiotherapy and chemistry in men with germ cell cancer. Fertil Steril 41(2):281–285

Bishop DW (1968) Testicular enzymes as fingerprints in the study of spermatogenesis. In: Diamond M (ed) Perspectives in reproduction and sexual behaviour. Bloomington, Indiana University Press, pp 261–286

Erickson RP, Spielmann H, Mangia F, Tennenbaum D, Epstein CJ (1975) Studies on lactate dehydrogenase isozymes in gametes and early development of mice. In: Markert CL (ed) Isozymes. Academic Press, pp 313–324

Fukutani K, Ishida H, Shinohara M, Minowada S, Niijima T, Nijikata K, Izawa Y (1981) Suppression of spermatogenesis in patients with Burchet's disease treated with cyclophosphamide and colchicine. Fertil Steril 36(1):76–80

Goldberg E, Hawtrey C (1970) The effect of experimental cryptorchism on the isozymes of lactate dehydrogenase in mouse testis. J Exp Zool 1967:411–418

Meistrich ML, Finch M, daCunha MF, Hacker U, Au WW (1978) Gradual regeneration of mouse testicular stem cells after exposure to ionizing radiation. Radiat Res 74:349–362

Searle AG, Beechey CV (1974) Sperm-count, egg-fertilization and dominant lethality after irradiation of mice. Mutat Res 22:63–72

Wheat TE, Goldberg E (1975) LDH-X the sperm-specific C_4 isozyme of lactate dehydrogenase. In: Markert CL (ed) Isozymes. Academic Press, pp 325–345

Mechanisms and Models in Toxicology
Arch. Toxicol., Suppl. 11, 277–280 (1987)
© by Springer-Verlag 1987

Comparative Effects of Mitozolomide (M & B 39125, NSC 353451 and a Series of Standard Anticancer Drugs on Mouse Testis

I. Wahed [1], M. C. Bibby [2], and T. G. Baker [1]

[1] School of Biomedical Sciences, University of Bradford, Bradford, BD7 1DP, UK
[2] School of Clinical Oncology, University of Bradford, Bradford, BD7 1DP, UK

Introduction

Cytotoxic agents are being widely used in man for the treatment of neoplastic and non-neoplastic diseases. With recent improvements in cancer chemotherapy, sterility has become one of the problems related to the toxicity of anticancer drugs (Etteldorf et al. 1976). The aim of this study is to compare the toxicity on mouse testicular germ cells of a new agent (mitozolomide) shown to have considerable experimental antitumour activity, with four standard anticancer drugs, methyl CCNU (MeCCNU), thioTepa, 5-fluorouracil (5-FU) and cyclophosphamide.

Materials and Methods

Groups of 5 NMRI mice from an inbred colony were killed at 5, 12, 23, 31, 48, 76 and 152 days after i.p. injection with cyclophosphamide (300 mg/kg, and at 5, 22, 32, 42 and 53 days after injection with thioTepa (20 mg/kg), mitozolomide (40 mg/kg), MeCCNU (15 mg/kg) and 5-FU (120 mg/kg). These are maximum tolerated single doses for these drugs. MeCCNU was a gift from the National Cancer Institute (NCI) USA; mitozolomide from Professor M. G. F. Stevens, University of Aston, UK; thioTepa from Lederle Laboratories, Gosport, Hants, UK; 5-FU from Roche, Welwyn Garden City, UK; and cyclophosphamide from Boehringer, London, UK. ThioTepa, 5-FU and cyclophosphamide were dissolved in 0.9% saline, mitozolomide was suspended in arachis oil and MeCCNU was dissolved in 10% ethanol/arachis oil. The testes were removed and weighed, fixed in Bouin's fluid, and then subjected to routine histological processing. Sections were cut at 5 μm and stained with haematoxylin and eosin (H&E) or periodic acid–Schiff (PAS). The seminiferous tubule diameter was measured by means of an ocular micrometer.

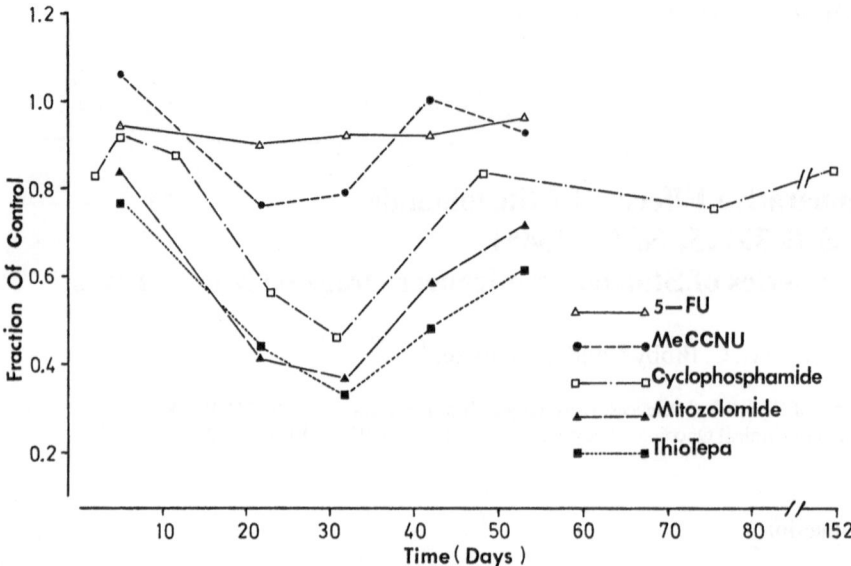

Fig. 1. Effects of mitozolomide, thioTepa, 5-FU, MeCCNU and cyclophosphamide on weight of mice testes

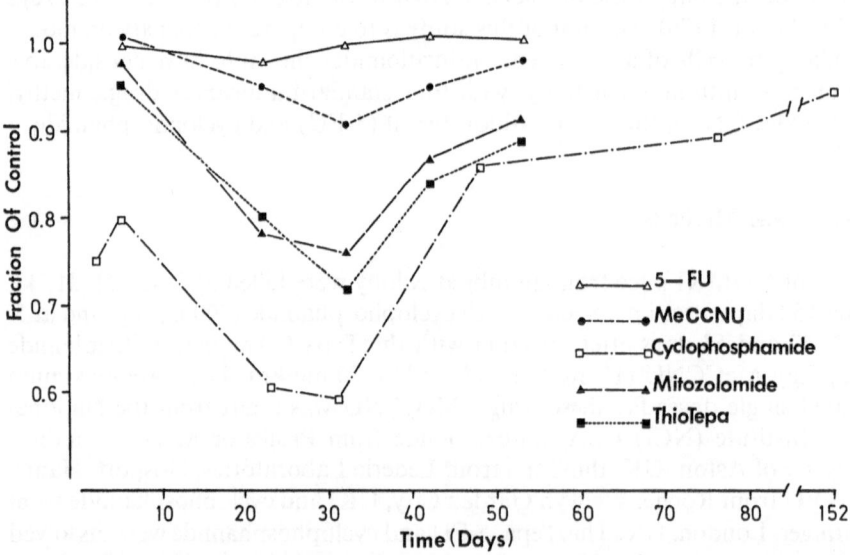

Fig. 2. Effects of mitozolomide, thioTepa, 5-FU, MeCCNU and cyclophosphamide on the diameters of seminiferous tubules in mice testes

Results

Figure 1 shows that a significant decrease in testicular weight was evident at 23 and 31 days after injection with cyclophosphamide. The same results occurred following thioTepa or mitozolomide treatment at 22 and 32 days after injection,

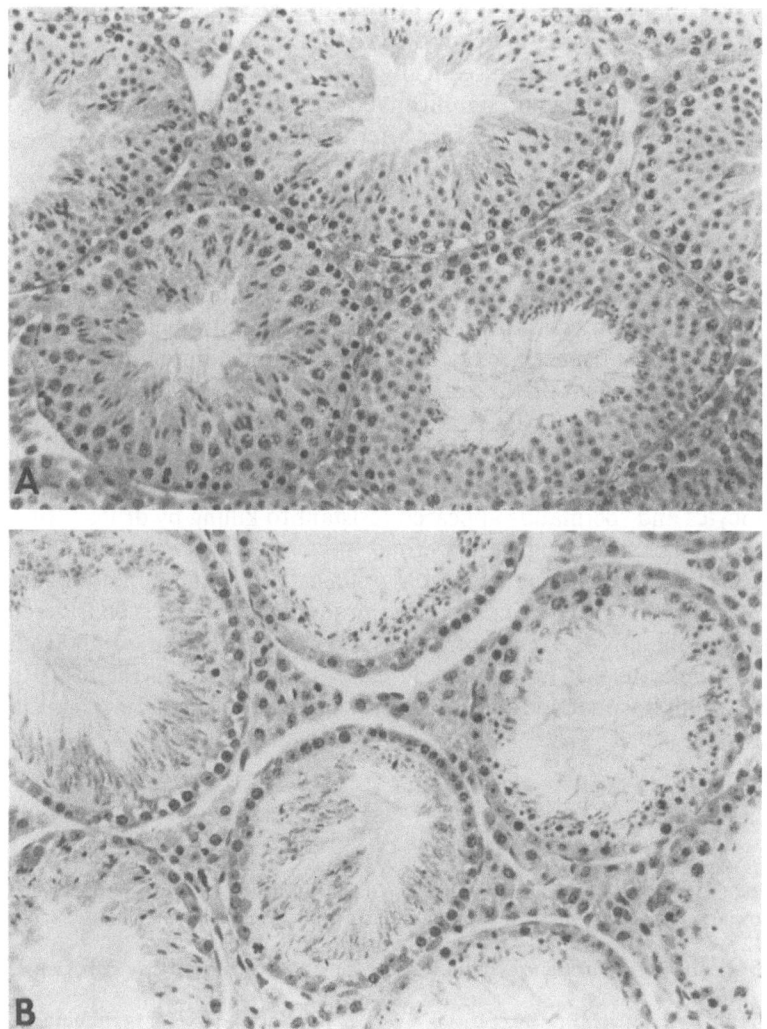

Fig. 3. Cross section of mouse testis (H & E). **a** Control, × 500. **b** Mitozolomide (40 mg/kg), × 700

but not following treatment with MeCCNU or 5-FU. The diameter of the seminiferous tubules of the testes of mice treated with cyclophosphamide showed an apparent decrease at 23 and 31 days (Fig. 2). There was a significant depression in the diameter of seminiferous tubules in mice treated with mitozolomide and thioTepa at 22 and 32 days after injection. No significant depression was seen in the tubule diameters in mice treated with MeCCNU and 5-FU.

The most significant damage with cyclophosphamide treatment was at 23 days. There was disorganization of the spermatogenic epithelium and dislodgement of different cell types which concentrate in the lumen of the tubules. The single layer attached to the basement membrane consisted of Sertoli cells and some stem cells. At day 22 thioTepa and mitozolomide (Fig. 3) caused a depletion in spermatogonia, spermatocytes and early spermatids, resulting in a decrease in germinal epithelial size. Sertoli cells appeared to be unaffected and stem cells only marginally affected. By contrast, 5-FU only caused a slight decrease in the number of late spermatids, while MeCCNU had no significant effect. All damaged testes showed signs of recovery by approximately 7 weeks after treatment.

Discussion

Anticancer drugs are known to produce germinal epithelial damage (Schilsky et al. 1980). The results presented in this study are consistent with such reports and show clearly that three anticancer drugs, cyclophosphamide, mitozolomide and thiotepa, have cytotoxic effects on the testis, while MeCCNU and 5-FU have only slight effects.

The differentiated spermatogonia were the most sensitive cells to the drugs, a finding similar to previous studies (Lu and Meistrich 1979; Meistrich et al. 1982). Late spermatocytes and spermatids appeared resistant to killing by drugs. Mitozolamide is a new anticancer drug, with a broad spectrum of activity against murine tumours, which is at present undergoing clinical trials. The predominant mechanism by which this group of compounds produces cell death is considered to be alkylation of the DNA. This observation is confirmed by the results from this study which indicate that mitozolomide has similar effects on the testis to those seen with cyclophosphamide and thioTepa, suggesting a similar mechanism of action.

References

Etteldorf JN, West CD, Pitcock JA, Williams DL (1976) Gonadal function, testicular histology and meiosis following cyclophosphamide therapy in patients with nephrotic syndrome. J Pediatr 88(2):206–212
Lu CL, Meistrich ML (1979) Cytotoxic effects of chemotherapeutic drugs on mouse testis cells. Cancer Res 39:3575–3582
Meistrich ML, Finch M, daCunha MF, Hacker U, Au WW (1982) Damaging effects of 14 chemotherapeutic drugs on mouse testis cells. Cancer Res 42:122–131
Schilsky RL, Lewis BJ, Sherins RJ, Young RC (1980) Gonadal dysfunction in patients receiving chemotherapy for cancer. Ann Intern Med 93(1):109–114

Mechanisms and Models in Toxicology
Arch. Toxicol., Suppl. 11, 281–284 (1987)
© by Springer-Verlag 1987

1,3-Dinitrobenzene: Toxicity and Metabolism in Rat Testicular Cell Cultures

S. C. Lloyd and P. M. D. Foster

Central Toxicology Laboratory, Imperial Chemical Industries plc, Alderley Park, Macclesfield, Cheshire, SK10 4TJ, UK

Introduction

1,3-Dinitrobenzene (DNB) is a testicular toxicant in rats (Cody et al. 1981), the initial response being located in the Sertoli cell (Blackburn et al. 1985; Foster et al. 1986). DNB in rabbits is metabolised principally by nitroreduction (Parke 1961). The purpose of these experiments was to study the effects of DNB and several putative metabolites in Sertoli-germ cell co-cultures of rat testis. Having established a morphological response by addition of DNB, further metabolic studies with radiolabelled compound were conducted in vitro.

Materials

DNB was purchased from Aldrich Chemical, Gillingham, Dorset, UK, and recrystallised to >99% purity as assessed using gas chromatography mass spectroscopy. Ring [^{14}C]DNB (>99% pure) was purchased from ICI Physics and Radioisotope Service, Billingham, Teeside, UK. Putative metabolites [as indicated by Parke (1961) for the rabbit], viz. m-nitroaniline (m-NA), m-phenylenediamine (m-PD), 2,4-dinitrophenol (DNP), 2,4-diaminophenol (DAP), 4-amino-2-nitrophenol (4A2NP), and 2-amino-4-nitrophenol (2A4NP) were purchased from Aldrich and used as supplied.

Methods

Sertoli-germ cell co-cultures were prepared according to Gray and Beamand (1984) using testes from 28-day-old Alpk:AP (Wistar-derived) rats. Following incubation for 24 h, serum-free medium was added containing appropriate concentrations of DNB or other compounds. Previous tissue distribution studies had indicated that peak blood and testis concentrations of radiolabel following a single oral dose of 50 mg DNB/kg b.w. were approximately 5 and 2×10^{-5} M, respectively.

[^{14}C]DNB (specific activity 51.6 mCi/mmol) was added to Sertoli-germ cell cultures at 10^{-6}, 10^{-5} and 10^{-4} M and radiolabel was monitored in medium, attached cells and detached cells over a 24-h period. Aliquots of fractions (10 µl) were spotted on thin-layer chromatography (TLC) plates and developed in toluene:ethyl acetate (5:1, v/v). Metabolites obtained from medium were extracted and concentrated; their identities were assigned following GCMS. As a control DNB was incubated at 32 °C in culture medium in the absence of cells.

Results

Addition of DNB to the cultures resulted in a significant increase in germ cell detachment from the Sertoli cell monolayer in a dose-related manner at DNB concentrations of 5×10^{-6} M to 10^{-4} M. The viability of detached cells varied from 96% to 66% (control 91%), suggesting that the germ cell release was not due to cytotoxicity. The morphological pattern of response was analogous to that reported for DNB in vivo (Foster et al. 1986) and similar to that previously observed in vitro with other Sertoli cell toxicants (Gray and Beamand 1984). None of the putative metabolites at concentrations of 10^{-5} or 10^{-6} M showed a morphological pattern of response similar to DNB, although some showed a general cytotoxicity at 10^{-4} M.

Metabolism studies indicated some incorporation of radiolabel into plated cells (maximally 1% of dose) and detached cells (maximally 0.1% of dose). Polar metabolites were produced in culture medium (Fig. 1). These were noted as two major spots (M1 and M2) each of which by 24 h constituted 3% of the total radiolabel present in the medium, with a further 3% remaining at the origin. M1 and

Table 1. Effect of DNB and some of its postulated metabolites on Sertoli-germ cell culture morphology

Agent	Concentration (M)	Culture morphology
DNB	5×10^{-4}–10^{-6}	Dose-related germ cell loss, vacuolated Sertoli cell monolayer, presence of "included" germ cells
	10^{-6}	Minimal cell loss, some Sertoli cell vacuolation
	10^{-7}	As control
m-NA	10^{-4}–10^{-6}	As control
m-PD	10^{-4}–10^{-6}	As control
DNP	10^{-4}	Monolayer disruption, patches of Sertolic cells with normal germ cell complement
	10^{-5}, 10^{-6}	As control
2A4NP	10^{-4}–10^{-6}	As control
4A2NP	10^{-4}	Same focal disruption of Sertoli cell monolayer
	10^{-5}, 10^{-5}	As control
DAP	10^{-4}	Complete cytotoxicity
	10^{-5}, 10^{-6}	As control

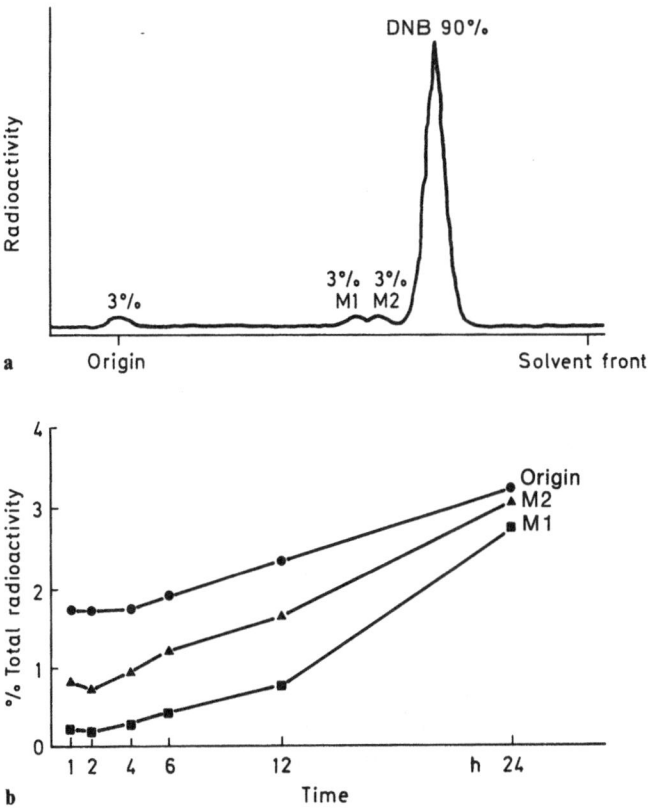

Fig. 1. a Radiochromatogramm of culture medium 24 h after exposure to 10^{-4} M DNB. M1 and M2 refer to polar metabolites. **b** Time course for the development of radioactivity associated with metabolites

M2 have been identified as *m*-nitroacetanilide and *m*-nitroaniline (*m*-NA), respectively. These compounds were without toxicity when returned to the culture system at doses up to 10^{-4} *M*. A similar pattern of metabolites has since been obtained from Sertoli cell cultures with no degradation of DNB in culture medium incubated in the absence of cells. The scheme shown in Fig. 2 is proposed for the metabolism of DNB in Sertoli cells; it is based on Mason and Josephy (1984).

Conclusions

1. The in vivo effects of DNB can be effectively modelled using a Sertoli-germ cell culture system.
2. The in vitro response with DNB occurred at and below concentrations equimolar with peak levels of radioactivity seen in blood and testis after a single, testicular toxic dose of DNB.
3. The response could not be reproduced with putative metabolites of DNB.
4. The culture system(s) is capable of xenobiotic metabolism.

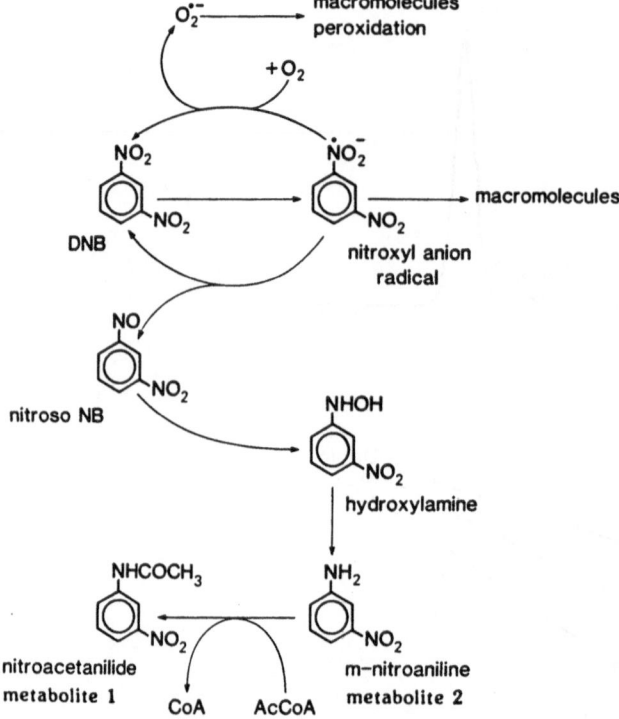

Fig. 2. Proposed scheme for the metabolism of DNB in Sertoli cells (after Mason and Josephy 1984)

5. DNB or a Sertoli cell metabolite (probably a reactive intermediate of nitroreduction produced in situ) is responsible for the observed testicular damage.

References

Blackburn DM, Lloyd SC, Gray AJ, Foster PMD (1985) Testicular toxicity of 1,3-dinitrobenzene in
    the rat. Toxicologist 5:121
Cody TE, Witherup S, Hastings L, Stemmer K, Christian RT (1981) 1,3-Dinitrobenzene: toxic effects
    in vivo and in vitro. J Toxicol Environ Health 7:829–847
Foster PMD, Sheard CM, Lloyd SC (1986) 1,3-Dinitrobenzene: a Sertoli cell toxicant? Excerpta Med
    Int Congr Ser (to be published)
Gray TJB, Beamand JA (1984) Effect of some phthalate esters and other testicular toxins on primary
    cultures of testicular cells. Fd Chem Toxicol 22:123–131
Mason RP, Josephy PD (1984) Free radical mechanism of nitroreductase. In: Rickert DE (ed) Toxicity
    of nitroaromatic compounds. Hemisphere, Washington, pp 121–140
Parke DV (1961) Studies in detoxication. 85. The metabolism of m-dinitro[^{14}C]benzene in the rabbit.
    Biochem J 78:262–271

Mechanisms and Models in Toxicology
Arch. Toxicol., Suppl. 11, 285–287 (1987)
© by Springer-Verlag 1987

Collagen Synthesis in Rats with Silica-Induced Pulmonary Fibrosis

A. Poole

Department of Toxicology, Smith Kline and French Research Ltd., The Frythe, Welwyn, Herts., AL6 9AR, UK

Introduction

Fibrotic disease in a complex phenomenon involving increases in the synthesis, accumulation and deposition of collagen (Prockop et al. 1979). Although much effort has been expended in studying the biochemistry of fibrotic lung disease (Laurent 1982), it has proven difficult to correlate histological observations with biochemical determinations or to find sensitive, quantitative bioassays for detecting (pre)-fibrotic changes. It has been suggested that elevations in the levels of enzymes involved in collagen biosynthesis, e.g. prolyl hydroxylase and lysyl oxidase, can be used as indicators of early changes in fibrosis (Counts et al. 1981; Chichester et al. 1981). In a series of experiments the relationship between alterations in the activities of three enzymes involved in collagen biosynthesis, the accumulation of collagen measured as hydroxyproline and histological changes occurring during the development of silica-induced pulmonary fibrosis were investigated.

Materials and Methods

Animals

Fischer F344 rats, originally from Charles River Breeding Laboratories, Wilmington, USA, bred under barrier-maintained conditions and free from pulmonary infection were used in the study.

Treatment

Male rats (10 weeks old) were randomly allocated to silica-treated and control groups. They were anaesthetized with ether and 0.5 ml of a sterile suspension of silica [DQ12 standard sample of silica as prepared by Robock (1973)] in phosphate-buffered saline (PBS; 25 or 50 mg/ml) was instilled by tracheotomy. Control animals received 0.5 ml sterile PBS. At 24 h and 3, 6, 12 and 24 weeks after treatment six control and six treated animals were anaesthetized and bled out of the right ventricle into heparinized tubes. The samples were centrifuged and the plasma was removed and frozen for later enzyme analysis. The lungs were perfused with PBS and then processed for histology or assayed for hydroxyproline content and lysyl oxidase, prolylhydroxylase and galactosylhydroxylysyl glucosyltransferase (GGT) activities. Techniques have been described in detail elsewhere (Poole et al. 1985). Student's t test was used to assess the significance of the differences between the means of the various groups of data.

Results and Discussion

The results show that the levels of the three enzymes in the treated animals were significantly higher than the controls at each time point (Fig. 1). Total lung collagen determined as mean hydroxyproline content showed an increase as the animals reached maturity, but differences between treated and control rats only reached significance at week 24 (Fig. 2). The lung sections showed cellular infiltrates and alveolar lipoproteinosis, which increased in extent and severity with time, but it was not until 12 and 24 weeks after treatment that the silica-exposed animals showed evidence of frank pulmonary fibrosis, i.e. areas of conglomerate completely acellular fibrosis. Circulatory levels of lysyl oxidase and GGT, although increased in the silica-exposed animals, often failed to achieve statistical significance. Investigators studying the acute effects of silica-induced pulmonary fibrosis have reported increased rates of collagen synthesis as early as 5 and 2 weeks following treatment (Halme et al. 1970; Reiser et al. 1982). The results of the studies reported here, however, show that it is possible to demonstrate qualitative and quantitative differences in the activities of collagen-synthesising enzymes in the lungs of silica-treated animals as early as 24 h after exposure. Thus, measurements of these enzymes may be used as a sensitive method for detecting (pre)fibrotic changes occurring in the lungs of animals with experimental fibrosis. Because the time scale of changes is so short, it is possible that such measurements

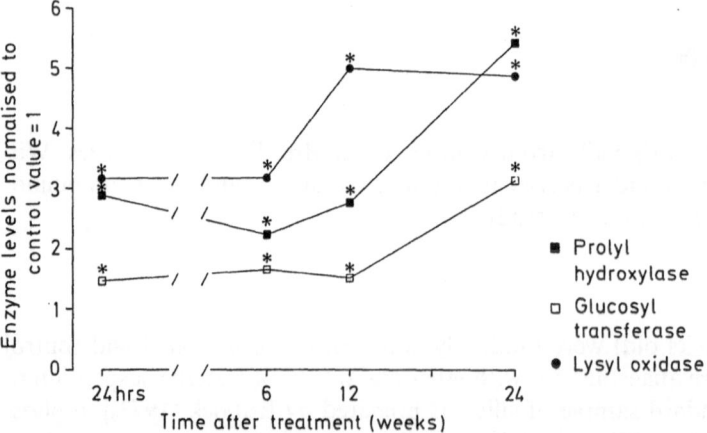

Fig. 1. Sequential changes in the lung activities of GGT, prolyl 4-hydroxylase and lysyl oxidase in rats exposed to a single intratracheal dose of silica (DQ12) or saline. Data are expressed as means of six animals per treatment group at each time. *, $p < 0.05$; assessed using Student's t test

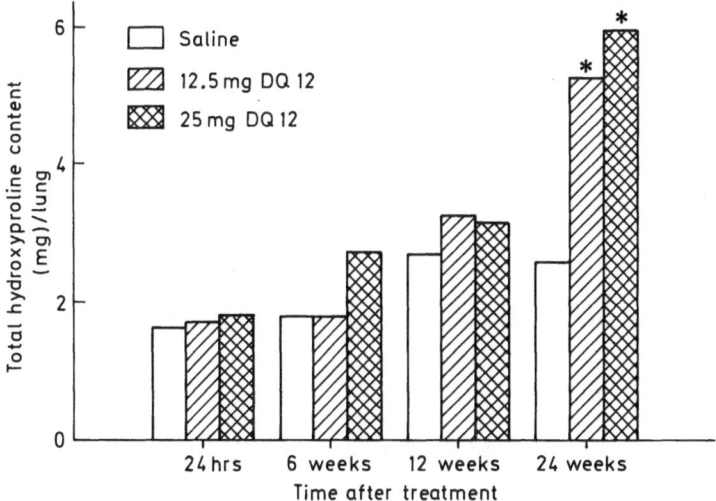

Fig. 2. Fischer F344 rats received a single intratracheal instillation of saline, silica (12.5 mg) or silica (25 mg). At various time points animals ($n = 6$) were killed and the total lung collagen was determined from hydroxyproline content. *, $p < 0.05$; assessed by using Student's t test

could provide sensitive, quantitative and rapid indications of shifts in collagen production which may prove useful for the development of short-term bioassays for the detection of potential fibrogenic materials.

In conclusion, the results of these studies demonstrate that, in experimental lung fibrosis, excess collagen deposition and accumulation is due to the increased synthesis of collagen and that the biosynthesis of the protein occurs rapidly, preceding by many weeks any histological evidence of disease.

References

Chichester CL, Palmer KC, Hayes JA, Kagan HM (1981) Lung lysyl oxidase and prolyl hydroxylase increases induced by calcium chloride inhalation and the effect of β-aminoproprionitrile in rats. Am Rev Respir Dis 124:709–713

Counts DF, Evans JM, Dipetrillo TA, Sterling KM, Kelley JR, Jason K (1981) Collagen lysyl oxidase activity in the lung increases during bleomycin-induced lung fibrosis. J Pharmacol Exp Ther 219:675–678

Halme J, Uitto J, Kahanpaa K, Karhunen P, Lindy S (1970) Protocollagen proline hydroxylase activity in experimental pulmonary fibrosis in rats. J Lab Clin Med 75:535–541

Laurent GJ (1982) Collagen in normal lung and during pulmonary fibrosis. In: Cumming G, Bonsignore G (eds) Proceedings of the fifth course of the international school of thoracic medicine. Plenum, New York, p 311

Poole A, Myllyla R, Wagner JC, Brown RC (1985) Collagen biosynthesis enzymes in lung tissue and serum of rats with experimental silicosis. Br J Exp Pathol 66:567–575

Prockop DJ, Kivirikko KI, Tuderman L, Guzman NA (1979) The biosynthesis of collagen and its disorders (second of two parts). N Engl J Med 301:77–85

Reiser KM, Hesterberg TW, Haschek WM, Last JA (1982) Experimental silicosis I. Acute effects of intratracheally instilled quartz on collagen metabolism and morphological characteristics of rat lungs. Am J Pathol 107:176–185

Robock K (1973) Standard quartz for experimental pneumoconiosis research projects in the Federal Republic of Germany. Am Occup Hyg 16:63–66

Mechanisms and Models in Toxicology
Arch. Toxicol., Suppl. 11, 288–291 (1987)

Pulmonary Toxicity of Naphthalene Derivatives in the Rat

D. Dinsdale and R. D. Verschoyle

MRC Toxicology Unit, Woodmansterne Road, Carshalton, Surrey SM5 4EF, UK

Introduction

The intraperitoneal administration of naphthalene (N) or N-derivatives damages the bronchiolar epithelium of mice (Rasmussen et al. 1986). The bronchiolar epithelium of rats is unaffected by naphthalene (O'Brien et al. 1985), but Clara cell necrosis has been described after administration of 1-nitronaphthalene (1NN; 100 mg/kg) to Sprague-Dawley rats (Johnson et al. 1984).

Materials and Methods

Female Wistar-derived rats (LAC:P) were injected, intraperitoneally, with a single dose of 0.5 mmol/kg body weight of 1NN, or 1mmol/kg body weight of 2-nitronaphthalene (2NN), 1-methylnaphthalene (1MN), or 2-methylnaphthalene (2MN), or 3 mmol/kg body weight of N. Compounds were obtained from Aldrich Chemical, Gillingham, UK and were 97% pure. The rats were killed 24 h later and sampled for microscopy (Dinsdale et al. 1984).

Results

The LD_{50} of 1NN was 150 mg/kg. A dose of 0.5 mmol (86.6 mg) 1NN/kg, in arachis oil, resulted in piloerection and respiratory distress within 4 h. At 24 h the rats had lost weight, their coats had become poor and they were panting. Pulmonary lesions were restricted to the bronchiolar epithelium (Fig. 1a), but damage was equally severe in all generations of bronchioles. Both ciliated and non-ciliated cells were injured and their detachment (Fig. 1b) resulted in discrete areas of exposed basement membrane (Fig. 1c). Ciliated cells had particularly contorted nuclei and their electron-dense, autophagosomes (Fig. 1d) were more numerous and much larger (up to 5 µm in diameter) than those found in control animals. Many of these cells contained focal concentrations of condensed apical cytoplasm rich

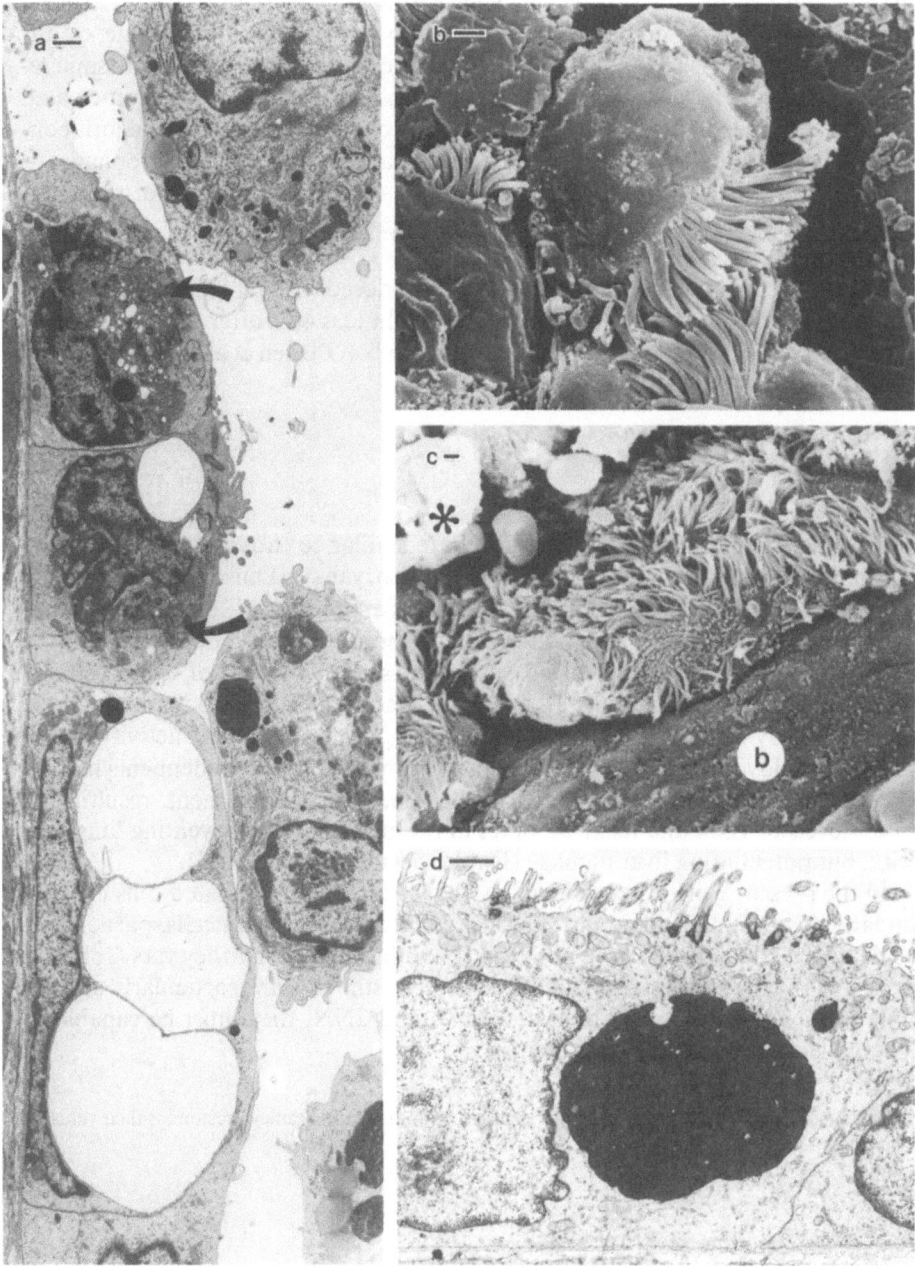

Fig. 1 a–d. Bronchiolar lining of a rat, 24 h after an intraperitoneal dose of 86.6 mg 1-nitronaphthalene/kg body weight. **a** Exposure of the basement membrane and vacuolation of the epithelial cells with focal concentrations of cytoplasm (*arrows*) in two ciliated cells. **b** Ciliated cells, detached from the basement membrane, lying on the surface of the epithelium. **c** The edge of an exposed area of basement membrane (**b**) with injured epithelial cells and part of the overlying "raft" (*) of cell debris and mucus. **d** Ciliated cell containing an electron-dense autophagosome. *Bars*, 1 μm

in cilia and cytoplasmic axonemes, which were not membrane-limited. Severe damage was often found adjacent to apparently normal cells of the same, or different, type. Lesions usually involved vacuolation of the smooth endoplasmic reticulum; few of the characteristic dense granules were retained in non-ciliated cells. The surviving bronchiolar epithelium was overlaid by a "raft" of debris containing little fibrin, but many damaged epithelial cells and a few macrophages.

Rats dosed with 2NN lost weight, without obvious respiratory distress, but produced lesions throughout the epithelium similar to those found after administration of 1NN.

Lesions were not detected in the lungs of rats dosed with N, 1MN or 2MN. The animals appeared normal except for slight weight loss 48 h after dosing. Necrotic Clara cells have been reported in mice after both N (O'Brien et al. 1985) and 2MN (Buckpitt et al. 1986).

Discussion

The changes found after 1NN and 2NN are similar to those reported after the inhalation of some toxic gases, notably methyl isocyanate (Dinsdale et al. in press).

The development of these lesions within cells exposed to different xenobiotics, via different routes, indicates a non-specific response to injury. Epithelial cells are in immediate contact with inhaled gases, but selective injury of Clara cells by many xenobiotics is commonly attributed to the intracellular production of toxic metabolites by the high level of cytochrome P_{450} mono-oxygenase activity within these cells (Boyd 1980). The metabolism of 1NN by P_{450}-dependent enzymes, in the liver, is indicated by the effect of phenobarbital pretreatment, resulting in lower levels of 1NN and its metabolites in rat lung, thereby preventing lung toxicity, but potentiating liver damage (Dankovic and Cornish 1982).

In the present work it seems unlikely that the damage to ciliated cells is a secondary effect of toxic metabolites produced by adjacent Clara cells, particularly as damaged ciliated cells have not been found in Sprague-Dawley rats (Johnson et al. 1984). Thus, unless the ciliated cells of Wistar rats are particularly susceptible to the circulating metabolites of 1NN and 2NN, they must be capable of metabolising these compounds themselves.

Acknowledgements. We are grateful to Jane Ingham, Brian Biles and Stanley Preston for their valuable assistance.

References

Boyd MR (1980) Biochemical mechanisms of chemical-induced lung injury. CRC Crit Rev Toxicol 7:103–176
Buckpitt AR, Bahnson LS, Franklin RB (1986) Comparison of the arachidonic acid and NADPH-dependent microsomal metabolism of naphthalene and 2-methylnaphthalene and the effect of indomethacin on the bronchiolar necrosis. Biochem Pharmacol 35:645–650
Dankovic D, Cornish HH (1982) Phenobarbital alterations of 1-nitronaphthalene levels in target organs of toxicity. Toxicologist 2:129

Dinsdale D, Nemery B, Sparrow S (1987) Ultrastructural changes in the respiratory tract of rats following methyl isocyanate inhalation. Arch Toxicol 59:385–390

Dinsdale D, Verschoyle RD, Ingham JE (1984) Ultrastructural changes in rat Clara cells induced by a single dose of O,S,S-trimethyl phosphorodithioate. Arch Toxicol 56:59–65

Johnson DE, Riley MGI, Cornish HH (1984) Acute organ toxicity of 1-nitronaphthalene in the rat. J Appl Toxicol 4:253–257

O'Brien KAF, Smith LL, Cohen GM (1985) Differences in naphthalene-induced toxicity in the mouse and rat. Chem Biol Interact 55:109–122

Rasmussen RE, Do DH, Kim TS (1986) Comparative cytotoxicity of naphthalene and its monomethyl- and mononitro-derivatives in the mouse lung. J Appl Toxicol 6:13–20

Mechanisms and Models in Toxicology
Arch. Toxicol., Suppl. 11, 292–294 (1987)

Toxicology Information for the Canadian Workforce

W. J. Louch, R. Whiting, and D. M. Halton

3 Material Hazards Section, Canadian Centre for Occupational Health and Safety,
250 Main Street East, Hamilton, Ontario, Canada, L8N 1H6

Introduction

Non-technical people in government and industry often need to know, understand, and apply toxicology information. The complexity of this information has impeded its utilization in the workplace. Existing information systems such as bibliographic databases, scientific journals, educational and other texts are directed primarily at the toxicologist or occupational health professional and not to the workforce which may have little or no scientific background.

The Material Hazards Section of the Canadian Centre for Occupational Health and Safety uses several approaches to ensure that toxicology information, concepts and knowledge are expressed in terms appropriate for understanding and use by lay people.

Methods

The approaches presently used and under development are as follows:

One-to-One Contact

The Centre provides direct contact between a member of the workforce having a specific concern and a scientist with expertise in that area. The scientist reviews the data, highlights the present state of knowledge and selects the points of importance. Finally, a letter or phone call will convey an explanation, advice or opinion on any necessary course of action. Any correspondence is written in simple language using lay terminology. It is edited to ensure that scientific concepts and knowledge are adequately explained in terms that will be understood by the inquirer.

This one-to-one contact with the lay person provides valuable insight for the subject specialist into the types of concerns about workplace chemicals. This insight is the basis for developing new approaches to information dissemination.

Hazard Summaries

Documents are prepared presenting information on the hazards and precautions necessary when using particular industrial chemicals. The "Hazard Summaries" are in two parts. The first is a single page describing the major features and hazards of the chemical; the second part gives a more detailed review of the scientific literature relating to the chemical.

Databases

There is a great need to develop computerized resources containing toxicology information that can be understood and applied by workers. Substantial efforts in this area are presently underway. One database, called TN (trade names), provides manufacturers' information on the potential hazards to people working with a particular proprietary product and on the necessary safety precautions. TN duplicates the complete contents of Material Safety Data Sheets which are provided voluntarily by chemical producers. TN contains information on about 20000 products (as at April 1986). A second database, CHEMINFO, provides practical information on pure chemicals. It describes the properties, reactivity, exposure limits, toxicity, personal protection, storage, handling and first aid treatment in relatively non-technical language (Halton 1986).

Educational Documents

Several documents have been published as part of a projected series of educational modules that describe the basic principles and concepts of toxicology and how they apply to workplace exposures.

Videotex

Several of the printed educational documents have also formed the basis of videotex presentations. Videotex is the rapidly developing technology which uses computer graphics and animation to present information in clear, easily understood ways. This medium greatly enhances the educational material by presenting toxicological principles and concepts with attractive, illustrative graphics.

Results

Some of the products described are already available to the Canadian public and the demand for this kind of information has proved considerable. The numbers of requests made for one-to-one consultation with a chemical hazards subject expert rose from 1300 in 1983 to 3500 in 1985. The number of people requesting this service in 1985 showed an almost twofold increase from the previous year. The requests for Hazard Summaries and educational document publications increased dramatically from 1000 in 1983 to 3000 in 1984. In 1985, almost 17000 toxicology education and Hazard Summary documents were distributed to the Canadian workforce.

Discussion

Toxicology is a complex science. Its complexity has impeded its use in the work-place and has given rise to demands for easily understood, practical informa-tion.

In Canada, workplace chemical hazard information is now available in forms that are appropriate for use by workers. Experience with this kind of information indicates that careful explanation of technical concepts and data is an essential and important step in the distribution of toxicology knowledge for the benefit of workplace health and safety.

References

Halton DM (1986) Computerized information resources in toxicology and industrial health – a review. Toxicol Ind Health 2:113–125

Mechanisms and Models in Toxicology
Arch. Toxicol., Suppl. 11, 295–299 (1987)

Predicting the Safety of Medicines from Animal Toxicity Tests I. Rodents Alone

C. E. Lumley and S. R. Walker

Centre for Medicines Research, Woodmansterne Road, Carshalton, Surrey, SM5 4DS, UK

Introduction

New potential therapeutic candidates are evaluated for safety in several animal species to generate information that may alert clinicians to potential hazards, the implication being that particular animal species have significant predictive value for toxicity in man. Surprisingly, few published studies have attempted to examine the qualitative predictability of human side effects from animal tests. The most substantial data refer to anti-cancer drugs, which are designed to induce cellular damage, and these data cannot be made the basis for making generalisations to other pharmaceutical compounds. Studies reported in the literature for drugs other than anti-neoplastics are summarised in Table 1. The studies by Litchfield (1961), Suter (1983) and Laurence et al. (1984) are constrained by the small number of compounds, and those by Cuthbert (1974) and Griffin (1985) by dependence solely on the literature data. The study by Bein et al. (1971) compares the results of animal tests carried out between 1959 and 1962 with data obtained from subsequent clinical trials; as testing procedures and criteria of assessment have changed considerably since that time, the relevance of this study to the current situation is debatable.

The Centre for Medicines Research (CMR) has already established a toxicology databank comprising detailed information from repeated-dose animal studies obtained from pharmaceutical companies in Europe (Lumley and Walker 1985 a). Results of analyses of these data show that there is little, if any, value in continuing studies beyond 6 months as, providing they are carefully designed, all salient effects are observed within this time period (Lumley and Walker 1985 b, 1986 a, 1986 b). In order to assess how well these animal safety evaluations predict adverse effects observed in man, the CMR has initiated a project to compare data from repeated-dose animal toxicity studies with clinical adverse findings at both the pre- and post-marketing stages. This paper reports the first stage of the project, an investigation of a possible methodology.

Table 1. Published studies comparing findings in animal studies with ADRs in man

Number of compounds	Therapeutic class	Source of data	Conclusions	Reference
6	Various	Author's laboratory	Several serious clinical effects were not foreseeable from studies in dogs or rats	Litchfield (1961)
113	Various	5 Pharmaceutical companies	In 84% of studies, clinical trials confirmed predictions of animal studies conducted 1959–1962	Bein et al. (1971)
11	NSAID	Literature	Animal tests predicted GI toxicity but were of limited value in detecting toxicity in several other body organ systems	Cuthbert (1974)
45	Various	CTC and PL applications	There were correlations between toxic effects in animals and ADRs in man, but the analyses are open to criticism	Fletcher (1978)
6	Various	Author's laboratory	One-third of clinically relevant side effects were not detected in animals	Suter (1983)
7	CVS	Literature, yellow cards	For some drugs all ADRs were predicted in animal studies; in others there was almost total failure of animal studies to predict human ADRs	Griffin (1985)
7	Various	4 Pharmaceutical companies	For 3 drugs, animal studies accurately predicted the absence of major toxicity in humans; for 1 data from animal studies were useful in predicting the human response. For 2 drugs, some side effects were not predicted and for 1 animal studies did not predict a major side effect	Laurence et al. (1984)

ADRs, adverse drug reactions; CTC, clinical trial certificates; CVS, cardiovascular system; GI, gastrointestinal system; NSAID, non-steroidal anti-inflammatory drug; PL, product licence.

Methodology

The CMR databank contains information from repeated-dose toxicity studies for 82 compounds with extensive clinical experience, including 54 marketed compounds. Twenty-nine of these have been identified to the CMR and relevant details are shown in Table 2. In order to establish a possible methodology for a larger study, the 29 compounds were grouped together, irrespective of therapeutic class, duration of rat studies or years on the market. Clinical side effects, compiled from the ABPI Data Sheet Compendium 1985–1986 (Anonymous 1985) and from Myler's Side Effects of Drugs (Dukes 1980), were tabulated by body system, together, with the findings from the rat studies. Six body systems were chosen for comparison: central nervous (CNS), cardiovascular (CVS), gastrointestinal (GI),

Table 2. Details of the 29 compounds included in the study

Therapeutic class	Study compound	Maximum duration of rat tests (months)	Years on UK market
Non-steroidal anti-inflammatories (5)	1	6	8.5
	2	6	17
	3	24	7
	4	24	4
	5	12	12.5
Other central nervous system agents (3)	1	12	17
	2	24	8
	3	24	3
Anti-infectives (8)	1	6	8
	2	6	12
	3	6	4
	4	6	14
	5	3	7
	6	6	17
	7	3	?
	8	6	4
Cardiovascular system agents (3)	1	24	11
	2	18	9
	3	6	6
Respiratory drugs (2)	1	6	17
	2	6	19
Skin (1)	1	24	2
Cytotoxics/immunosuppressants (2)	1	24	3
	2	18	23
Endocrine agents (1)	1	24	10
Gastrointestinal system drugs (3)	1	18	4.5
	2	12	9.5
	3	18	3.5
Anti-allergics (1)	1	18	18

liver, respiratory (RS) and urinary (US). Correlations between the rat and man were divided into four categories, as defined by Schein et al. (1970): true positive (TP, toxicity observed in both animals and man); false positive (FP, toxicity observed in animals, but not in man); true negative (TN, no toxicity observed in animals or man), false negative (FN, toxicity not observed in animals, but found in man). While specific effects were not compared for a given compound, any effect on a body system in rats was considered a true positive if any adverse effect on that body system had been noted in man.

Results

To examine underprediction by the animal studies, the number of compounds with a false negative correlation was related to the total number of compounds

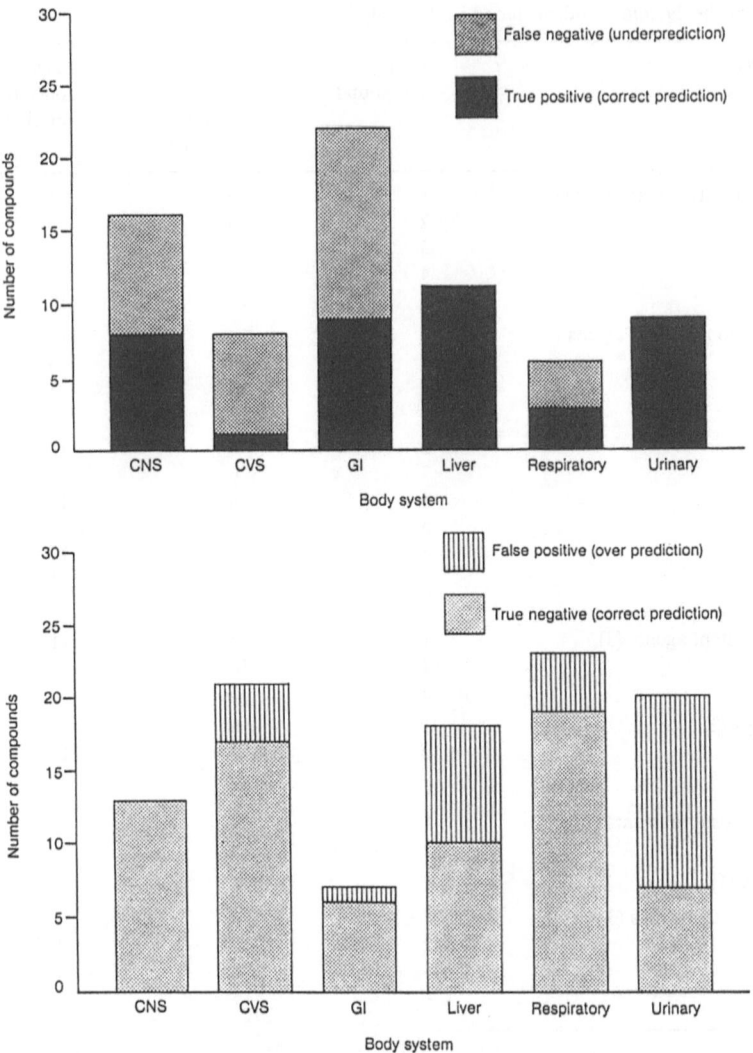

Fig. 1. Under- and overprediction in 29 rat studies. *%UP*, percentage underprediction; *%OP*, percentage overprediction; *CNS*, central nervous system; *CVS*, cardiovascular system; *GI*, gastrointestinal system

with a clinical side effect on each body system and the percentage underprediction (%UP) was calculated as:

%UP = [FN/(FN+TP)] × 100

The number of compounds with a false positive result was related to the total number without a clinical side effect on each body system and the percentage overprediction (%OP) was calculated as:

%OP = [FP/(FP+TN)] × 100

Under- and overprediction are shown in Fig. 1.

Discussion

Due to the small number of compounds in this study and the diverse therapeutic classes and duration of tests, it is not possible to draw definitive conclusions regarding the ability of repeated-dose toxicity tests in rats to predict clinical effects in each of the body systems examined. However, within these limitations, the rat correctly predicted all the compounds with clinical effects on the liver or urinary system, with some overprediction. Only half of the compounds with effects on the central nervous, gastrointestinal or respiratory systems and one of eight compounds with clinical side effects on the cardiovascular system were identified, although account has not been taken of animal pharmacology studies or other investigative tests which may well have identified these effects.

This methodology will be utilised to examine whether a change in study design or tests in a second species would improve the predictive value of animal studies. However, this study illustrates that it is inadequate to rely solely on repeated-dose toxicology and data sheet information. In a major study, all relevant toxicological data and pre- and post-marketing clinical ADRS will be collected directly from pharmaceutical companies.

Acknowledgements. The authors are grateful to the following companies for providing repeated-dose animal toxicity data for this study: Beecham Pharmaceuticals, The Boots Company PLC, Ciba-Geigy AG, Fisons Pharmaceuticals, Glaxo Group Research Ltd, Reckitt & Colman, F. Hoffman-LaRoche & Co, Sandoz Ltd, Smith Kline & French Research Ltd, Syntex (USA) Inc, Thomae GmbH and The Wellcome Research Laboratories

References

Anonymous (1985) ABPI Data sheet compendium 1985–1986. Datapharm, London

Bein HJ et al. (1971) Comparison of experimental and clinical findings: an analysis of clinical trial preparations. Proc Eur Soc Study Drug Toxicol 12:179–183

Cuthbert MF (1974) Adverse reactions of non-steroidal antirheumatic drugs. Curr Med Res Opin 2:600–609

Dukes MNG (1980) Myler's side effects of drugs, 9th edn. Excerpta Medica, Amsterdam

Fletcher AP (1978) Drug safety tests and subsequent clinical experience. J R Soc Med 71:693–696

Griffin JP (1985) Predictive value of animal toxicity studies. ATLA 12:163–170

Laurence DR, McLean AEM, Weatherall M (1984) Safety testing of new drugs. Academic, London

Litchfield JT (1961) Forecasting drug effects in man from studies in laboratory animals. JAMA 177:104–108

Lumley CE, Walker SR (1985a) A toxicology databank based on animal safety evaluation studies of pharmaceutical compounds. Human Toxicol 4:447–460

Lumley CE, Walker SR (1985b) The value of chronic animal toxicology studies of pharmaceutical compounds: a retrospective analysis. Fundam Appl Toxicol 5:1007–1024

Lumley CE, Walker SR (1986a) The questionable value of long-term animal toxicology studies – a regulatory dilemma. Arch Toxicol 59:237–239

Lumley CE, Walker SR (1986b) A critical appraisal of the duration of chronic animal toxicity studies. Regul Toxicol Pharmacol 6(1):66–72

Schein PS, Davis RD, Carter S, Newman J, Schein DR, Rall DP (1970) The evaluation of anti-cancer drugs in dogs and monkeys for the prediction of qualitative toxicities in man. Clin Pharmacol Ther 11:3–40

Suter KE (1983) Relevance of standard toxicological tests: comparison of the experimental and clinical data of six pharmaceutical preparations. In: Zbinden et al. (eds) Current problems in drug toxicology. Libbey, London

Mechanisms and Models in Toxicology
Arch. Toxicol., Suppl. 11, 300–304 (1987)

Predicting the Safety of Medicines from Animal Toxicity Tests II. Rodents and Non-Rodents

C. E. Lumley and S. R. Walker

Centre for Medicines Research, Woodmansterne Road,
Carshalton, Surrey SM5 4DS, UK

Introduction

Toxicity tests are routinely conducted in both a rodent and a non-rodent species before new medicines are administered to man, based on the assumption that these studies will predict any toxicity a clinician may subsequently encounter. In order to assess the ability of repeated-dose animal toxicity tests to predict adverse effects observed in man, the Centre for Medicines Research (CMR) has initiated a project to compare data from these animal tests with clinical adverse effects. The first stage, which investigated a possible methodology, is reported in the preceding paper. This methodology has been studied further to determine whether it is capable of demonstrating changes in under- and overprediction resulting from the utilisation of a second animal species.

Methodology

Of the 29 marketed compounds in the toxicology databank identified to the CMR, 20 were studied in both the rat and the dog, while 11 were investigated in the rat and a primate. Relevant details of the compounds and studies are shown in Table 1.

Clinical side effects for the two groups, those tested in rats/dogs and those tested in rats/primates, were compiled from the ABPI Data Sheet Compendium 1985–1986 (Anonymous 1985) and Myler's Side Effects of Drugs (Dukes 1980). These were compared with findings in the repeated-dose animal toxicology studies for six body systems: central nervous (CNS), cardiovascular (CVS), gastrointestinal (GI), liver, respiratory (RS) and urinary (US). Specific effects were not compared. Correlations were divided into the four categories defined by Schein et al. (1970): true positive (TP), false positive (FP), true negative (TN), and false negative (FN).

Table 1. Details of the compounds included in the study

Therapeutic class	Study	Maximum duration of animal tests			Years on UK market
		Rat	Dog	Primate	
I. Rat and dog					
NSAID (2)	1	6	6		17
	2	24	10		4
Other CNS drugs (3)	1	12	6		17
	2	24	12		8
	3	24	12		3
Anti-infectives (6)	1	6	6		8
	2	6	6		12
	3	6	6		4
	4	6	6		14
	5	3	3		7
	6	6	6		4
CVS agents (3)	1	24	12		11
	2	18	12		9
	3	6	6		6
Respiratory drugs (2)	1	6	12		17
	2	6	12		19
Cytotoxic/immunosuppressant (1)	1	24	12		3
Endocrine (1)	1	24	12		10
Gastrointestinal (2)	1	18	12		4.5
	2	12	12		9.5
II. Rat and primate					
NSAID (5)	1	6		12	8.5
	2	6		12	17
	3	24		12	7
	4	24		18	4
	5	12		12	12.5
Other CNS drugs (1)	1	24		6	8
Anti-infectives (2)	1	6		6	17
	2	3		3	?
Cytotoxic/immunosuppressant (1)	1	24		3	3
Endocrine (1)	1	24		3	10
Anti-allergic (1)	1	18		1	18

CNS, central nervous system; CVS, cardiovascular system; NSAID, non-steroidal anti-inflammatory drug

Results

The percentage underprediction (%UP) and overprediction (%OP) were calculated for the rat and the dog alone and for both together (Fig. 1). Of the 11 compounds tested in both rats and primates, six or more had clinical side effects on only the central nervous and gastrointestinal systems. Over- and underprediction in these two systems is shown in Fig. 2.

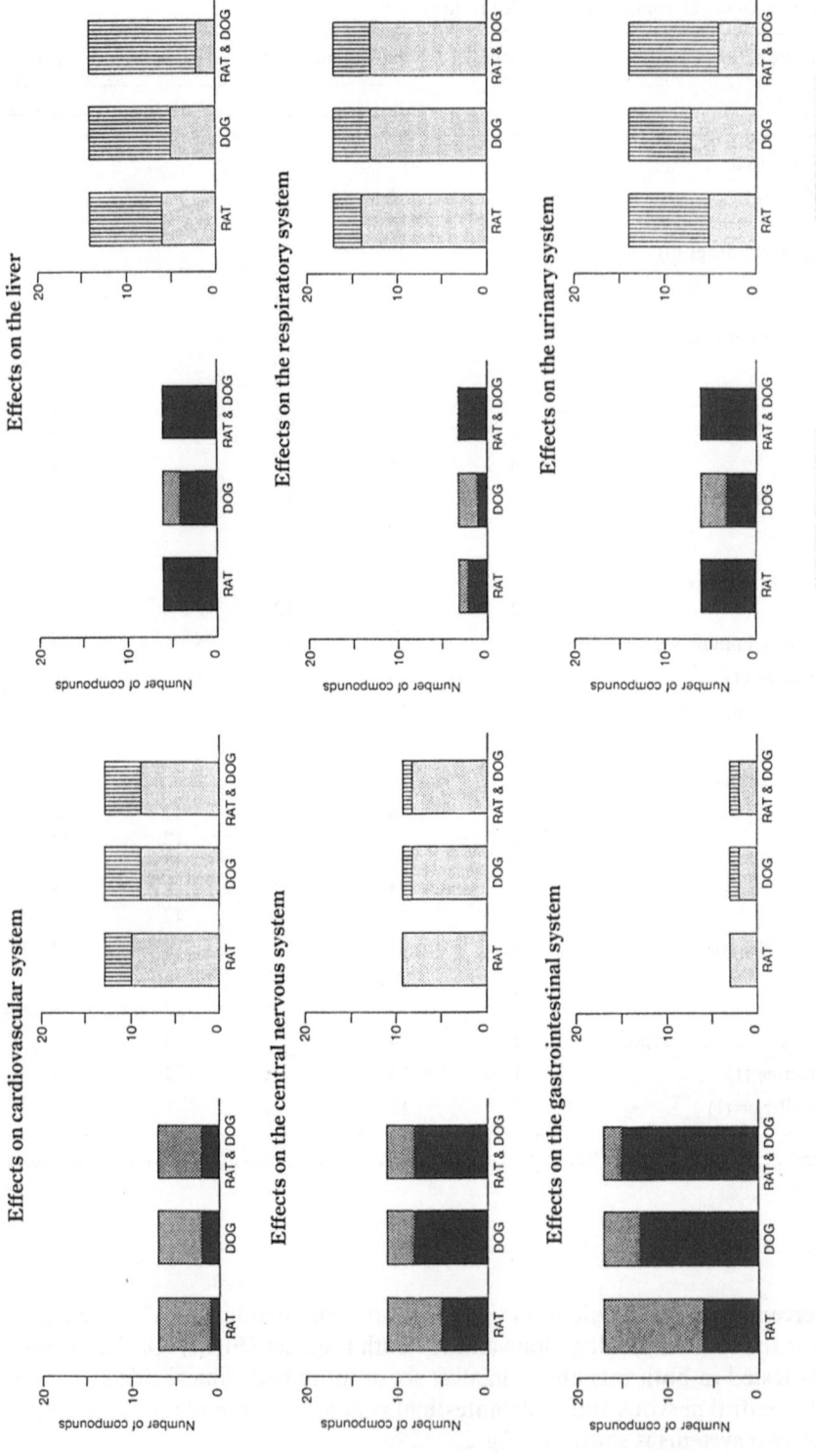

Fig. 1. Under- and overprediction in 20 studies in rats and dogs

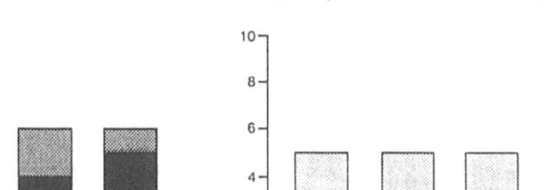

Effects on the central nervous system

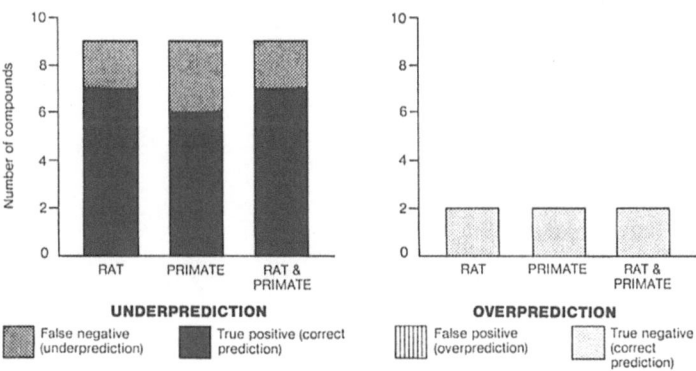

Fig. 2. Under- and overprediction in 11 studies in rats and primates

Discussion

Due to the small number of compounds included and the diversity of therapeutic classes and study durations, definitive conclusions cannot be drawn regarding the effect of a second species on the predictive value of rat tests. However, these results illustrate the approach that will be employed in a major study, which will include clinical data collected directly from pharmaceutical companies rather than from the literature. This study will endeavour to assess the predictive value of:

1. Rodent and non-rodent species with regard to specific effects
2. Animal tests within specific therapeutic classes of compounds
3. Animal tests of differing durations
4. Animal tests carried out between 10 and 20 years ago as compared to current tests

Studies such as this should provide valuable information for refining the available methodology for animal toxicity tests, with a view to improving their predictive value for man.

Acknowledgements. The authors are grateful to the following companies for providing repeated-dose animal toxicity data for this study: Beecham Pharmaceuticals, The Boots Company PLC, Ciba-Geigy AG, Fisons Pharmaceuticals, Glaxo Group Research Ltd, Reckitt & Colman, F. Hoffman-LaRoche & Co, Sandoz Ltd, Smith Kline & French Research Ltd, Syntex (USA) Inc, Thomae GmbH and The Wellcome Research Laboratories

References

Anonymous (1985) ABPI data sheet compendium 1985–1986. Datapharm, London

Dukes MNG (1980) Myler's effects of drugs 9nd edn. Excerpta Medica, Amsterdam

Schein PS, Davis RD, Carter S, Newman J, Schein DR, Rall DP (1970) The evaluation of anti-cancer drugs in dogs and monkeys for the prediction of qualitative toxicities in man. Clin Pharmacol Ther 11:3–40

Mechanisms and Models in Toxicology
Arch. Toxicol., Suppl. 11, 305–309 (1987)
© by Springer-Verlag 1987

Comparative Activation of Paracetamol in the Rat, Mouse and Man

C. E. Seddon, A. R. Bobois, and D. S. Davies

Department of Clinical Pharmacology, Royal Postgraduate Medical School, Du Cane Road, London, W12 0HS, UK

Introduction

The minor analgesic paracetamol is relatively non-toxic at normal therapeutic doses. In overdose it is hepatotoxic in a number of species, including man, due to its conversion to a highly reactive intermediate, N-acetyl-p-benzoquinoneimine (NABQI), by the hepatic mixed function oxidase system (reviewed in Prescott 1983). There are marked differences in susceptibility to the hepatotoxicity of paracetamol, both within and between species (Davis et al. 1974). The causes of this variation are largely attributable to differences in the extent to which paracetamol is converted to NABQI, i.e. to differences in the activity of cytochrome P_{450} (Davis et al. 1974; Green et al. 1984). However, the factors responsible for regulating the forms of cytochrome P_{450} involved in this reaction have yet to be identified. Certainly, environmental factors play some role. For example, chronic ingestion of ethanol alters the activation and hence the toxicity of paracetamol in laboratory animals (Peterson 1983) and possibly in man (Prescott 1983). The extent to which genetic factors contribute to interindividual differences in this reaction is still far from clear. The present study was conducted to investigate some of the possible causes of inter- and intraspecies differences in paracetamol activation and also to attempt to identify the specific forms of cytochrome P_{450} involved.

Methods

Reduced glutathione (GSH), NADPH, 3-methylcholanthrene (3-MC), metyrapone, isoniazid (INH) and paracetamol were purchased from Sigma Chemical, Poole, Dorset. Aniline hydrochloride was purchased from Aldrich Chemical, Gillingham, Dorset. Phenobarbitone (PB) sodium and phenacetin were supplied by McArthy's, London. Ketoconazole was a gift from Janssen Pharmaceutica, Beerse, Belgium. Cimetidine and proadifen (SKF 525A) were generously provided by Smith, Kline and French, Welwyn Garden City. Pregnenalone 16α-carbonitrile (PCN) was generously provided by G. D. Searle, Skokie, Ill. 3-S-Gluta-thionyl paracetamol, the mercapturic acid of paracetamol and its L-cysteine, glucuronide and sulphate conjugates were all generous gifts from D. Johnson, Sterling Winthrop, Newcastle-upon-Tyne. [Ring U-^{14}C]Paracetamol, specific activity 19.5 mCi/mmol (98% pure) was obtained from Amersham International, Amersham, Bucks. Solvents used for high pressure liquid chromatography (HPLC) were of HPLC grade. All other reagents were of analytical reagent grade or better.

Human liver samples were obtained as previously described (Boobis et al. 1980). The use of such tissue in these studies was with the permission of the local Research Ethics Committee. Male Wistar rats (180–250 g) and male MF1 mice (18–25 g) were obtained from Olac, Bicester, Oxon. The maintenance of animals and the isolation of hepatic microsomal fractions were as previously described (Sesardic et al. 1986).

The microsomal activation of paracetamol was determined by trapping NABQI as its adduct with exogenously added GSH and quantifying the product by radiometric HPLC as previously described (Tee et al. 1986).

Paracetamol metabolism was investigated in vivo in man. Healthy, normal volunteers agreed to ingest 1 g paracetamol and provide a 2-h urine sample collected between 6 and 8 h after dosing. Subjects gave written informed consent for the study, which had local Research Ethics Committee permission. The metabolites of paracetamol in these samples were quantified by UV-HPLC using a C8 column and a mobile phase of 0.1 M sodium acetate buffer, pH 4.0: 0.1% ethyl acetate: 0.2% methoxyethanol: 0.2% methanol: 0.2% propanol, with reference to authentic standards. Free paracetamol was measured by extracting 1 ml urine, buffered to pH 7.0, with ethyl acetate, using acetanilide as internal standard. The organic phase was blown to dryness under nitrogen and reconstituted in 500 µl mobile phase (30 mM sodium acetate buffer: 0.06% propan-2-ol: 0.06% methanol: 0.06% methoxyethanol: 3.5% acetonitrile). Paracetamol was analysed by HPLC using a Nova-Pak C18 column (flow 2 ml/min).

Results

The kinetics of paracetamol activation by hepatic microsomal fractions were determined for humans, the rat and the mouse. The mouse had the lowest K_m and the highest V_{max}, while humans and the rat had similar values (Table 1). The calculated intrinsic clearance to NABQI in the mouse was 10- to 15-fold greater than in the other two species.

The forms of cytochrome P_{450} involved in paracetamol activation were investigated with selective inducers and inhibitors. In the rat, activation of paracetamol was increased by 3-MC, PB, isoniazid and PCN, the greatest induction occurring with PCN (Table 1). Activation by microsomes from isoniazid-treated rats was competitively inhibited by aniline ($k_i = 275 \pm 78$ µM), a substrate for cytochrome P_{450} form j, whereas in the control rat aniline was a weaker, non-competitive inhibitor ($k_i = 890$ µM). Inhibition of paracetamol activation was compared in control mouse and human microsomes (Table 2). In the mouse, the most potent inhibitor was metyrapone, which was at least 40 times less potent in

Table 1. Michaelis-Menten parameters for the in vitro oxidation of paracetamol to its glutathione adduct

Species	Treatment	K_m	V_{max}	Intrinsic clearance
		(μM)	(pmol/mg/min)	(μl/min/mg)
MF1 mouse	None	448	900	2.01
Human	None	952	115	0.12
Wistar rat	None	1 570	291	0.19
Wistar rat	INH	2 435	570	0.23
Wistar rat	3-MC	1 607	525	0.33
Wistar rat	PB	664	336	0.50
Wistar rat	PCN	731	572	0.78

Values are means from two to four liver samples per group. Treatment of rats was as follows: INH, 1 mg/ml in drinking water for 11 days, followed by 50 mg/kg b.w. by i.p. injection 3 h prior to being killed; 3-MC, 80 mg/kg b.w. in corn oil by i.p. injection 51 h prior to being killed; PB, 80 mg/kg b.w. in saline by i.p. injection daily for 4 days, the animals being killed 24 h after the last injection; PCN, 100 mg/kg b.w. in corn oil by i.p. injection daily for 3 days, the last injection being given 30 h prior to being killed.

Table 2. Inhibition of the in vitro activation of paracetamol by microsomal fractions from human and mouse liver IC_{50} (μM)

Inhibitor	IC_{50} (μM) Mouse	IC_{50} (μM) Human
Ketoconazole	75	120
Cimetidine	300	>1 000
Phenacetin	150	600
Metyrapone	25	>1 000
Aniline	200	450
SKF 525A	200	>1 000

man. Similarly, SKF 525A, phenacetin and cimetidine were more potent inhibitors in the mouse than in humans. In contrast, ketoconazole and aniline showed similar inhibitory potency in both species.

The metabolism of paracetamol in vivo was studied in 179 healthy human volunteers. The range for the percentage of the recovered dose excreted as oxidation products (the sum of the amount of mercapturic acid and cysteine conjugate, estimated separately) was 10-fold. The frequency distribution curve was not normal, with a significant skew to lower values (Fig. 1). A small number of individuals had higher activity than would be predicted from a normal distribution of the data.

Discussion

There is an increasing impression from clinical experience that not all subjects taking an overdose of paracetamol are equally susceptible to its hepatotoxic ef-

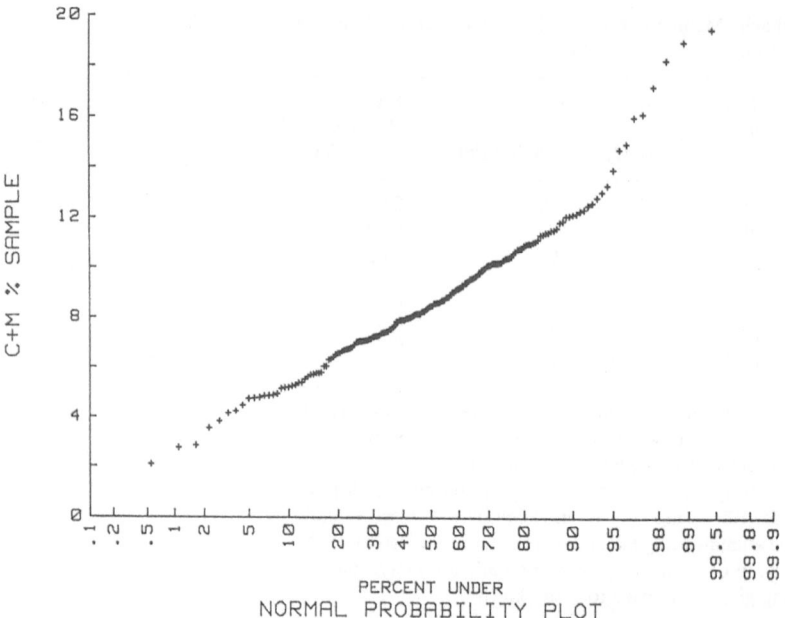

Fig. 1. Probit plot for the percentage of the recovered dose of paracetamol in urine excreted as oxidation products (cysteine conjugate, C, + mercapturic acid, M) in 179 healthy volunteers

fects (Prescott 1983). In studies performed in isolated hepatocytes, it has been demonstrated that this is not due to any intrinsic difference in sensitivity to the effects of the putative toxic metabolite, NABQI (Boobis et al. 1986). Thus, the likeliest explanation is a difference in the extent of activation of paracetamol. In the present study the microsomal activation of paracetamol by mouse and rat liver agreed very closely with the relative toxicity of paracetamol in these species (Davis et al. 1974). The results with human liver support those of previous studies (Boobis et al. 1986) suggesting that human liver is generally poor at activating paracetamol, with an activity closer to that of the rat than the mouse. There is increasing evidence that only a small number of forms of cytochrome P_{450} can catalyse the activation of paracetamol. One of these forms (form j) is inducible by ethanol and isoniazid in laboratory animals (Morgan et al. 1983; Ryan et al. 1986), and there is evidence for enhanced toxicity of paracetamol in subjects chronically ingesting alcohol (Prescott 1983). Results of the present study implicate a number of different forms of cytochrome P_{450} in the rat, including form j, 3-MC and PB inducible forms and, in particular, a form inducible by PCN. However, inhibition studies with aniline show that the form(s) of cytochrome P_{450} catalysing paracetamol activation in control rats is different from that in isoniazid-induced animals (form j).

A comparison of the effects of inhibitors on the activation of paracetamol in the mouse and in humans reveals major differences in specificity, and shows that the mouse is not an appropriate model in which to study the individual forms of cytochrome P_{450} that might be responsible for this activity in man. In particular, cimetidine has been shown to protect mice from paracetamol toxicity (Rudd et al. 1980), but this compound has no effect on the formation of the oxidation products of paracetamol in vivo in man (Mitchell et al. 1984). The present study shows that this could well be due to a difference in the sensitivity of cytochrome P_{450} in the two species to inhibition by cimetidine.

The amount of paracetamol oxidised in man shows considerable variation, with a range of over 10-fold. In addition, the amount of oxidised product formed is not normally distributed in man and spans the range between the mouse, a sensitive species, and the rat, a resistant species, with the majority of people oxidising only a small percentage of a dose of paracetamol to NABQI. The causes of this variation are currently under investigation.

Acknowledgements. We wish to express our thanks to Dr. Chris Speirs of this department for liaising with Dr. K. H. M. Young, OBE, who made the volunteer study possible. We are particularly grateful to Sister Pati Nolan and Dr. Young's staff at the Department of Occupational Medicine at Shellmex House, London, for all their hard work in recruiting and instructing the volunteers, and for ensuring safe delivery of the samples. We also wish to express our gratitude to all 179 volunteers at Shellmex who took part. Parts of this study were supported by a project grant from the Medical Research Council.

References

Boobis AR, Brodie MJ, Khan GC, Fletcher DR, Saunders JH, Davies DS (1980) Monooxygenase activity of human liver in microsomal fractions of needle biopsy specimens. Br J Clin Pharmacol 9:11–19

Boobis AR, Tee LBG, Hampden CE, Davies DS (1986) Freshly isolated hepatocytes as a model in which to study the toxicity of paracetamol. Food Chem Toxicol 24:731–736

Davis DC, Potter WZ, Jollow DJ, Mitchell JR (1974) Species differences in hepatic glutathione depletion, covalent binding and hepatic necrosis after acetaminophen. Life Sci 14:2099–2109

Green CE, Dabbs JE, Tyson CA (1984) Metabolism and cytotoxicity of acetaminophen in hepatocytes isolated from resistant and susceptible species. Toxicol Appl Pharmacol 76:139–149

Mitchell MC, Schenker S, Speeg KV (1984) Selective inhibition of acetaminophen oxidation and toxicity by cimetidine and other histamine H_2-receptor antagonists in vivo and in vitro in the rat and in man. J Clin Invest 73:383–391

Morgan ET, Koop DR, Coon MJ (1983) Comparison of six rabbit liver cytochrome P-450 isozymes in formation of a reactive metabolite of acetaminophen. Biochem Biophys Res Commun 112:8–13

Peterson FJ, Holloway DE, Erickson RR, Duquette PH, McClain CJ, Holtzman JL (1980) Ethanol induction of acetaminophen toxicity and metabolism. Life Sci 27:1701–1711

Prescott LF (1983) Paracetamol overdosage. Pharmacological considerations and clinical management. Drugs 25:290–314

Rudd GD, Donn KH, Grisham JW (1980) Prevention of acetaminophen-induced necrosis by cimetidine in mice. Res Commun Chem Pathol Pharmacol 32:369–372

Ryan DE, Koop DR, Thomas PE, Coon MJ, Levin W (1986) Evidence that isoniazid and ethanol induce the same microsomal cytochrome P-450 in rat liver, an isozyme homologous to rabbit liver cytochrome P-450 isozyme 3a. Arch Biochem Biophys 246:633–644

Sesardic D, Boobis AR, McQuade J, Baker S, Lock EA, Elcombe CR, Robson RT, Hayward C, Davies DS (1986) Inter-relatedness of some isozymes of cytochrome P-450 from rat, rabbit and human determined with monoclonal antibodies. Biochem J 236:569–577

Tee LBG, Davies DS, Seddon CE, Boobis AR (1986) Species differences in the hepatotoxicity of paracetamol are due to differences in the rate of conversion to its cytotoxic metabolite. Biochem Pharmacol 36:1041–1052

Mechanisms and Models in Toxicology
Arch. Toxicol., Suppl. 11, 310–312 (1987)
© by Springer-Verlag 1987

Nisoldipine, a New Calcium Antagonist, Elevates Plasma Levels of Digoxin

W. Kirch, J. Stenzel, S. R. Santos, and E. E. Ohnhaus

I. Medical Department, Christian Albrechts University, D-2300 Kiel, FRG

Introduction

Several studies have been published reporting an elevated bioavailability and an altered hemodynamic effect of digoxin during simultaneous ingestion of calcium channel blockers such as nifedipine, verapamil, and gallopamil (Belz et al. 1983; Kirch et al. 1984, 1986; Pedersen et al. 1983). Nisoldipine is a new dihydropyridine substance, which does not exert an electrophysiological effect on sinus and AV node, but has a marked peripheral vasodilating activity (Pasanisi et al. 1985). Therefore, this calcium antagonist appears to be specifically indicated for patients with heart failure and/or arterial hypertension and it may be frequently given concurrently with digitalis glycosides. The aim of the present study was to elucidate a possible pharmacokinetic and hemodynamic interaction between nisoldipine and digoxin.

Patients and Methods

The study was performed in 10 patients (7 female, 3 male) aged from 21 to 74 years (61.3 ± 5.1; $\bar{X}$ ± SEM) with cardiac insufficiency, NYHA (New York Heart Association) stage II–III). The patients, who had all been on digoxin therapy for at least 3 months previously, had given their written, informed consent to participate in the study. In a placebo-controlled double-blind study, the patients were treated in a randomized order for 7 days, first with digoxin (Lanicor, Boehringer, Mannheim, FRG) 0.25 mg twice daily as monotherapy or digoxin 0.25 mg twice daily combined with nisoldipine 10 mg twice daily. Thereafter, the crossover to the corresponding therapy period, lasting again 7 days, was performed. Plasma samples for determination of digoxin were collected during each treatment week on days 5, 6 and 7, before and 4 h after the morning dose. The plasma levels of digoxin were estimated using a commercially available radioimmunoassay (RIA; Diagnostic Products). Systolic time intervals were determined on day 7 of each treatment week, before the morning dose and 3 and 8 h afterwards. Statistical analysis of the data was performed using the Wilcoxon test for paired differences.

Results

In Fig. 1 mean plasma concentrations of digoxin ($\bar{X} \pm$ SEM) of 9 patients are shown during monotherapy with digitalis glycoside and under combined treatment with nisoldipine. One patient failed to complete the study and therefore is not included in the control data (digoxin monotherapy).

Plasma Levels of Digoxin

Digoxin through levels were distinctly increased by nisoldipine administration – from 0.98 ± 0.15 ng/ml on day 7 under monotherapy (digoxin alone) to 1.33 ± 0.21 ng/ml on day 7 under simultaneous nisoldipine ingestion ($p < 0.05$). Comparing mean values of digoxin plasma levels from days 5, 6 and 7 under monotherapy with those from days 5, 6 and 7 when nisoldipine was given concurrently also yields a significant difference (1.16 ± 0.14 ng/ml in monotherapy vs 1.35 ± 0.14 ng/ml in combined treatment; $p < 0.02$). The digoxin plasma concentrations 4 h after the morning dose were also significantly elevated by nisoldipine coadministration; mean values of days 5, 6 and 7 were 1.53 ± 0.16 ng/ml for digoxin alone and 1.92 ± 0.16 ng/ml when nisoldipine was given concurrently.

Systolic Time Intervals

A significant shortening of preejection period (PEP), from 139 ± 11 ms under monotherapy to 129 ± 11 ms was found ($p < 0.05$), 8 h following simultaneously ingestion of nisoldipine with digoxin. Also the ratio PEP/LVET was significantly decreased from 0.395 ± 0.037 to 0.356 ± 0.036 ms ($p < 0.05$).

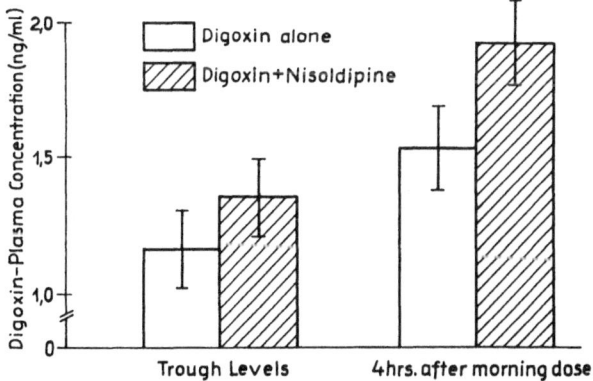

Fig. 1. Mean plasma concentrations of digoxin ($\bar{X} \pm$ SEM) during monotherapy and combined treatment with nisoldipine (mean values of treatment days 5, 6, and 7)

Discussion

As has been found for other calcium channel blockers such as verapamil, gallo-pamil, nifedipine, and nitrendipine, in the present study the new calcium antagonist nisoldipine was also observed to increase plasma levels of digoxin significantly. The rise of the digoxin plasma concentrations under concurrent therapy with calcium channel blockers has been speculated to be due to a reduction of renal excretion of digoxin caused by these drugs (Belz et al. 1983). In accordance with data described by Belz et al. (1983) for nifedipine, verapamil, and gallopamil, the systolic time intervals under digoxin treatment, in the study reported here were also altered by nisoldipine coadministration. The PEP and the ratio of PEP/ LVET were significantly shortened in comparison with the values for digoxin monotherapy 8 h following the last concurrent ingestion of digoxin and nisoldipine. Such a spectrum of behavior of the systolic time intervals is indicative of an afterload reduction, accompanied by some increase in contractility. Therefore, these changes appear to be mainly due to the calcium antagonist itself, accompanied by some effect of the increasing plasma digoxin concentration. In conclusion, data reported in this study indicate a significant pharmacokinetic interaction between nisoldipine and digoxin. In individual patients this effect of nisoldipine on plasma concentrations of digoxin may be of clinical relevance.

References

Belz GG, Doering E, Munkes R, Matthews J (1983) Interaction between digoxin and calcium antagonists and antiarrhythmic drugs. Clin Pharmacol Ther 33:410–417

Kirch W, Hutt HJ, Heidemann H, Rämsch K, Janisch HD, Ohnhaus EE (1984) Drug interactions with nitrendipine. J Cardiovasc Pharmacol 6:S982–S985

Kirch W, Hutt HJ, Dylewicz P, Gräf KJ, Ohnhaus EE (1986) Dose dependence of the nifedipine/digoxin interaction. Clin Pharmacol Ther 39:35–39

Pasanisi F, Meredith PA, Reid JL (1985) The pharmacodynamics and pharmacokinetics of a new calcium antagonist nisoldipine in normotensive and hypertensive subjects. Eur J Clin Pharmacol 29:21–24

Pedersen KE, Tayssem P, Klitgaard NA, Christiansen BD, Nielsen-Kudski F (1983) Influence of verapamil on the inotropism and pharmacokinetics of digoxin. Eur J Clin Pharmacol 25:199–206

Mechanisms and Models in Toxicology
Arch. Toxicol., Suppl. 11, 313–315 (1987)

Influence of Inhibitors on the Thrombogenicity and Toxicity of Prothrombin Complex Concentrates

H.-P. Klöcking, G. Dornheim, and H. Schulze-Riewald

Institute of Pharmacology and Toxicology, Medical Academy Erfurt, Nordhäuser Str. 74, 5010 Erfurt, GDR

Introduction

Patients treated with prothrombin complex concentrates (PCCs) have frequently been found to develop arterial thrombosis, venous thromboembolism or disseminated intravascular coagulation (Kasper 1975). Consequently, PCCs must be regarded as potentially thrombogenic substances (Elödi 1977). Within the framework of studies of a new PCC (Klöcking et al. 1984), the influence of heparin, pentosan polysulphate and synthetic thrombin inhibitors on the thrombogenicity of PCCs was examined. Furthermore, the effect of heparin, pentosan polysulphate or aprotinin was studied on the acute toxicity of PCC and on that observed after 7 days.

Materials and Methods

The following substances were used: PCC (District Institute for Blood Transfusion, Suhl, GDR); pentosan polysulphate (SP$_{54}$, Benechemie, München, FRG); heparin (Heparin "Richter", Gedeon Richter, Budapest, Hungary); aprotinin (Contrykal, VEB Arzneimittelwerk, Dresden, GDR); APPA (4-amidinophenylpyruvic acid ester hydrochloride, VEB Arzneimittelwerk, Dresden, GDR); Tos-(mAm)Phe-Pip ($N\alpha$-tosyl-3-amidinophenylalanine piperidide, Lehrstuhl Pharmazeutische Chemie, Sektion Biowissenschaften, Karl-Marx-Universität, Leipzig, GDR); βNas-Gly-(pAm)Phe-Pip ($N\alpha$-(2-naphthylsulphonyl-glycyl)-4-amidinophenylalanine piperidide, VEB Arzneimittelwerk, Dresden, GDR); Tos-(pAm) Phe-Pip ($N\alpha$-tosyl-4-amidinophenylalanine piperidide; Lehrstuhl Pharmazeutische Chemie, Sektion Biowissenschaften, Karl-Marx-Universität, Leipzig, GDR).

Thrombogenicity studies were carried out in female Wistar rats (body mass 227 ± 31 g; $n = 243$) applying the stasis model according to Wessler (1955) to produce venous clotting thrombi, the thrombogenic PCC was administered instead of heterologous serum.

The amount of clot formed was scored on a scale from 0 to 4; a score of 0 represented no clot; a score of 1, a few macroscopic strands of fibrin; a score of 2, several small thrombi; a score of 3, two or more large thrombi; and a score of 4 represented a single thrombus forming a cast of the isolated segment.

For toxicity studies, female ICR mice were used (body mass 28 ± 6 g; $n = 223$). LD_{50} values were calculated according to Litchfield and Wilcoxon (1949).

Results and Discussion

The thrombogenicity of PCC (200 U factor IX/kg), as determined in rats using the stasis model according to Wessler (1955), may be reduced or suppressed by administration of heparin, pentosan polysulphate, and the synthetic thrombin inhibitors βNas-Gly-(pAm)Phe-Pip, Tos-(mAm)Phe-Pip, Tos-(pAm)Phe-Pip, and APPA. Doses that prevented thrombus formation in 50% of rats (ED_{50}) are summarized in Table 1. Comparison of ED_{50} values ($\mu mol/kg$) showed that heparin was most potent. The amount of clot formed (expressed as mean score) may be reduced by administration of different doses of βNas-Gly-(pAm)Phe-Pip

Table 1. Influence of inhibitors on the thrombogenicity of prothrombin complex concentrates (200 units factor IX/kg; Wessler stasis model)

Substance	ED_{50} ($\mu mol/kg$)[a]
Heparin	0.05 (0.05– 0.05)
Pentosan polysulphate	0.32 (0.28– 0.35)
βNas-Gly-(pAm)Phe-Pip	1.05 (0.87– 1.31)
Tos-(pAm)Phe-Pip	10.78 (8.27–17.97)
Tos-(pAm)Phe-Pip	18.33 (1.79–22.16)
APPA	24.38 (22.90–26.23)

[a] Dose that prevented thrombus formation in 50% of the animals under the test conditions described.

Table 2. Effect of i.v. application of heparin, pentosan polysulphate (SP_{54}), and aprotinin on the acute toxicity of prothrombin complex concentrates (PCCs) in mice (charge, 070380)

	Dose	Toxicity of PCC		
		LD_{50} (F IX/kg)	Confidence limit	Effect and confidence limit
PCCs	–	1585	922–2726	1.0
Heparin	200 IU/TU	1585	1229–2045	1.0 (0.58–1.74)
SP_{54}	2 mg/TU	1413	1082–1843	0.89 (0.51–1.56)
Aprotinin	25000 ATrU/TU	1585	1229–2045	1.0 (0.58–1.71)

TU, transfusion unit.

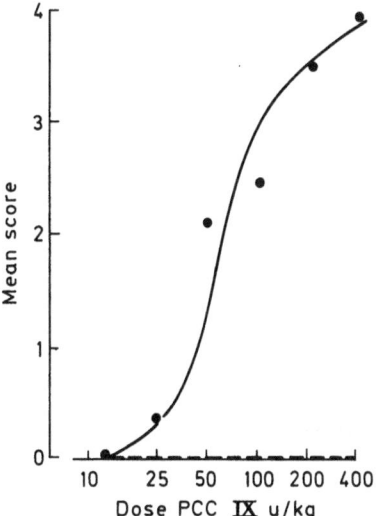

Fig. 1. Influence of heparin (1.5 mg/kg; –––) on the thrombogenicity of prothrombin complex concentrate (●—●). The formation of thrombi in the isolated segment of the jugular vein of rats was determined after 10 min using the scoring system described by Wessler

(0.046 mg/kg, 0.23 mg/kg) or pentosan polysulphate 0.115 mg/kg, 0.23 mg/kg, 0.46 mg/kg). Addition of heparin (10 U/ml reconstitution volume) to PCC totally suppressed thrombogenicity of PCC (Fig. 1). This is the recommended amount of heparin to counteract the thrombogenicity of PCCs (Menarche 1975).

The addition of heparin, pentosan polysulphate or aprotinin had no significant influence on the acute toxicity (Table 2) or on that observed after 7 days. This is consistent with the results obtained by Magner and Aronson (1979), who found that the toxicity of PCC was not influenced by enzyme inhibitors (diisopropyl-fluorophosphate, soybean trypsin inhibitor and heparin). Therefore, it appears reasonable to assume that factors other than thrombogenicity play a role in causing death.

References

Elödi S (1977) Thrombogenic properties of prothrombin complex concentrates. Blood 50:961–965

Kasper CK (1975) Thromboembolic complications. Thrombos Diathes Haemorrh 33:640–644

Klöcking H-P, Kleßen Ch, Jablonowski Ch, Meerbach W, Dornheim G (1984) Untersuchungen zur Thrombogenität eines neuen Prothrombinkomplexkonzentrates. Folia Haematol 111:645–661

Litchfield JT, Wilcoxon P (1949) A simplified method of evaluating dose-effect experiments. J Pharmacol Exp Ther 96:99–113

Magner A, Aronson DL (1979) Toxicity in mice of factor IX concentrates. Thrombos Haemostas 42:200

Menarche D (1975) Factor IX concentrates. Thrombos Diathes Haemorrh 33:600–605

Wessler S (1955) Studies in intravascular coagulation. The pathogenesis of serum-induced venous thrombosis. J Clin Invest 34:647–653

Mechanisms and Models in Toxicology
Arch. Toxicol., Suppl. 11, 316–318 (1987)

Lipid Parameters of a Non-Human Primate Following Administration of a High Fat Diet

P. Hudson and A. McCraw

Inveresk Research International Ltd., Musselburgh, EH21 7UB, Scotland, UK

Methods

Normal levels of lipid parameters were established for baboon (*Papio* species), cynomolgus monkeys (*Macaca fascicularis*) and man.

Total cholesterol (Baker Test Kit, Ref 219000), free cholesterol (Boehringer Test Kit, CHOD-PAP, Ref 310328), HDL cholesterol (Boehringer Test Kit, Ref 543004), phospholipids [Boehringer Test Kit (enzymatic), Ref 691844], and triglycerides (Baker Test Kit, Ref 30-012-100) were assayed on a Centrifichem 500 centrifugal analyser (Baker Instruments, UK). Lipoprotein electrophoresis was performed on a Corning System (Corning Medical and Scientific, UK) using agarose plates stained with Fat Red B. Agarose plates were scanned on a Helena Densitometer (Helena Laboratories, USA); α/β lipoprotein ratios were calculated from the integrator traces.

Twelve cynomolgus monkeys were treated for the first 56 days with high fat diet, consisting of butter 25.5%, cholesterol 0.5%, sucrose 43.0%, casein 25.0%, and vitamin-mineral supplement 6.0% (Malinow et al. 1977). This preparation has been said to approximate to the level of fat taken in a standard USA diet. Between days 56 and 84 the high fat diet was modified by the addition of normal primate feed at a ratio of 1:1. Animals were offered 200 g of diet daily.

Blood samples were collected at days 0, 28, 42, 56, 70 and 84 into lithium heparin and the plasma was separated by centrifugation.

Aortas were removed and examined macroscopically at post mortem. Histological examinations were performed following staining of sections with haematoxylin/eosin and elastic Van Gieson.

Results

The normal plasma levels of total cholesterol, free cholesterol, HDL cholesterol, triglycerides, phospholipids and α/β lipoprotein ratio were established for cynomolgus monkeys, baboons and man (Table 1).

Table 1. Circulating plasma lipid levels in normal human and nonhuman primates. All units are mmol/l (except α/β ratio)

	Total choles- terol	Free choles- terol	HDL choles- terol	Tri- glycerides	Phospho- lipids	α/β ratio
Human	3.9–7.7	1.27–1.74	0.90–1.42	0.85–2.00	2.04–3.66	0.32–0.83
Macaca fascicularis (Cynomolgus monkey)	2.3–5.3	0.65–1.76	0.69–1.79	0.33–0.83	2.92–4.19	0.30–1.70
Papio species (Baboon)	2.0–4.8	0.69–1.69	0.56–1.30	0.31–1.56	1.99–3.35	0.36–1.66

A summary of the changes in lipid parameters for the cynomolgus monkey is included in Fig. 1.

At day 0 all cynomolgus monkeys were shown to be within the expected limits for the species for all lipid parameters. By day 28, following administration of high fat diet, animals had shown a marked increase in total cholesterol and free cholesterol. Phospholipids, which were measured at day 28 only, showed a notable but less marked increase while triglycerides were similar to baseline levels.

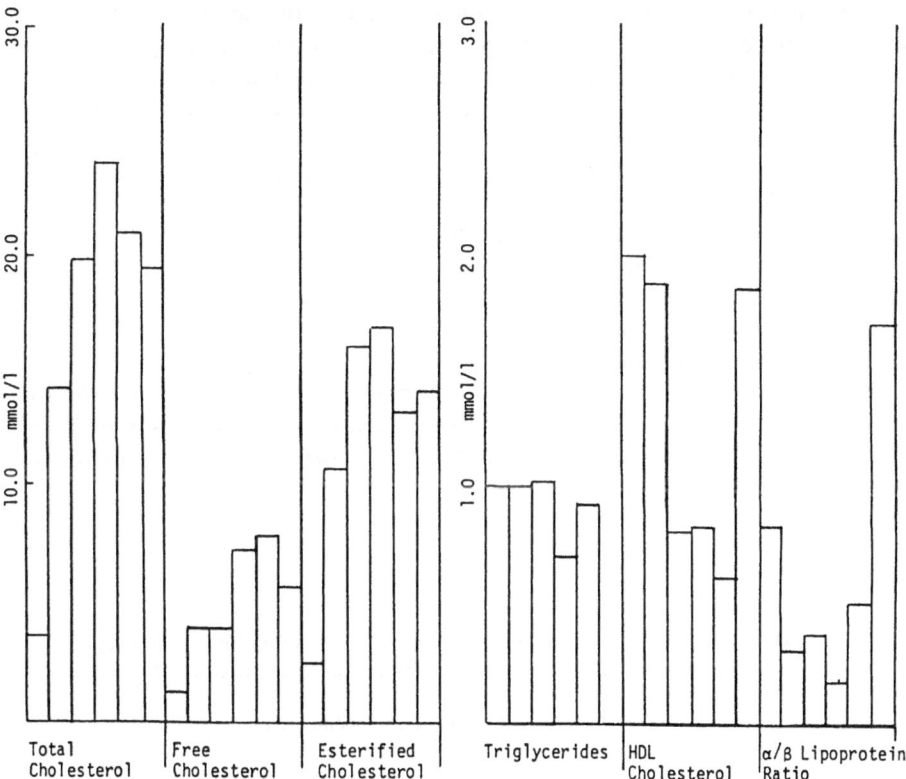

Fig. 1. Plasma lipid profile of cynomolgus monkey treated with high fat diet for 56 days. Modified diet days 56–84. Histogram shows data at days 0, 28, 42, 56, 70 and 84

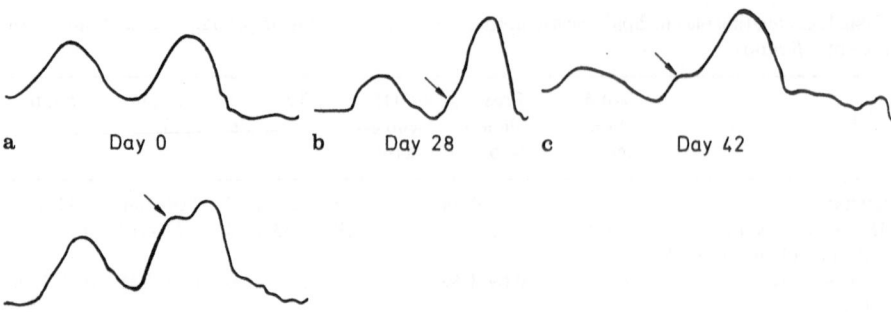

a   Day 0   b   Day 28   c   Day 42

d   Healthy human

Fig. 2. The α/β ratio lipoprotein electrophoretic pattern of a cynomolgus monkey at 3 points over 42 days' administration of high fat diet (**a, b, c**) in comparison with a human pattern (**d**). An increase in the LDL fraction and the development of a pre-β band corresponding to the VLDL fraction in man (*arrowed*) can be seen

HDL cholesterol was lower than at day 0. Calculation of the α/β lipoprotein ratio showed a reduction compared to day 0 correlating with the increase in total cholesterol and the reduction in HDL cholesterol.

At days 42 and 56 the increase in total cholesterol continued to a level > 20.0 mmol/l. HDL cholesterol was further reduced to a level at which the tolerance of the cholesterol assay method became questionable. Triglycerides were reduced between days 42 and 56, possibly as a result of palatability problems with the diet. Until day 42, α/β lipoprotein ratios continued to fall, followed by a steady low level between days 42 and 70.

Following modification of the diet, from day 56 onwards, there was a decrease in total cholesterol and free cholesterol. HDL cholesterol and consequently α/β lipoprotein ratios increased during the period between days 56 and 84.

Lipoprotein electrophoresis traces showed a modification of lipid bands during the study. On day 28 there was an increase in the β fraction (LDL, IDL) together with a reduction in the α band (HDL). By day 42 a small pre-β band (VLDL) was detected between the α and β bands (Fig. 2).

Macroscopic examination at post mortem showed aortic, atherosclerotic plaques in streaks on the tissue surface. Histological examination showed smooth muscle proliferation and cell multiplication precursors of fibrofatty plaques (Sim 1983).

References

Malinow R, McLaughlin D, Papworth L, Natio HK, Lewis L, McNulty WP (1977) Effect of alfalfa meal on shrinkage (regression) of atherosclerotic plaques during cholesterol feeding in monkeys. Adv Exp Med Biol 67:3

Sim AK (1983) Proc 17 Kitzbühel angiological symposium. Schattauer, Stuttgart, p 51

Mechanisms and Models in Toxicology
Arch. Toxicol., Suppl. 11, 319–320 (1987)

Immunological Studies in Asthmatics Exposed to Allergens

M. Maheshwari, M. Jaju, P. S. Devi, K. J. R. Murthy, P. V. R. Rao, S. N. Jain, and P. B. Sattur

Medical Mycology and Allergy Research Centre, Mahavir Hospital, A C Guards, Hyderabad 500004 (A-P), India

Introduction and Method

Environmental factors, both abiotic (house dust, house dust mite) and biotic (pollen and fungal spores, food ingestants and drugs), are known to cause allergic asthma in hypersensitive individuals with an altered immune system. However, allergens responsible for causing allergy differ from region to region, with variations in ecogeographic and climatic conditions (Hobday and Stewart 1973; Annand and Agashe 1984).

Allergic patients have increased IgE levels in their blood. Production of IgE is controlled by the T-lymphocyte subsets which also regulate cell-mediated immunity. In the present study, it was intended to assess the response of allergens on the immune status of exposed asthmatics. A total of 40 patients with asthma were screened. A detailed history of exposure to allergens was recorded with the help of a printed form containing a list of the allergens of the area (e.g. house dust, house dust mite, various types of pollen and fungal allergens like *Amaranthus spinosus, Parthenium, Cyperus rotandus, Candida albicans, Aspergillus flavus, Aspergillus fumigatus, Helminthosporium*), degree of exposure, family history of the disease and the clinical symptoms. Whether the disease was allergic in nature was established by intradermal skin testing with 20 predominant allergens in accordance with the history taken. Blood was drawn from each subject without and with anticoagulant for serum and cells, respectively.

The parameters studied were: (a) IgE quantitation – levels were determined using the ELISA technique; (b) cell-mediated immune response, evaluated in vivo using purified protein derivative (PPD) and dinitrochlorobenzene (DNCB), in vitro by LMI with PPD and PHA; and (c) quantitation of T and B lymphocytes, by E rosettes and EAC rosettes. Concurrently, 12 control subjects were also studied.

Table 1. Percentage of T and B lymphocyte population using the Rosette technique

	N	T lymphocytes	B lymphocytes
Controls	12	63.12 ± 3.68	22.68 ± 3.15
Patients	40	59.58[a] ± 2.98	25.75[a] ± 3.57

[a] $P < 0.05$.

Results and Discussion

All subjects showed positive reactivity to PPD and DNCB. There was no difference in LMI index in the controls (area of migration <0.8) and the patient population (area of migration <0.8) with PPD and PHA. The reason could be that these antigens are non-specific stimulants of lymphocytes. It is likely that the response may be depressed with specific allergens to which patients are sensitive. Valverde et al. (1984) also did not find a depressed response with non-specific antigens.

IgE levels in controls were found to be less than 110 U/ml. Of the 40 patients, 17% had IgE values in the normal range, while 87% had increased IgE values, i.e. more than 110 IU/ml.

There was a significant reduction in the T-lymphocyte population and a significant increase in the B-lymphocyte population (Table 1) in the patients as compared with the controls. These findings of low levels of T-lymphocyte population are in agreement with the findings of Strannegard and Strannegard (1979) and Valverde et al. (1984). Reduction in T lymphocytes may allow increased production of IgEs, which in turn may cause sensitivity to different allergens in asthmatics.

References

Anand P, Agashe SN (1984) Immunological approaches to extra mural environmental nasobronchial allergy. Int J Otolaryngol 30:39–44

Hobday JD, Stewart AJ (1973) Relationship between daily asthma attendance, weather parameters, spore and pollen counts. Aust NZ J Med 3:552–556

Strannegard O, Strannegard IL (1979) In vitro differences between the lymphocytes of normal subjects and atopics. Clin Allergy 9:637

Valverde E et al. (1984) Cells mediated in perennial allergic rhinits. Ann Allergy 52:187–193

Mechanisms and Models in Toxicology
Arch. Toxicol., Suppl. 11, 321–324 (1987)
© by Springer-Verlag 1987

The In Vitro Effects of Trichothecenes on the Immune System

K. Miller and H. A. C. Atkinson

Immunotoxicology Department, British Industrial Biological Research Association, Woodmansterne Road, Carshalton, Surrey, SM5 4DS, UK

Introduction

The trichothecene deoxynivalenol (DON), a *Fusarium* mycotoxin, has been identified as a major contaminant of crops in temperate climates (Ueno 1985). All trichothecenes have been shown to inhibit protein and DNA synthesis and are therefore generally considered to have immunosuppressive properties.

Several recent publications have shown that the production of interleukins, which exert fine control over immune responses, may be superinduced by protein synthesis inhibitors (Bendtzen 1983). The present study was undertaken to investigate whether low concentrations of DON could affect production of interleukins in a similar manner.

Materials

DON, nivalenol (Alpha Laboratories) and cyclohexamide (CHX, Sigma) were dissolved in RPMI 1640 (Gibco), filtered and stored at $-20\,°C$.

Methods

Lymphocyte Blastogenesis Assay

PVG rat peripheral blood lymphocytes (PBL) were purified and cultured according to a previously described standard protocol (Atkinson and Miller 1984). Briefly, lymphocytes were cultured for 48 h together with 7.5 µg/ml phytohaemagglutinin (PHA) and various concentrations of DON and nivalenol. Tritiated thymidine was added for the last 6 h of culture.

Interleukin-1 (IL-1) Assay

Thioglycollate-elicited PVG rat peritoneal macrophages (12×10^{-6}) were incubated with DON or CHX for 24 h followed by 20 h culture in fresh medium either with or without concanavalin A (Con A) present. This conditioned medium was dialysed and filter-sterilised. IL-1-like activity was determined by incubating mouse (C3H) thymocytes together with 25% CM and PHA for 48 h. Thymidine incorporation in this co-mitogenic assay was measured over the final 6 h of culture.

Rosetting Assay

Macrophages were cultured on glass coverslips and incubated with 0–2.4 μg/ml DON for 24 h. The cultures were then washed and incubated for 30 min with a 3% suspension of sheep red blood cells (SRBC, Oxoid) previously sensitised with 1:100 rabbit anti-sheep haemolysin (Flow) at 37 °C for 1 h. The adherence of 3 or more SRBCs to a macrophage constituted a rosette.

Results

Lymphocyte cultures exposed to low levels of DON demonstrated enhanced stimulation of PHA-induced blastogenesis. This was evident at concentrations of 0.005–1.0 ng/ml, whereas concentrations above 50 ng/ml inhibited proliferation as previously reported (Fig. 1). When DON was present at these low levels incorporation of [3H]thymidine was increased by an average of 30%. Nivalenol caused

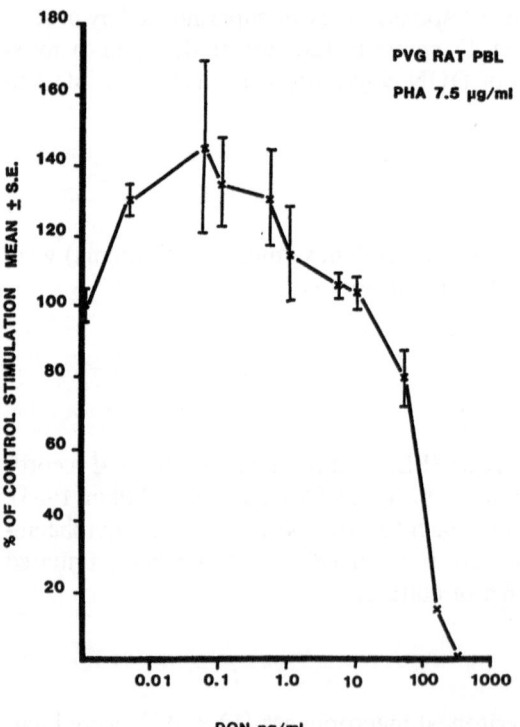

Fig. 1. Effect of DON on mitogen-induced blastogenesis in rat peripheral blood lymphocytes

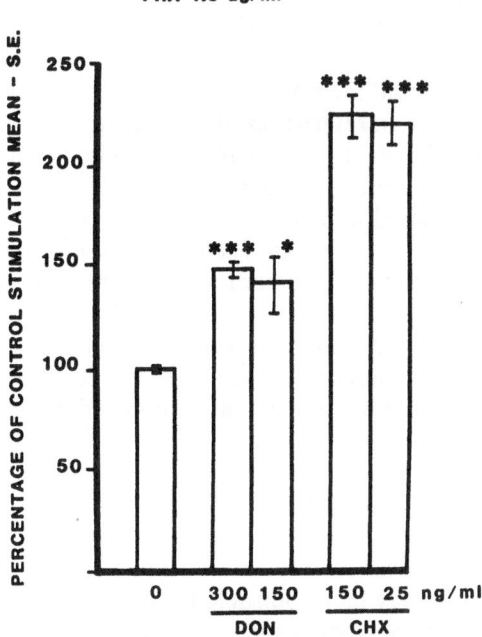

PHA 1.0 ug/ml

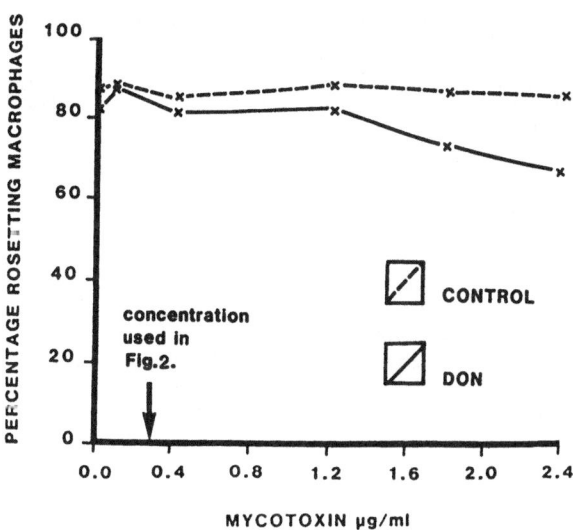

Fig. 2. Comitogenic effect of DON- and CHX-macrophage conditioned medium on thymocyte proliferation. *, $p < 0.05$; ***, $p < 0.001$

Fig. 3. Effect of DON on macrophage Fc rosetting capacity

total inhibition of thymidine incorporation in PBL cultures when present at levels above 150 ng/ml. There was some enhanced proliferation with a concentration of 25 ng/ml.

To further investigate whether DON induced the release of mitogenic proteins such as the interleukins, monolayers of adherent rat peritoneal macrophages were cultured for 24 h with either media alone, DON, or the protein synthesis inhibitor CHX. Treatment of supernatants from macrophages treated with DON contained increased IL-1-like activity as measured in a co-mitogenic assay system. DON was less active in this respect than CHX (Fig. 2). The concentrations of DON used did not inhibit the rosetting capacity of peritoneal macrophages (Fig. 3).

Macrophages were also incubated with ConA which is a known stimulator of IL-1 synthesis. When macrophages were incubated with DON in the presence of ConA, further release of IL-1 into the medium was evident, as determined in the thymocyte co-stimulator assay.

Discussion

Increased release by macrophages of IL-1 may be responsible for the enhanced proliferation observed in PHA-activated lymphocytes exposed to low concentrations of DON.

Macrophages are also known to synthesise and secrete IL-1 after stimulation with ConA. In this study, addition of ConA to macrophage cultures increased secretion of IL-1 and this increase was not affected by DON. On the contrary, medium from macrophages incubated with ConA and DON further enhanced the PHA response of mouse thymocytes. This suggests that the increased amounts of IL-1 synthesised in response to ConA are no longer under intracellular control (Lester and Cooper 1985) and demonstrates that DON may act as an immunostimulator precisely because of its ability to inhibit protein synthesis.

Acknowledgment. This work was supported by the UK Ministry of Agriculture, Fisheries and Food to whom our thanks are due. The results of the research are the property of the Ministry of Agriculture, Fisheries and Food and are Crown Copyright

References

Atkinson HAC, Miller K (1984) Inhibitory effect of deoxynivalenol, 3-acetyldeoxynivalenol and zearalenone on induction of rat and human lymphocyte blastogenesis. Toxicol Lett 23:215–221
Bendtzen K (1983) Biological properties of interleukins. Allergy 38:219–226
Lester EP, Cooper HL (1985) Lymphocyte blastogenesis: post-transcriptional controls of protein synthesis. Biochim Biophys Acta 824:365–368
Ueno Y (1985) The toxicology of mycotoxins. CRC Crit Rev Toxicol 14:99–132

Mechanisms and Models in Toxicology
Arch. Toxicol., Suppl. 11, 325–328 (1987)

Macrophage Migration Inhibition Test to Evaluate the Sensitizing Potential of Drugs in the Guinea Pig

A. Laschi-Loquerie [1], P. Tachon [2], C. Veysseyre [1], and J. Descotes [3]

[1] Department of Immunology, Pasteur Institute, Lyons, France
[2] Hazleton-Institut Français de Toxicologie, L'Arbresle, France
[3] Immunotoxicology Section, Department of Pharmacology, INSERM U80-CNRS UA1177-UCB, Faculty of Medicine Alexis Carrel, Lyons, France

Introduction

Drug-induced hypersensitivity reactions are frequently encountered in clinical practice. The availability of reliable predictive methods in this regard would be most helpful to devise adequate preventive measures in patients being treated. Contact sensitization testings are commonly used in the guinea pig to assess the allergenic potential of drugs and chemicals (Guillot et al. 1983). However, some limitations do persist particularly regarding the detection of weak allergens.

Macrophage migration inhibition factor (MIF) is a lymphokine released by primed T lymphocytes following challenge with the corresponding antigen. Cell migration is therefore an in vitro correlate of delayed hypersensitivity (George and Vaughan 1962) and the leukocyte migration test has been proposed for the diagnosis of drug allergy (Ponvert et al. 1977).

This study was undertaken to determine whether a combination of in vivo testing, i.e., contact sensitization, with in vitro testing, i.e., assessment of migration inhibition, in the same guinea pigs would prove more instrumental than current procedures to detect the allergenic potential of drugs.

Material and Methods

Animals

Male and female adult albino Dunkin-Hartley guinea pigs purchased from Iffa Credo (L'Arbresle, France) and weighing 300–400 g at the beginning of the study were used throughout. They were kept in plastic cages and given free access to food and water. The sensitizing protocol was started after a 1-week quarantine.

Contact Skin Sensitization

Contact sensitization testings were performed according to Guillot et al. (1983): after determining the maximal nonirritating concentration of each test substance, guinea pigs were injected intradermally with 0.1 ml Freund's complete adjuvant (Difco) diluted to 50% in isotonic saline, followed by a 48-h occlusive topical application of 0.5 ml of the test substance in ethanol, on the right flank. The animals were then given one 48-h occlusive topical application of 0.5 ml of the test substance in ethanol at days 2, 4, 7, 9, 11 and 14, on the same flank. Following a rest period of 11 days, a 48-h occlusive topical application of 0.5 ml of the maximal nonirritating concentration of the test substance was given on the left flank. After removal of the occlusive patch, macroscopic reactions were read according to Draize et al. (1944); positive or doubtful reactions were followed by a histological examination. Only histologically confirmed reactions were considered positive.

Migration Inhibition Testing

Cell migration inhibition was assessed as follows (David et al. 1964): peritoneal exudates were elicited by injecting 15 ml mineral oil intraperitoneally at the end of the skin sensitization procedure. The animals were bled 4 days later and mononuclear cells obtained from peritoneal exudates were centrifuged and washed twice in 199 medium (Serva, Heidelberg, FAG). Cell migration in 199 medium enriched with 15% foal serum (Pasteur Institute, Paris, France) was measured at the end of an 18-h incubation period at 37 °C in capillary tubes (Thor et al. 1968). At least three different concentrations of each drug were tested. Each measurement was done in triplicate. Migration inhibition was expressed as the mean migration index, calculated from the average migration of each guinea pig's cell population in the presence of the three drug concentrations as compared to control migrations.

Chemicals

Six drugs were chosen for their known potential for inducing or not inducing allergic reactions in humans (Dukes 1984): penicillin, phenindione, nitrofurantoin, phenobarbital, phenazone, and naftidrofuryl. They were obtained from French commercial sources. The maximal nonirritating concentration was determined prior to the contact sensitization process. The following concentrations were used for in vitro studies: penicillin (0.1, 1, 10, 100 and 200 IU/ml), phenindione (1, 10, 100 μg/ml), nitrofurantoin (0.5, 5, 50 μg/ml), phenobarbital (0.3, 3, 30 μg/ml), phenazone (10, 100, 1000 μg/ml), naftidrofuryl (1, 10, 100 μg/ml).

Results

The results of this study are presented in Table 1. Penicillin caused the highest level of positive reactions in the contact sensitization testing (38%), followed by phenindione (13%) and nitrofurantoin (8%). No positive reactions were noted with either phenobarbital, phenazone, or naftidrofuryl.

Mean migration index was similar with penicillin, phenindione and nitrofurantoin: 22%–25%. Phenobarbital and phenazone led to a small inhibition, i.e., 6%. Naftidrofuryl exerted no effect at all.

Table 1. Comparison of the contact sensitizing potential, migration inhibition and incidence of human allergic reactions with six test substances

Test drug	Skin sensitization[a]	MMI[b]	Allergenicity rating[c]
Penicillin	6/16 (38%)	25%	+ + +
Phenindione	2/15 (13%)	22%	+ +
Nitrofurantoin	1/13 (8%)	23%	+ +
Phenobarbital	0/17 (0%)	6%	+
Phenazone	0/19 (0%)	6%	+
Naftidrofuryl	0/19 (0%)	0%	0

[a] Only histologically confirmed positive reactions are considered.
[b] MMI (mean migration index) was calculated as the average migration inhibition observed in each individual guinea pig following incubation with each concentration of the test drug.
[c] "Allergenicity rating" was tentatively determined from the available medical literature (Dukes 1984).

Discussion

The six drugs tested in this study were chosen owing to their known potential for inducing allergic reactions in humans (Dukes 1984). The allergenicity of penicillin is well established, whereas phenindione and nitrofurantoin use may be associated with kidney and lung immunoallergic complications, respectively. Allergic reactions are seldom encountered following phenobarbital and phenazone intake. Finally, no such reactions have been yet reported with naftidrofuryl. When comparing the percentage of histologically confirmed skin positive reactions, the mean migration index and the "allergenic rating" (derived from available information in the literature), a good correlation could be suggested as shown in Table 1.

Interestingly, penicillin, which certainly is the most allergenic drug among the six tested here, was associated with the highest percentage of positive results in both testing procedures, whereas naftidrofuryl, which is devoid of any allergic potential, gave consistent negative results. Phenindione and nitrofurantoin, the therapeutic use of which is sometimes associated with immunoallergic systemic reactions, produced only limited skin sensitization, but a level of migration inhibition similar to that of penicillin. Accordingly, phenobarbital and phenazone, which seldom induce allergic reactions in man, gave positive results in the migration test only. It is therefore tempting to offer the conclusion that the migration inhibition test might prove more sensitive to detect weak allergens.

Due to the lack of extensive validation, conclusions drawn from these preliminary results must remain cautious. It is, however, felt that the combination of both in vivo and in vitro methods might substantially improve current procedures to predict drug allergenicity.

Acknowledgement. The technical assistance of R. Tedone is warmly acknowledged.

References

David JR, Askari AL, Lawrence HS, Thomas L (1964) Delayed hypersensitivity in vitro. I. The specificity of inhibition of cell migration by antigens. J Immunol 93:263–273

Draize JH, Woodgard G, Calvery HO (1944) Methods for the study of irritation and toxicity of substances applied topically to the skin and mucous membranes. J Pharmacol Exp Ther 82:377

Dukes MNG (1984) Meyler's side-effects of drugs, 10th edn. Elsevier Science, Amsterdam

George M, Vaughan JH (1962) In vitro cell migration as a model for delayed hypersensitivity. Proc
Soc Exp Biol Med 111:514–521

Guillot JP, Gonnet JF, Clement C, Faccini JM (1983) Comparative study of methods chosen by the
Association Française de Normalisation (AFNOR) for evaluating, sensitizing potential in the albino guinea-pig. Fd Chem Toxicol 21:795–805

Ponvert C, Saurat JH, Scheinmann P, Geloppin L, Paupe J (1977) Leukocyte migration test and penicillin. Clin Exp Dermatol 2:345–350

Thor DC, Dray S (1968) The cell migration inhibition correlate of delayed hypersensitivity conversion
of human nonsensitive lymph-node cells to sensitive cells with an RNA extract. J Immunol
101:469–480

Mechanisms and Models in Toxicology
Arch. Toxicol., Suppl. 11, 329–333 (1987)
© by Springer-Verlag 1987

An Evaluation of the Toxichromotest, a Bacterial Toxicity Bioassay, and an Assessment of its Potential Use in Human Poisoning

P. Lympany, S. L. Cassidy, and J. A. Henry

National Poisons Unit, Guy's Hospital, London, SE1 9RT, UK

Introduction

A novel bacterial toxicity bioassay, the Toxichromotest, has recently been proposed (Reinhartz et al., in press). It is based on the ability of toxic materials to inhibit the de novo synthesis of an inducible enzyme, β-galactosidase, in a mutant strain of *Escherichia coli* (*E. coli*) after lyophilic stress.

The aims of the present study were to further evaluate the test with other agents, particularly pharmaceuticals and to assess whether the test could be shortened and adapted to assay toxicity in the biological fluids of poisoned patients.

This research group has a particular interest in human poisoning by drugs or chemicals which possess membrane stabilising activity, i.e. whose non-specific membrane activity is related to their lipophilicity and other molecular descriptors.

Methods

The chemicals and drugs used in the study are shown in Table 1. The purity was greater than 96% in all cases except: acebutolol HCl (90%), promethazine HCl ($>89\%$), and erythromycin (>920 units/mg). All chemicals were dissolved in distilled water for use in this test. The Toxichromotest (Orgenics, Israel) was used according to kit instructions (using the method described in detail by Reinhartz et al., in press). Briefly, two-fold dilutions of toxic chemicals with bacterial reaction mixture were incubated in a multiwell titration plate at 37 °C to produce a colour from hydrolysis of a chromogenic substrate by β-galactosidase (the marker enzyme). The colour (optical density) was measured photometrically. For all UV absorbance readings, either the Unicam SP1800 UV spectrophotometer or a Labsystems Uniskan 1 microtitration plate reader was used at the appropriate wavelength for the colour of substrate; the wavelengths were 615 nm for bromochloroindoxyl-beta-D-galactoside (the blue substrate) and 405 nm for *O*-nitrophenyl-beta-D-galactoside (the yellow substrate). There was no detectable difference in

Table 1. Results using full incubation time

	MIC		EC_{50}		PC	MSA
	mg/l	Molarity	mg/l	Molarity		
β-Adrenergic receptor blockers						
D-L-Propranolol HCl	170	5.75×10^{-4}	340	1.15×10^{-3}	20.2	+ +
LabetalolHCl	220	6.03×10^{-4}	360	9.87×10^{-4}	11.5	+
OxprenololHCl	440	1.46×10^{-3}	1600	5.3×10^{-3}	2.28	+
Timolol maleate	80	1.85×10^{-4}	980	2.27×10^{-3}	1.16	−
Metoprolol tartrate	1700	2.48×10^{-3}	4300	6.38×10^{-3}	0.98	+/−
Acebutolol HCl	2100	5.63×10^{-3}	5200	0.014	0.68	+/−
Sotalol HCl	150	4.86×10^{-4}	4400	0.014	0.039	−
Nadolol	860	2.78×10^{-3}	1700	5.49×10^{-3}	0.066	−
Atenolol	540	2.01×10^{-3}	1600	6.0×10^{-3}	0.015	−
Local anaesthetics						
Procaine HCl	2100	7.70×10^{-3}	4600	0.02	1.01	
Tetracaine HCl	37	1.23×10^{-4}	230	7.65×10^{-4}	9.99	
Dibucaine HCl	76	2.0×10^{-4}	150	3.95×10^{-4}	33.92	
Antibiotics						
Flucloxacillin Na	0.0072	1.46×10^{-8}	0.03	6.07×10^{-8}		
Benzylpenicillin Na	0.052	1.46×10^{-7}	0.18	5.05×10^{-7}		
Tetracycline	0.011	2.29×10^{-8}	0.38	7.90×10^{-7}		
Chloramphenicol Na succinate	0.062	1.39×10^{-7}	0.15	4.04×10^{-7}		
Erythromycin	0.05	6.81×10^{-8}	0.36	4.91×10^{-7}		
Antidepressants and neuroleptics						
Amitriptyline HCl	2.8	8.92×10^{-6}	6.8	2.17×10^{-5}	74.6	
Trazodone HCl	120	2.94×10^{-4}	210	5.14×10^{-4}	63.27	
Chlorpromazine HCl	3.3	9.29×10^{-6}	15	4.22×10^{-5}	79.8	
Lofepramine HCl	19	4.17×10^{-5}	33	7.25×10^{-5}	−	
Analgesics						
Dextropropoxyphene HCl	48	1.28×10^{-4}	94	2.5×10^{-4}	25.87	
Acetylsalicylic acid	40	2.0×10^{-4}	170	9.43×10^{-4}	11.69	
Pesticides and antiprotozoal agents						
Metronidazole	20	1.17×10^{-4}	125	7.30×10^{-4}		
2,4-D	13	5.88×10^{-5}	37	1.67×10^{-4}		
Paraquat chloride	190	7.39×10^{-4}	700	2.72×10^{-3}		
Heavy metals						
Thallium nitrate	28	1.05×10^{-4}	64	2.4×10^{-4}		
Mercury chloride	0.103	3.70×10^{-7}	0.34	1.26×10^{-6}		
Histamine receptor antagonists						
Cimetidine	600	2.38×10^{-3}	420	1.67×10^{-2}		
Ranitidine HCl	24	6.84×10^{-5}	52	1.48×10^{-4}		
Promethazine HCl	22	6.86×10^{-5}	82	2.56×10^{-4}		
Chlorpheniramine maleate	105	2.69×10^{-4}	760	1.94×10^{-3}		

MIC, minimum inhibitory concentration, i.e. 20% toxicity; EC_{50}, 50% toxicity; PC, *n*-octanol/water partition coefficient; MSA, membrane stabilising activity: + positive MSA, − negative MSA, +/− intermediate MSA.

Table 1. (continued)

	MIC		EC$_{50}$		PC	MSA
	mg/l	Molarity	mg/l	Molarity		
Steroids						
Cortisol	10	2.75×10^{-5}	not estimable			
Cortisone acetate	No detectable toxicity up to 20 mg/l					
β-Sitosterol	No detectable toxicity up to 20 mg/l					
Cholesterol	No detectable toxicity up to 20 mg/l					
Miscellaneous						
Ethyl alcohol	9000	0.19	20,300	0.44		
n-Octanol	508	3.91×10^{-3}	1200	9.23×10^{-3}		
KCN	0.34	5.23×10^{-6}	0.96	1.48×10^{-5}		
Humic acid	8.4	–	37	–		
Cyclophosphamide	78	2.79×10^{-4}	340	1.22×10^{-3}		
Formaldehyde	3.7	1.23×10^{-4}	5.8	1.93×10^{-4}		
Hexane ⎫ Heptane ⎬ Octane ⎭	All showed 80%–100% toxicity at the lowest dilutions (i.e. 0.016 M for hexane, 0.008 M for heptane and 0.004 M for octane)					

the toxicity results between the two photometers or the two substrate colours when the results were compared for mercury chloride, the standard toxicant.

The full incubation times recommended for the test, 90 min (before substrate addition) and 40 min (after substrate addition) for the blue substrate, and 90 min and 20 min for the yellow substrate, were used for all chemicals, but for some drugs the test was repeated at reduced incubation times (70 min and 25 min using the blue substrate).

A minimum of two columns per chemical were used to obtain the percentage toxicity which could be calculated from the absorbance values as follows:

$$\text{Percentage toxicity} = \left\{ 1 - \frac{\text{Opt D}_{\text{test well}}}{\text{Opt D}_{\text{control}}} \right\} \times 100 \quad (\text{Opt D} = \text{optical density}).$$

From these values, a dose-response curve was obtained and the minimum inhibitory concentration (20% toxicity) and the EC$_{50}$ (50% toxicity) were determined.

For 17 drugs, the results were compared with the n-octanol/phosphate-buffer partition coefficients (pH 7.4, 37 °C). For the nine β-adrenergic receptor antagonists, published data were used (Woods and Robinson 1981); for the remaining chemicals, the partition coefficients were determined in this laboratory.

Results

The results of the assay on the 41 drugs, heavy metals, pesticides and other chemicals are shown in Table 1, together with their octanol/water partition coefficients (where known) and, for the β-adrenergic receptor antagonists, an indication of membrane-stabilising potency.

Table 2. Results using reduced incubation times of 70 min (pre-substrate addition) and 25 min (post-substrate addition)

	MIC		EC_{50}	
	mg/l	Molarity	mg/l	Molarity
2,4-D	3	1.36×10^{-5}	29	1.31×10^{-4}
Formaldehyde	2.6	8.67×10^{-5}	5.2	1.73×10^{-4}
Ethyl alcohol	2000	0.04	10,400	0.23
Atenolol	410	1.54×10^{-3}	1300	4.88×10^{-3}
Acebutolol HCl	860	2.30×10^{-3}	4200	0.011
Paraquat chloride	34	1.32×10^{-4}	360	1.40×10^{-3}
Nadolol	1600	5.17×10^{-3}	6800	0.022
Oxprenolol	840	2.78×10^{-3}	2400	7.95×10^{-3}
D,L-Propranolol	48	1.62×10^{-4}	210	7.10×10^{-4}
D-Propranolol	30	1.01×10^{-4}	160	5.41×10^{-4}

When the test was repeated for 10 chemicals using the reduced incubation times (see Table 2) no consistent increase or decrease in sentivitity was observed. However, on several occasions, the tests failed completely due to lack of colour development; consequently it is concluded that the incubation times cannot be reduced without loss of reliability. Drug-free samples of human plasma and urine and phosphate-buffered saline (PBS, Dulbecco 'A', Oxoid) all showed a high toxicity ($> 80\%$) at the highest concentration which decreased with dilution, with the exception of lower toxicity (0%–40%) for PBS at pH 7.0-pH 8.0. Inactivation of complement in the plasma (by incubation at 56 °C for 30 min) reduced the toxicity to 35%–45%. Distilled water had no toxicity between pH 4 and pH 11 and it was therefore used as the solvent for all chemicals; for three steroids only, the testing was limited by lack of aqueous solubility. Similar results for distilled water, PBS, plasma and urine were obtained in experiments using the reduced incubation times.

Three chemicals (ethanol, formaldehyde and mercuric chloride) already tested by Reinhartz et al. (in press) produced similar results in this laboratory, showing good reproducibility for this test.

Discussion

Comparison of the toxicity of drugs in this assay both within and between different classes of drug show that toxicity could be correlated with lipid solubility (partition coefficient), with the notable exception of the anomalously high toxicity of atenolol and the antibiotics which were toxic at much lower concentrations than the other pharmaceuticals. Exceptional results may be explained by differences in pH of the drug/bacterial suspension mixture and the pH used in the partition coefficient determination (7.4). The pH of the bacterial suspension/reaction mixture combination alone was 5.1, thus the pH of the tests for each chemical may differ.

The concentrations of pharmaceuticals required to produce toxicity in the Toxichromotest are rather higher (in some cases 100-fold higher) than those found in the body fluids of severely poisoned patients.

This lack of sensitivity, together with the toxicity of the biological fluids themselves and the relatively long run time for the test (ca. 2½ h) tend to exclude it from clinical detection of toxicity in human patients, although it may still be of use for the laboratory determination of potential toxicity of membrane-stabilising drugs.

It is concluded that the Toxichromotest would not be suitable for the quantitative measurement of toxicity in human biological fluids, but it may be useful in a preclinical laboratory assessment of the non-specific toxicity of lipid-soluble drugs. The assay appears to be primarily of use for the detection of general environmental contaminants (e.g. heavy metals, industrial/agricultural chemicals and naturally occurring toxins), as originally proposed by Reinhartz et al. (in press), but it cannot be recommended for chemicals which have a specific toxicity for either bacteria or higher organisms including mammals.

It is suggested that two modes of action can be ascribed to bacterial toxicity tests such as the Toxichromotest: (a) a non-specific interaction of lipophilic substances with bacterial lipid phases, and (b) a specific interaction of a given toxicant with bacterial metabolic processes. The second would give positive results at relatively low concentrations of the toxicant, and would detect substances such as antibiotics, heavy metals and known metabolic poisons. Some of these interactions would be very poorly representative of mammalian toxicity (e.g. the antibiotics, whose mode of action involves selective bacterial toxicity).

Acknowledgements. We are indebted to Dr. John Speight and Miss Martine Jones of Cambio Diagnostics, Science Park, Cambridge, CB4 4BH, England for the supply of the Toxichromotest kits which were manufactured by Orgenics, PO Box 360, Yavne 70650, Israel. We thank Pfizer Laboratories, Smith Kline and French, Roussel Laboratories, and Squibb Europe for financial assistance.

References

Reinhartz A, Lampert I, Herzberg M, Fish F (1987) A new, short-term, sensitive bacterial assay kit for the detection of toxicants. Toxicity Assessment 2(2):in press for may 1987

Woods PB, Robinson ML (1981) An investigation of the comparative liposolubilities of beta-adrenoceptor blocking agents. J Pharm Pharmacol 33:172–173

Mechanisms and Models in Toxicology
Arch. Toxicol., Suppl. 11, 334–337 (1987)
© by Springer-Verlag 1987

Cell Membrane Toxicity
Detected with the Chromium-51 Release Test

U. Eichhorn[1], R. Klöcking[1], H. Schweizer[1], and H.-P. Klöcking[2]

[1] Institut für Medizinische Mikrobiologie der Medizinischen Akademie Erfurt, Nordhäuser Str. 74, 5010 Erfurt, GDR
[2] Institut für Pharmakologie und Toxikologie der Medizinischen Akademie Erfurt, Nordhäuser Str. 74, 5010 Erfurt, GDR

Introduction

A great number of chemicals and naturally occurring substances cause toxicity in cells in the form of an increase of cell membrane permeability. This kind of pathological cell alteration can be sensitively detected in vitro by measuring the accelerated chromium-51 release of suitable target cells (Zawydiwski and Duncan 1978).

The aim of this study was to evaluate the cell membrane toxicity of various chemical compounds, bioproducts, pesticides, drugs and disinfectants by detecting their influence on the chromium-51 release of Fogh and Lund (FL) cells and to classify them according to their maximum tolerable concentrations (MTC).

Materials and Methods

Chemicals used were: dimethylsulphoxide (DMSO) purchased from Reachim (Moscow, USSR), pentosan polysulphate (SP_{54}) from Benechemie (Munich, FRG), heparin and ouabain from Spofa (Prague, CSSR), chloramine (sodium tosyl chloramide) from VEB Fahlberg-List (Magdeburg, GDR), formamide from Merck (Darmstadt, FRG), phenol from VEB Laborchemie Apolda (GDR), sodium dodecyl sulphate from Serva (Heidelberg, FRG), and digitoxin from VEB Philopharm Quedlinburg (GDR).

Lignosulphonic acid was a gift from VEB Papierfabrik Heidenau (GDR), dimethoate, 2,4-dichlorophenoxyacetic acid (2,4-D) and diquat from Prof. Beitz, Institut für Pflanzenschutzforschung Kleinmachnow (GDR), and lysolecithin from Prof. P. Nuhn, Sektion Pharmazie der Martin-Luther-Universität Halle-Wittenberg (GDR). Platelet activating factor (PAF) was kindly supplied by Prof. H. K. Mangold, Institut für Biochemie und Technologie Münster (FRG).

The preparation of PAF has been described by Muramatsu et al. (1981). Humic acid-like polymers were synthesised by oxidation of o- and p-diphenolic compounds with periodic acid, according to Helbig et al. (1985). Stable analogues of PAF have been synthesized by Kertscher et al. (1985).

Cells

FL cells, a continuous line of human amnion epithelial cells (Fogh and Lund 1957) were grown to confluence in Roux flasks using Eagle's minimum essential medium (MEM) supplemented with 10% bovine serum, lactalbumin hydrolysate (100 µg/ml) and antibiotics.

Test Procedure

For cytotoxicity experiments, 2×10^5 cells/ml were seeded into tubes, supplied with 1.5 ml MEM containing 18.5 kBq/ml $Na_2{}^{51}CrO_4$ (Institute of Isotopes, Budapest, Hungary) and 5% bovine serum. After an incubation at 37 °C for 24 h, the radioactive medium was replaced with 1.5 ml maintenance medium containing the test substances in two-fold serial dilutions. Control cells received the maintenance medium without test substances. All experiments were carried out on five cell culture tubes for each substance concentration. To measure chromium-51 release after an incubation time of 24 h, tubes were centrifuged at 800 g for 5 min and 1 ml of each supernatant was transferred into tubes for γ-counting. The cpm values of quintuplicates were averaged and the substance-induced specific chromium-51 release was calculated using the formula:

$$\% \text{ spec. release} = \frac{\text{cpm test release} - \text{cpm spontaneous release}}{\text{cpm maximum release}} \times 100,$$

where cpm test release is the cpm in the presence of test substance, cpm spontaneous release is the cpm of control cell cultures, and cpm maximum release is the

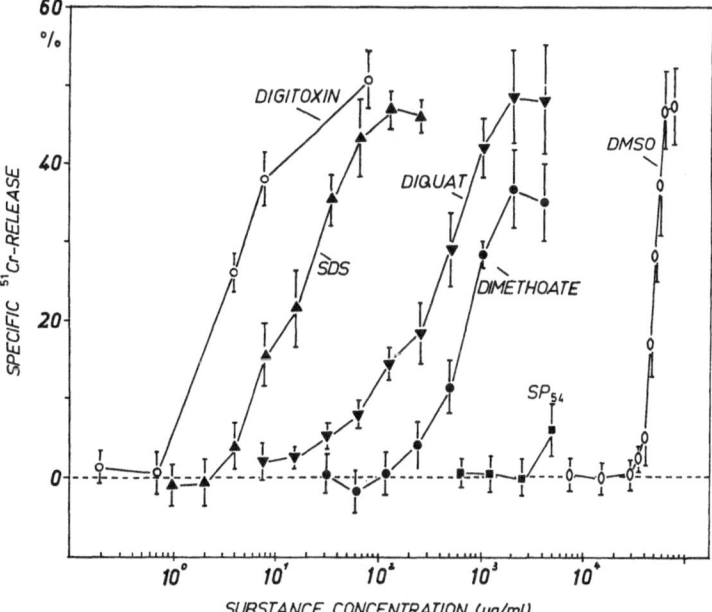

Fig. 1. Dose-response relationships between the specific chromium-51 release of FL cells and the concentration of various chemical compounds

total chromium-51 label incorporated by the cells. This value is calculated as the difference between the radioactivity in the labelling medium at the beginning and at the end of the labelling period.

For determination of maximum tolerable concentration (MTC) of test compounds in FL cell cultures, the highest concentration that does not induce specific chromium-51 release was read from the semilogarithmic graph shown in Fig. 1.

Results and Discussion

The results of testing 26 substances in the chromium-51 release test are shown in Table 1. According to their influence on the chromium-51 release of FL cells, the

Table 1. Results of testing various chemical compounds in the chromium-51 release test

Test substance	Maximum tolerable concentration, MTC (μg/ml)	Classification of cell membrane toxicity
Dimethylsulphoxide (DMSO)	33 000	Low ($MTC \geq 10^3$)
Formamide	5 000	
Lignosulphonic acid	2 500	
Pentosan polysulphate (SP$_{54}$)	2 500	
Humic acid-like polymers		
PYROP	2 000	
HYKOP	1 000	
CHOP	1 000	
GENOP	1 000	
KOP	500	Low-moderate
3,4-DHPOP	250	($10^2 \leq MTC < 10^3$)
Heparin	200	
Chloramine	175	
Dimethoate	164	
Phenol	125	
2,4-Dichlorophenoxyacetic acid (2,4-D)	64	Moderate
Diquat	13	($10^1 \leq MTC < 10^2$)
Lysolecithin	7.5	Moderate-high
Platelet activating factor	7.0	($10^0 \leq MTC < 10^1$)
Sodium dodecyl sulphate (SDS)	2.7	
Stable analogues of platelet activating factor (Alkyl-PPC)		
Methyl-PPC	1.6	
Ethyl-PPC	1.6	
Propyl-PPC	1.6	
Butyl-PPC	1.7	
Pentyl-PPC	3.5	
Digitoxin	0.76	High ($MTC < 10^0$)
Ouabain	0.58	

PYROP, HYKOP, CHOP, GENOP, KOP, and 3,4-DHOP are humic acid-like polymers synthesized by oxidation of pyrogallol, hydrocaffeic acid, chlorogenic acid, gentisinic acid, caffeic acid, and 3,4-dihydroxyphenylacetic acid, respectively. Alkyl-PPC: 1-O-hexadecyl-2-n-alkylpropandiol-3-phosphocholin.

substances may be classified into five groups ranging from substances with low (MTC $\geq 10^3$ µg/ml) to substances with high (MTC $< 10^0$ µg/ml) membrane toxicity. As expected, the inhibitors of Na^+K^+-ATPase digitoxin and ouabain possess high cell membrane toxicity, followed by SDS, lysolecithin, and the PAF. Pesticides belong to the groups with low–moderate and moderate cell membrane toxicity. The highest MTC values were found for dimethylsulphoxide and for the polyanionic substances, such as humic acid-like polymers, pentosan polysulphate and lignosulphonic acid. Figure 1 shows examples for the dose-response relationships of six substances tested in this study.

References

Fogh J, Lund RO (1957) Continuous cultivation of an epithelial cell strain (FL) from human amniotic membrane. Proc Soc Exp Biol Med 94:532–537

Helbig B, Hartung J, Klöcking R, Sprössig M, Gräser H (1985) Reduktiver Abbau einer Huminsäure-Modellsubstanz: Nachweis der Abbauprodukte mittels Chromatographie. Geoderma 36:255–261

Kertscher HP, Ostermann G, Lang A, Weissflog W, Gawrisch K (1985) Synthese und biologische Aktivität einiger stabiler Strukturanaloga des Plättchenaktivierenden Faktors. Pharmazie 40:702–704

Muramatsu T, Tomani N, Mangold HK (1981) A facile method for the preparation of 1-O-alkyl-1-O-2-O-acetoyl-sn-glycero-3-phosphocholines (platelet activating factor). Chem Phys Lipids 29:121–127

Zawydiwski R, Duncan CR (1978) Spontaneous ^{51}Cr release by isolated rat hepatocytes: an indicator of membrane damage. In Vitro 14:707–714

Mechanisms and Models in Toxicology
Arch. Toxicol., Suppl. 11, 338–343 (1987)

An Inert Mixture for Solubilizing Lipophilic Drugs in Cell Culture Assays

M. Carrara, S. D'Ancona, and L. Cima

Department of Pharmacology, University of Padova, Largo E. Meneghetti 2, 35131 Padova, Italy

Introduction

The search for inert solvent mixtures to assay lipophilic molecules in cell cultures has been carried out in order to test aquamimetic compounds such as dimethyl sulfoxide (DMSO) or nonionic surfactants such as sorbitan derivatives and macrogol esters in the absence or in the presence of ethanol or glycols. However, some cytotoxic effects have been reported for these solvent mixtures which are largely employed for pharmaceutical purposes. Polyoxyethyleneglycerol triricinoleate (Cremophor EL) holds an important role among the solubilizers best tolerated in vivo. For instance, it emulsifies fat soluble vitamins and cyclosporin A in aqueous-alcoholic solution, without producing any apparent cell injury. On the other hand, anaphylactoid reactions (Dye and Watkins 1980), transient hematological and biochemical disturbances (Padfield and Watkins 1977), and unusual hyperlipidemias (Forrest et al. 1977) have been reported when Cremophor EL was used as aqueous solution for intravenous injection of anesthetic drugs, e.g., Althesin (alphaxalone and alphadolone; Forrest et al. 1977) and propanidid (Watkins 1979).

By contrast, minor or no in vivo damage appears to occur if the emulsifier is employed in aqueous alcoholic mixtures, e.g., cyclosporin A 50 mg/ml in a mixture of Cremophor EL, 94% ethanol 1:0.42 (Sandimmune, Sandoz), concentrated solution for intravenous administration.

Materials and Methods

Chemicals

The main component of Cremophor EL (BASF) is glycerol polyethylenglycol ricinoleate which, together with fatty acid esters of polyethylenglycol, represents the hydrophobic part of the product. The smaller hydrophilic part consists of polyethylene glycols and ethoxylated glycerol.

Cells and Treatment

The experiments were performed using two types of cells, F10 metastatic cells of B16 murine melanoma (Fidler's source), and 3T3 fibroblasts. Cell cultures were seeded at $3 \cdot 10^4$ cells/ml in Dulbecco's modification of Eagle's medium (DMEM) plus 20% fetal calf serum, 1% 200 mM glutamine, 1% Hepes buffer (Flow), 100 units penicillin/ml, 500 µg/ml kanamycin (Farmitalia). Each experiment was performed in triplicate in small petri dishes. A Cremophor EL alcoholic solution 1:0.42 was diluted 1:20, 1:50, 1:100 and each mixture was finally diluted 1:10 in the culture medium. Cultures were maintained in an atmosphere containing 5% CO_2 at 37 °C. After 24 and 48 h of incubation the cells were detached from the culture surface by 0.25% trypsin and counted in a hemocytometer for evaluation of cell growth. All the results were expressed as percent of controls and statistically evaluated using Student's t test.

Cytological Examination

Optical Microscopy. Control and treated cells, cultured in duplicate on coverslips in petri dishes, were fixed after 24 and 48 h in Bouin's solution, stained with hematoxylin and eosin, serially dehydrated in alcohol, and cleared in xylene. They were then mounted in Canada balsam and observed by optical microscopy.

Scanning Electron Microscopy (SEM). After 24 and 48 h of incubation at 37 °C with the two lowest concentrations of Cremophor EL alcoholic solution, the cells were washed in normal medium and fixed in 2.5% glutaraldehyde in 0.1 M sucrose. The cells were kept in the fixative for 30 min at 37 °C, 2 h at room temperature and 2 days at 5 °C (Rickberg et al. 1984). The fixed cells were then washed in medium for 30 min at room temperature. Finally, the fixed cells were postfixed in 0.1% OsO_4 in pH 7.2 buffer for 1 h, washed several times in distilled water, dehydrated through a graded ethanol series, dried by CO_2 critical point procedure in Balzers Union and finally coated with gold using Edwards S150 A Sputter Coater and examined under a scanning electron microscope (SEM) (Cambridge Stereoscan 250).

Results

Effect on Growth

Following 24 h exposure of F10 cells to the three concentrations of Cremophor EL ethanol mixture (1:0.42) no statistically significant growth change was observed. After 48 h exposure to the 1:200 and 1:500 concentrations of the cmulsifying agent, statistically significant ($p < 0.01$) growth inhibition and growth delay occurred respectively. At 1:1000, neither exposure time caused any change in growth as compared to the control (Fig. 1 a).

Following 24 h exposure of 3T3 cells to the three concentrations of the mixture, a significant growth inhibition ($p < 0.01$) occurred only with the 1:200 concentra-

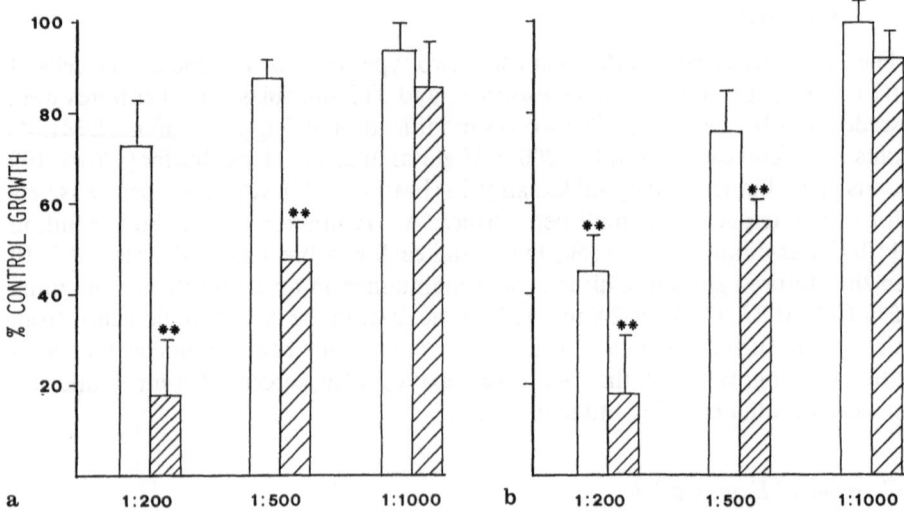

Fig. 1. Control growth (%) of F10 (**a**) and 3T3 (**b**) cells after 24 (□) and 48 h (■) exposure to 1:200, 1:500, and 1:1000 concentrations of Cremophor EL-ethanol mixture (1:0.42). **$p<0.01$

tion (Fig. 1b). The response to the other two concentrations after either 24 or 48 h exposure were not substantially different from those observed with F10 cells. Therefore, the murine fibroblasts seem to be more sensitive to the emulsifying agent, but at 1:1000, like F10 cells, they are not damaged.

Cytological Examination

No clear difference between controls and 3T3 or F10 cells exposed to 1:500 and 1:1000 concentrations for 24 or 48 h was observed at optical microscopy.

SEM of F10 cells exposed to 1:500 concentration for 24 h showed that the cells were more tapered with thinner microvilli in comparison to the control cells (data not shown); after 48 h exposure the microvilli were still thinner. With the 1:1000 concentration the microvilli were more scattered after 48 h exposure (Fig. 2).

SEM of 3T3 cells exposed to 1:500 and 1:1000 concentrations for 24 h showed no evident difference in comparison to the control cells (data not shown). After 48 h the exposed cells were less crowded and had fewer microvilli than the control cells (Fig. 3).

Therefore the SEM observation confirms that 1:1000 exposure causes no cytotoxic morphological changes in either cell line.

Discussion

These observations on the growth and morphology of two lines of cells seem to represent encouraging facts which suggest that an optimal mixture ratio has been obtained to assay lipophilic molecules in cell cultures. Of course, further studies are necessary to confirm the apparent biological inertness of the proposed mix-

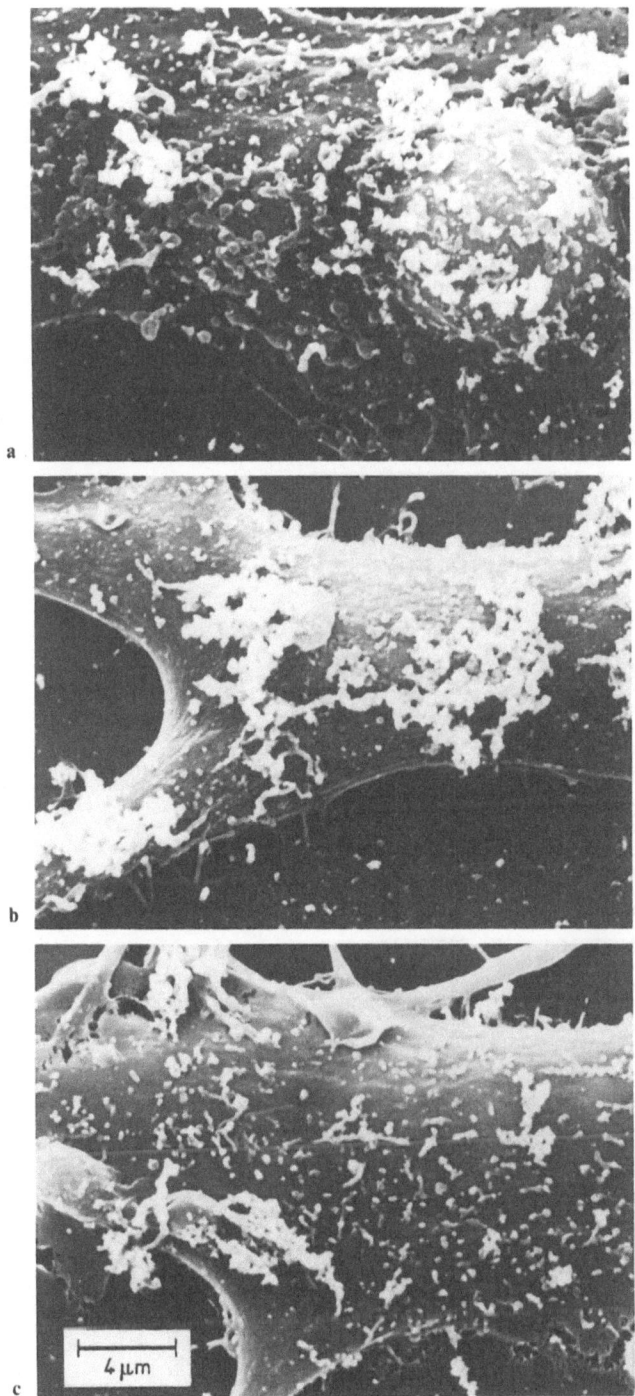

Fig. 2a–c. Scanning electron micrographs of F10 cell cultures for 48 h. **a** Control cells; **b** cells exposed to 1 : 500 and **c** 1 : 1000 concentrations of Cremophor EL–ethanol mixture (1 : 0.42) respectively

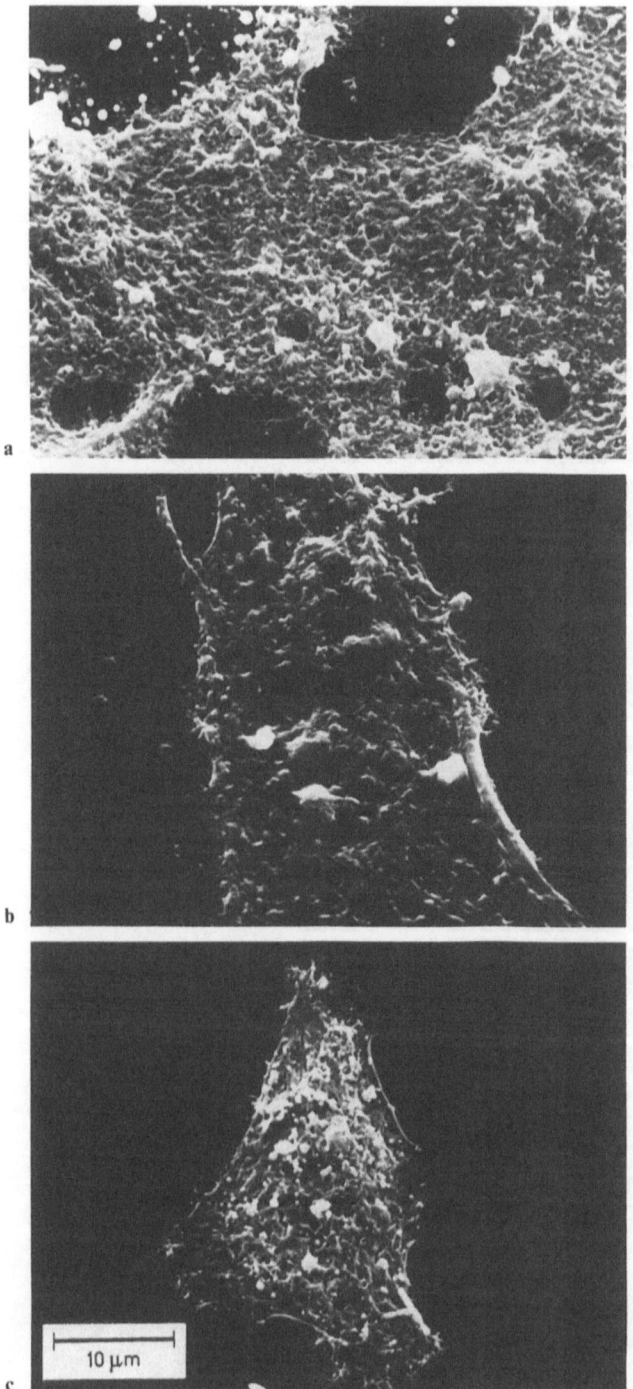

Fig. 3a–c. Scanning electron micrographs of 3T3 cells cultures for 48 h. **a** Control cells; **b** cells exposed to 1 : 500 and **c** 1 : 1000 concentrations of Cremophor EL–ethanol mixture (1 : 0.42) respectively

ture, e.g., the influence on membrane enzymes, colony forming assay, vital dyes exclusion, and enzyme release.

At present, the 1:1000 concentration appears to be the minimal acceptable dilution, although further dilutions are suitable for treating cell cultures with hydrophobic compounds, probably avoiding the cytotoxic effects of alternative solubilizing compounds such as dimethyl sulfoxide or nonionic surfactants in the absence or presence of ethanol or glycols.

Acknowledgements. This work was supported by a grant from the Italian National Research Council, Special Project "Oncology," contract No. 840043444.

References

Dye D, Watkins J (1980) Suspected anaphylactic reaction to Cremophor EL. Br Med J 280:1353

Forrest ARW, Watrasiewicz K, Moore CJ (1977) Long-term Althesin infusion and hyperlipidaemia. Br Med J 2:1357–1358

Padfield A, Watkins J (1977) Allergy to diazepam. Br Med J 1:575–576

Rickberg AB, Katsen AD, Chumak SM (1984) Precise method for identification and study of individual cells by light and scanning electron microscopy. Scanning 6:183–186

Watkins J (1979) Anaphylactoid reactions to i.v. substances. Br J Anaesth 51:51–60

Mechanisms and Models in Toxicology
Arch. Toxicol., Suppl. 11, 344–347 (1987)

Han/Wistar Rats Are Exceptionally Resistant to TCDD. II.

R. Pohjanvirta and J. Tuomisto

Department of Environmental Hygiene and Toxicology, National Public Health Institute, P.O.B. 95, SF-70701 Kuopio, Finland

Introduction

In previous studies from this laboratory, adult male Han/Wistar rats were shown to be very resistant to the lethal effect of a single dose of 2,3,7,8-tetrachlorodibenzo-p-dioxin (TCDD). Doses of 125–1400 µg/kg body weight caused a dramatic decrease in feed consumption and a consecutive decrease of 20%–25% in the body weight. Only 2/40 animals died, however, and none in the highest dose group. Hence, the lethal dose for 50% of the group (LD_{50}) must have been over 1400 µg/kg in this strain in contrast to Sprague-Dawley and Long-Evans strains, which have an LD_{50} of 50 µg/kg or lower. In the present study higher doses were tested to obtain an indication of the LD_{50} in the Han/Wistar strain.

Material and Methods

Twenty Han/Wistar rats weighing 300–350 g were given 1500–3000 µg/kg TCDD in corn oil and kept in metabolic cages for 39 to 40 days, as previously described (Pohjanvirta et al. 1987). Feed and water intake were recorded daily, with the cage construction allowing for the calculation of spillage; the animals were weighed every other day. At the termination of the experiment, the animals were killed by exsanguination under ether anesthesia, and the following organs were weighed during necropsy: brains, thymus, heart, lungs, liver, kidneys, adrenals, spleen, ventral prostate, testicles, and interscapular brown adipose tissue.

Results and Discussion

Only one animal died during the experiment (dose, 2000 µg/kg). Therefore, the LD_{50} could not be calculated, but it must be substantially over 3000 µg/kg, the highest dose used. Due to the low solubility, higher doses are not practicable, and increasing the dose was not continued. Even the present result demonstrates,

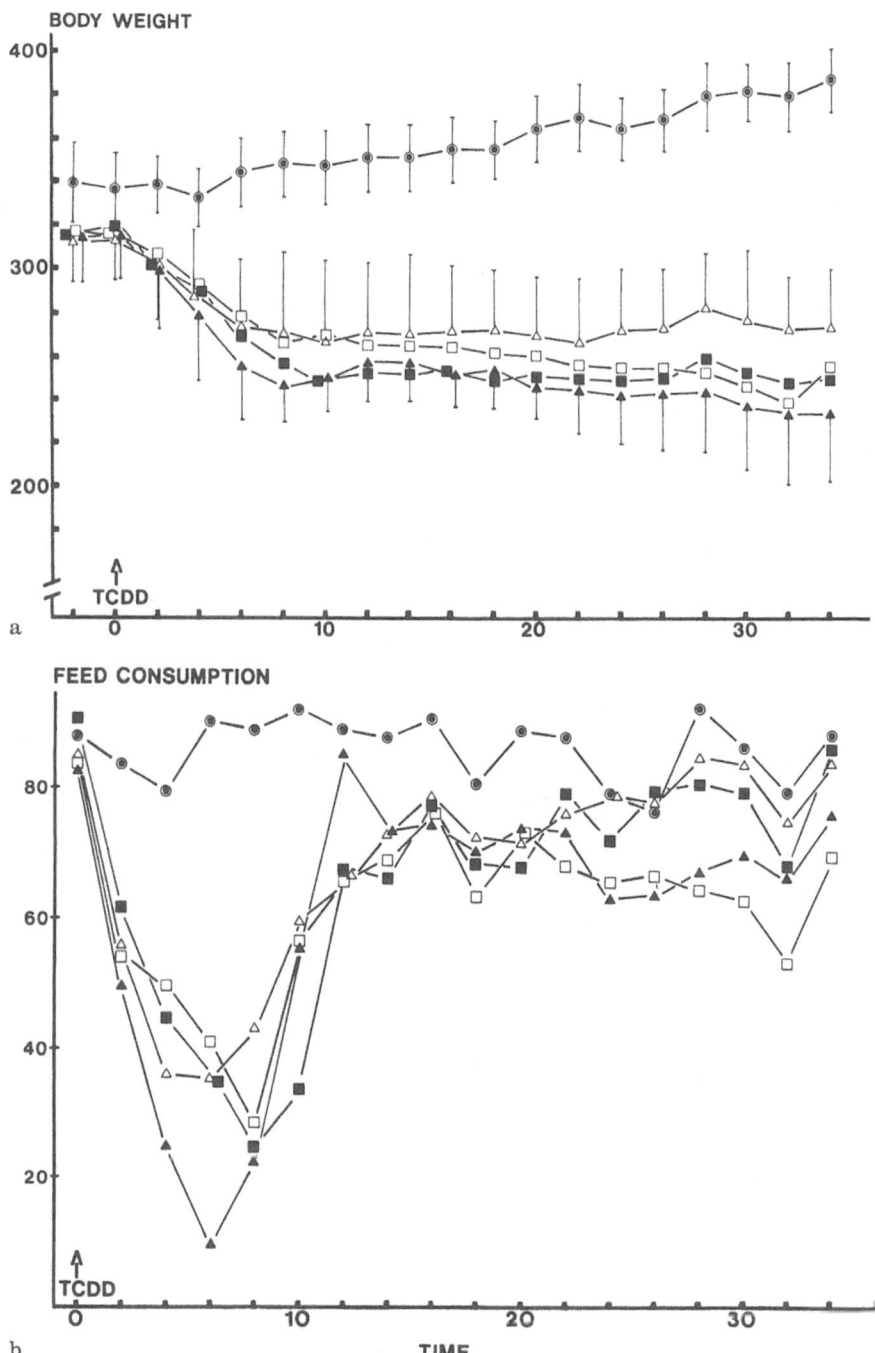

Fig. 1. a Body weights (*g*) of Wistar rats (*n* = 5 per group) after the administration of TCDD. Mean ± SD (for clarity some SDs were omitted). *Circled dots*, control; *open triangles*, 1500 µg/kg; *open squares*, 2000 µg/kg; *closed triangles*, 2500 µg/kg; *closed squares*, 3000 µg/kg. **b** Simultaneous feed consumption as calculated for metabolic body mass (body weight$^{0.75}$) in g kg^{-1} 2 days^{-1}

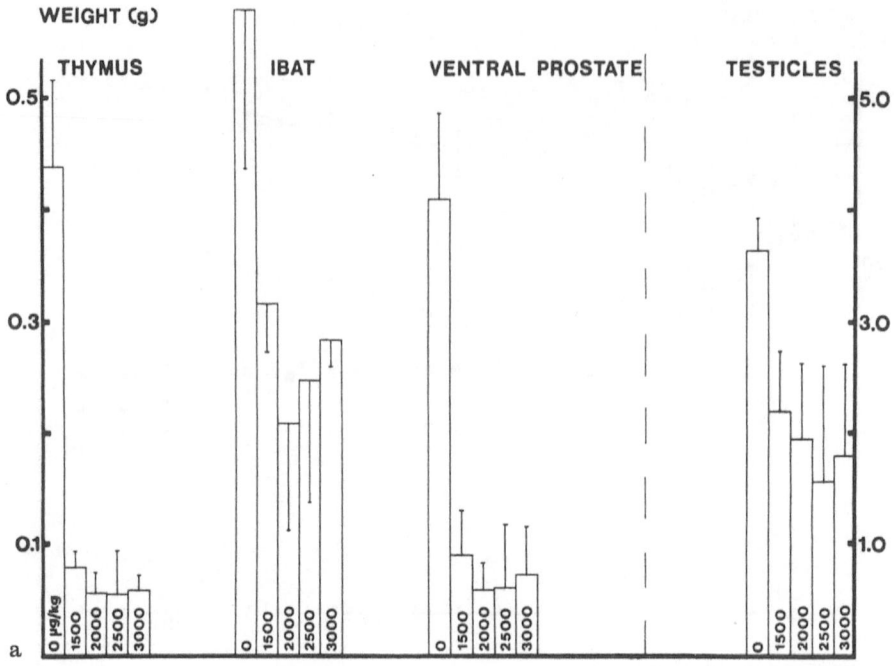

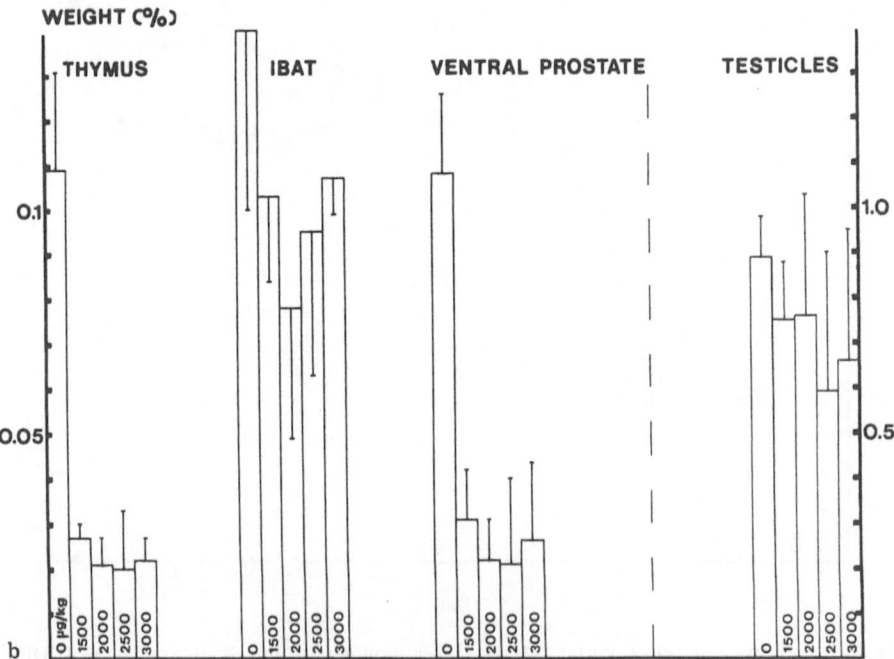

Fig. 2. a Absolute weights (g) of thymus, interscapular brown fat, ventral prostate and testicles, and **b** relative weights (% of body weight) of the same organs. Means ± SD

however, that this rat strain must be at least as resistant to TCDD as the hamster, the most resistant species hitherto known.

The body weights of the rats declined for about 10 days (15%–21%) and then became stable (Fig. 1 a). The weight loss was comparable to that after lower doses, and there was no clear dose response. Feed consumption as calculated per metabolic body mass (body weight$^{0.75}$) decreased notably during the first 4 days and returned thereafter gradually to the control level in 4 weeks (Fig. 1 b). Water intake decreased after day 4 and persisted for about 1 week.

In organ weights, the most striking finding was the atrophying of the thymus, testicles, prostate, and interscapular brown fat (Fig. 2). There were statistically significant changes in other organs as well, but only in these four were both absolute and relative weights decreased.

These and the previous results suggest that there is a maximal response to TCDD at a relatively low dose level (probably between 100 and 200 µg/kg), and most parameters do not show an increased response at dose levels higher than that. This maximal response does not necessarily cause lethality in all strains of rats. The mechanism of such saturable phenomena cannot be predicted on the basis of these results, but it is obvious that it cannot be a direct cellular toxicity. Rather, some kind of regulatory mechanism is implied. This could be searched for in the energy metabolism (Rozman et al. 1984; Potter et al. 1986), endocrinological changes (Peterson et al. 1984), Ah-receptor levels (Chapman and Schiller 1985), or disturbances of hypothalamic regulatory functions (Seefeld et al. 1984). It is noteworthy that the administration of TCDD led to a rapid and profound decrease of feed consumption, suggesting an involvement of a hypothalamic disturbance, either direct or indirect. The decrease correlated well with the wasting syndrome, and seems to explain it adequately. This serious fast must also contribute to the lethality, and it remains to be seen to what extent a different sensitivity to fast explains the different sensitivity to TCDD.

References

Chapman DE, Schiller CM (1985) Dose-related effects of 2,3,7,8-tetrachlorodibenzo-*p*-dioxin (TCDD) in C57BL/6J and DBA/2J mice. Toxicol Appl Phar 78:147–157

Peterson RE, Potter CL, Moore RW (1984) The wasting syndrome and hormonal alterations in 2,3,7,8-tetrachlorodibenzo-*p*-dioxin toxicity. In: Lowrance WW (ed) Public health risks of the dioxins. Kaufmann, Los Altos, pp 315–349

Pohjanvirta R, Tuomisto J, Vartiainen T, Rozman K (1987) Han/Wistar rats are exceptionally resistant to TCDD. I. Pharmacol and Toxicol 60:145–150

Potter CL, Menahan LA, Peterson RE (1986) Relationship of alterations in energy metabolism to hypophagia in rats treated with 2,3,7,8-tetrachlorodibenzo-*p*-dioxin. Fundam Appl Toxicol 6:89–97

Rozman K, Rozman T, Greim H (1984) Effect of thyroidectomy and thyroxine on 2,3,7,8-tetrachlorodibenzo-*p*-dioxin (TCDD) induced toxicity. Toxicol Appl Pharmacol 72:372–376

Seefeld MD, Keesey RE, Peterson RE (1984) Body weight regulation in rats treated with 2,3,7,8-tetrachlorodibenzo-*p*-dioxin. Toxicol Appl Pharmacol 76:526–536

Abstracts

Depletion of Hepatic Glutathione in the Guinea Pig after Administration of (±)-Buthionine Sulphoximine

C. M. Lazenby, E. S. Harpur, A. Gescher, and S. J. Lee

MRC Mechanisms of Drug Toxicity Research Group, Pharmaceutical Sciences Institute, Aston University, Birmingham, UK

Less is known about the metabolism of xenobiotics, or the status of hepatic glutathione (G), in the guinea pig than in many other species of laboratory animal. Despite this it is often the animal of choice in ototoxicological studies. 'Loop' diuretics are ototoxic but only one of these, ethacrynic acid (EA), is known to be conjugated with G, and it has been speculated that the cysteine adduct of EA is the ototoxic species. As part of a study of the role of metabolism in the ototoxicity of EA, the time course of depletion of hepatic G in guinea pigs was determined after administration of (±)-buthionine sulphoximine (BSO), an inhibitor of γ-glutamylcysteine synthetase. Male Hartley albino guinea pigs (253–836 g) were injected i. p. with 1,600 mg/kg body weight BSO in saline and were killed at eight time points up to 72 h later ($n=3$ at each time point). The livers were removed and total G (GSH + GSSG) was measured. Control values (mean, 7.13 µmol/g liver) were established using non-injected animals. Hepatic G stores were depleted by BSO administration with the nadir (mean value 14.2% of control mean) occurring after 24 h. The levels rose sharply between 48 h (24.9% of control) and 62 h (75.6% of control). By 72 h the G levels (84.1%) were not significantly different from control values. This time course of depletion of G in the guinea pig after BSO administration is markedly different to that observed in the mouse. This has clear implications for the use of the guinea pig for toxicological studies of compounds which may be either activated or detoxified by G conjugation.

Acute Effect of Buthionine Sulphoximine on the Glutathione Content of Mouse Liver

B. Bal, and A. Poole

Department of Toxicology, Smith Kline, and French Research Ltd., Welwyn, Herts., AL6 9AR, UK

The purpose of this study was to determine whether two commercially available forms of buthionine sulphoximine, i. e. L and DL-BSO, when given by intravenous (i. v.) injection to CD-1 mice, could deplete liver concentrations of reduced glutathione (GSH) without causing overt hepatotoxicity. Single i. v. injections of BSO at concentrations up to 400 mg/kg body weight depressed hepatic GSH in a dose-dependent manner, but higher treatment levels (up to 1,600 mg/kg) failed to produce further reductions. Repeated daily injections (every 24 h for up to 7 days) also failed to depress levels further than was seen following a single injection. Doses administered more frequently, i. e. every 2.5 h with up to three injections, were more effective in lowering GSH levels than the daily treatment. There were no treatment-related changes in plasma enzyme levels and microscopic examination of livers showed no evidence of abnormality.

How Much Can Arsenate Compete with Phosphate in Living Cells?

A. E. Peel[1], M. Imbenotte[1], G. Vermeersch[2], and F. Erb[1]

[1] Département Toxicologie-Hydrologie-Hygiène Faculté de Pharmacie, rue du Pr Laguesse, 59045 Lille Cedex, France
[2] Laboratoire de Physique, Faculté de Pharmacie, rue du Pr Laguesse, 59045 Lille Cedex, France

In a convenient culture medium, the cytotoxicity of arsenate 10–500 µg l^{-1} was studied by observing the cell growth and RNA synthesis rates. A stimulation was observed for 200 µg l^{-1} and over. Small amounts of trivalent inorganic arsenic and cacodylic acid were detected in the culture medium by an ion-exchange separation coupled to the atomic absorption spectrometry, whereas only arsenate could be detected in cell lysates. To check the controversial hypothesis of adenosine diphosphate-arsenate occurrence due to a direct molecular process, a ^{31}P NMR study of adenosine triphosphate (ATP) solutions supplemented with arsenate was performed under physiological conditions of pH and ionic strength. Formation of supramolecular associations could be related to a pertubation of ATP synthase-ligand interactions, possibly linked to the phosphorylation uncoupler properties of arsenic.

Effect of Exposure Time on the In Vitro Teratogenicity of Retinoic Acid

R. Marlow, L. Reilly, and C. E. Steele

Department of Toxicology, Smith Kline and French Research Ltd., The Frythe, Welwyn, Herts., AL6 9AR, UK

Retinoic acid (RA) has been shown to be teratogenic to rat embryos both in vivo and in vitro, causing neural tube defects and craniofacial abnormalities. The majority of in vitro studies have involved culture of embryos for 48 h in medium containing RA. Although this provides valuable information concerning vitamin A teratogenesis, it does not mimic the transient peaks in plasma vitamin A in vivo. Embryos cultured in medium containing RA were therefore removed 1 h or 2 h after the start of culture and replaced in fresh medium. The data indicate that only a short period of exposure is required to elicit typical RA malformations. If whole embryo culture is to be used as a screen, then an exposure period equal to the half-life of the compound would be appropriate.

The Effect of Organic Solvents on Human Erythrocyte Membrane Adenosinetriphosphatase Activities In Vitro

H. Tähti, and M. Korpela

Department of Biomedical Sciences, University of Tampere, BOX 607, SF-33101 Tampere, Finland

To study the effects of aromatic hydrocarbons, chlorinated aliphatic hydrocarbons, and alcohols on erythrocyte membrane, changes in the membrane-bound total ATPase activity were tested after solvent treatment in vitro. Human erythrocyte ghosts were used. A modified method of Lowry and Lopez was used to determine the ATPase activity. The ATPase activities of solvent-treated samples were expressed as a percentage of the activity of untreated controls. Benzene and toluene decreased the total ATPase activity markedly in concentrations of 2,000 ppm and 3,000 ppm. Styrene and o-xylene already had a clear effect in concentrations of 600 ppm. Of the chlorinated hydrocarbons, 1,1,2,2-tetrachloroethane and tetrachloroethylene decreased most the ATPase activity. Of the alcohols studied, methanol had no effect, while ethanol, propanol and butanol had a slight ATPase activity-increasing effect. The differences between the effects of various solvents may be due to their lipid solubilities. Organic solvents may, according to these results, cause membrane disorder through their effect on membrane-bound protein.

The Perchlorate Discharge Test
for Examining Thyroid Function in Rats

C. K. Atterwill, P. Collins, C. G. Brown, and R. F. Harland

Department of Toxicology, Smith Kline and French Research Ltd., The Frythe, Welwyn, Herts., AL6 9AR, UK

A perchlorate discharge test was developed for rats to detect changes in the thyroidal iodide accumulation and organification mechanisms. Rats were pretreated with two compounds which alter thyroid function by different mechanisms, SKF 93479 ($C_{21}H_{27}N_5O_2S$, 3HCl, an H_2-antagonist which enhances pituitary TSH drive) and propylthiouracil (PTU, an inhibitor of iodide organification). Six hours following administration of ^{125}I, either potassium perchlorate (10 mg/kg body weight × 2.5 min) or saline were given i. p. Perchlorate significantly reduced the thyroid : blood ^{125}I ratio in PTU-treated rats, but had no effect in those pretreated with SKF 93479, indicating an iodide-organification block in the former. At the same time thyroidal radio-iodide accumulation in SKF 93479-treated rats (no perchlorate) was enhanced, whereas that in PTU-treated animals (no perchlorate) was depressed.

Pathological Changes in the Livers of BALB/c Mice
Induced by *N*-Methylformamide

P. G. Pearson[1], I. S. Pratt[2], A. Gescher[1], and E. S. Harpur[1]

[1] MRC Mechanisms of Drug Toxicity Research Group, Pharmaceutical Sciences Institute, Aston University, Birmingham, UK
[2] Department of Pharmacology, University College, Blackrock, Co. Dublin, Ireland

As part of an investigation into the mechanism of hepatotoxicity of *N*-methyl formamide (NMF, OHCNHCH$_3$), liver sections from BALB/c mice were examined by light microscopy 24 h after i. p. administration of either saline, 100, 200 or 400 mg/kg NMF. The most marked changes, seen in the centrilobular region of the liver, were necrosis with moderate inflammatory (neutrophil) response, pooling of blood in sinusoids and deposition of pigments in hepatocytes and sinusoids. Periportal hepatocytes showed varying degrees of vacuolation, fatty changes and glycogen accumulation. The threshold dose for the appearance of centrilobular necrosis was between 100 and 200 mg/kg NMF, similar to the threshold dose for elevation of the activity of the liver enzymes sorbitol dehydrogenase (SDH), alanine aminotransferase (ALT) and aspartate aminotransferase (AST) in plasma. At 200 mg/kg NMF some animals showed centrilobular necrosis, while others showed a severe haemorrhagic lesion without necrosis. Periportal glycogen accumulation, without any centrilobular changes, was seen after 100 mg/kg NMF. Pretreatment of mice with *N*-acetyl-L-cysteine (1,200 mg/kg p. o.) greatly reduced the pathological changes in the liver and elevation in plasma of SDH, AST and ALT caused by administration of 200 or 400 mg/kg NMF. Conversely, depletion of hepatic glutathione by administration of ($\pm$)-buthionine sulphoximine (1,600 mg/kg i. p.) prior to NMF lowered the hepatotoxic dose threshold to below 100 mg/kg. These findings suggest that NMF causes liver toxicity through generation of reactive necrogenic species.

The Effect of 1,3-Dinitrobenzene and Mono-(2-ethylhexyl)phthalate on Lactate and Pyruvate Production by Rat Sertoli Cell Cultures

J. Williams, and P. M. D. Foster

Central Toxicology Laboratory, Imperial Chemical Industries plc, Alderley Park, Macclesfield, Cheshire, SK10 4TJ, UK

Lactate and pyruvate productions, as markers of Sertoli cell function in vitro, were studied using follicle-stimulating hormone (FSH), dibutyryl cyclic adenosine monophosphate (dbcAMP), 1,3-dinitrobenzene (DNB), and mono-(2-ethylhexyl)phthalate (MEHP). FSH and dbcAMP produced dose-related parallel increases in lactate and pyruvate concentrations in medium of Sertoli cell cultures. Both DNB and MEHP produced significant dose-related increases in lactate concentration. Dose-related increases in pyruvate concentrations were observed for DNB, but not for MEHP. DNB together with FSH or dbcAMP produced increases in lactate (as did MEHP with hormones) and pyruvate concentrations greater than those increases with each separately. However, with MEHP and hormone addition pyruvate levels were lower than with hormone addition alone. It appears that lactate: pyruvate ratio is a sensitive index of altered Sertoli cell function in vitro. DNB might act independently of hormone-stimulated lactate and pyruvate production, whereas MEHP interferes with hormone-stimulated pyruvate (but not lactate) production.

Toxicity of the Potential Antineoplastic Agent Ambazone

U. Horn, A. Härtl, J. Güttner, and H. Hoffmann

Academy of Sciences of the GDR, Central Institute of Microbiology and Experimental Therapy, Beutenbergstraße 11, 6900 Jena, GDR

The LD_{50} values of ambazone (1,4-benzochinone-guanylhydrazone-thiosemicarbazone) for adult male mice were calculated to be between 2,000 and 3,000 mg/kg body weight p.o. and 750 mg/kg body weight i.p. In rats th LD_{50} was 1,200 mg/kg p.o., and 200–400 mg/kg i.p. When ambazone was given orally to male rats at daily single doses of 15, 30 or 60 mg/kg for 28 days the non-effect dose level was found to be about 15 mg/kg. At the higher doses severe injury of the gastrointestinal tract, atrophy of the thymus, and reduced hemopoiesis in the bone marrow of the animals were histopathologically observable. The therapeutic index in mice calculated from both the maximum tolerated dose (MTD) and the antineoplastic efficacy (ED_{50}) of ambazone ranged between 2 and 4. This is remarkable for an antineoplastic agent and may be due to the mode of action of ambazone characterized by probable immunomodulating activity and the failure of marked cytotoxicity.

Reproduction Study of Rifaximin (L/105) in Rats

G. Borelli, and D. Bertoli

Alfa Ricerche S. p. a., Via Ragazzi del '99 n. 5, 40133 Bologna, Italy

This study evaluated the effects of Rifaximin, a new semisynthetic derivative of rifamycin, on reproduction of the rat. Rifaximin (L/105), 4-deoxy-4'-methyl-pyrido [1',2':1,2]imidazo[5,4 − c]rifamycin, is an antibiotic with a wide antibacterial activity and low gastroenteric absorption. Both male and female Sprague-Dawley rats were treated, by the oral route, before mating; the females alone were treated after mating until the end of the lactation period. Half of the females in each dose group were killed on days 11–14 of pregnancy and the uterine contents examined for live or dead fetuses and resorptions. The remaining dams were allowed to deliver and the physical and neuromuscular development of the pups was studied. This study was repeated up to the 2nd progeny. Histopathological examinations were performed on the testes, epididimes, seminal vesicles, and prostate of the parent animals. None of the parent males or females exhibited marked adverse effects which could be attributed to the treatment. There was no significant change in the fertility in the F_0, F_1 and F_2 matings, nor in gestation, as shown by the number of implantations, live and dead embryos, and resorption sites. There was also no evidence of changes in parturition or lactation. Rifaximin showed no toxic effects on the fetuses; the pups up to the 2nd progeny presented normal physical and neuromuscular development.

An Aid to the Maintenance of Disease-Free Animals

G. Clough [1], and J. R. Needham [2]

[1] Medical and Scientific Structures Ltd., New Lane, Huntington, York, Y03 9PT, UK
[2] The Microbiology Laboratories, 56, Northumberland Road, North Harrow, Middlesex, HA2 7RE, UK

Long-term studies require that experimental animals be kept disease-free for the duration of the experiment. The maintenance of microbiologically clean conditions within a confined space is facilitated by minimizing the survival of micro-organisms within it. One way of achieving this is to ensure that any part of the fabric of the building onto which organisms might fall does not support their growth or survival.

Clean samples of standard wall and ceiling finishes used in the buildings made by Medical and Scientific Structures Ltd. were inoculated with organisms representative of those likely to occur in biomedical laboratories and animal houses; these were *Bacillus species, Escherichia coli, Salmonella typhimurium* and *Staphylococcus aureus*. The samples were maintained under 'standard' laboratory conditions (21 °C, ca. 50% relative humidity).

Surface samples were collected using a moist, sterile swab at 0.5 h, 1 h and then hourly until 8 h after inoculation. The swabs were cultured overnight, then examined quantitatively for the presence of organisms. Controls of uninoculated samples and aliquots of each inoculum were maintained and assessed in a similar way. Seven materials were tested: 'Stelvetite', coving, corner pieces, PVC and silicone rubber sealants, polyurethane foam and lignum. By 7 h after inoculation very few *Bacillus species* were recovered, and only from the coving and lignum, showing that none of the materials per se supports the survival of the test organisms. All control samples were negative throughout and the bacterial dilution in each aliquot was within 15% of the initial count at the end of each test period. The sporadic recovery pattern of the *Bacillus species* shows that its ability to form spores enables it to survive better than the other organisms used.

The results demonstrate that the use of such materials in the fabrication of buildings facilitates the maintenance of clean conditions and hence healthy animals.

Author Index

Subject Index